Immunogenetics of Fungal Diseases

Agostinho Carvalho
Editor

Immunogenetics of Fungal Diseases

Springer

Editor
Agostinho Carvalho
Life and Health Sciences Research Institute (ICVS)
University of Minho, School of Medicine
Braga, Portugal

ISBN 978-3-319-50840-5 ISBN 978-3-319-50842-9 (eBook)
DOI 10.1007/978-3-319-50842-9

Library of Congress Control Number: 2017936194

Printed on acid-free paper

This Springer imprint is published by Springer Nature
The registered company is Springer International Publishing AG
The registered company address is: Gewerbestrasse 11, 6330 Cham, Switzerland

Preface

Fungal infections represent a worldwide healthcare problem. They are estimated to occur in over a billion people each year, and recent evidence suggests the rate is increasing. Vaccines are not available and, particularly in immunocompromised hosts and critically ill patients, the management of invasive fungal diseases (IFDs) is a challenging endeavor associated with unacceptable mortality and morbidity rates. Critical risk factors for IFD include hematologic malignancies, stem cell or solid organ transplantation, primary or acquired immunodeficiencies, and long-term intensive care treatment and immunosuppressive therapy. Despite the availability of a broad spectrum of antifungal drugs, successful treatment of IFD is often hampered by limitations in diagnostic approaches that do not allow a rapid and reliable identification of infection, and in the assessment of host-derived biomarkers of susceptibility. Of note, the risk of IFD and its clinical outcome vary remarkably even among patients with similar predisposing clinical conditions and microbiological exposure. Since there is no evidence for geographical or genomic factors influencing fungal virulence, susceptibility to IA is thought to depend mainly on genetic predisposition and degree of pathogen exposure, with interactions between the two likely contributing substantially to the risk of infection.

The inter-individual variability in the development and progression of IFD raises fundamental questions about their actual pathogenesis. Clinical and epidemiological studies have reported an increasing number of both monogenic defects and common polymorphisms associated with susceptibility to fungal disease. The study of genetic variation regulating the immune response provides important insights into the human immunobiology by pinpointing directly relevant immune molecules and pathways. Genetic studies of susceptibility to infection have typically focused on defects of antibody production, lack of T cells, phagocytes, natural killer cells, or complement, each of which can cause a classic immunodeficiency syndrome. More recently, genetic defects that impair pathogen recognition by the innate immune system and increase susceptibility to selected fungi have also been reported.

This book responds to a pressing demand for timely and authoritative information offering a comprehensive overview of the current state of the art of immunogenetics of fungal diseases. Worldwide leading experts in the field address ongoing developments in the elucidation of the genetic bases regulating the molecular and cellular processes that contribute to human susceptibility to fungal disease in both patients with primary and acquired immunodeficiencies. Moreover, genetics of susceptibility to fungal disease is discussed within possible strategies aimed at decoding the host-fungus dialogue and at its exploitation towards personalized medical interventions. The discovery of accurate and reliable genetic markers of susceptibility may be a turning point towards innovative clinical tools to predict risk and severity of disease, efficacy of antifungal prophylaxis and therapy, and eventually contribute to the successful design of antifungal vaccines and patient-tailored immunotherapy.

Braga, Portugal Agostinho Carvalho

Contents

Fungal Infections in Primary and Acquired Immunodeficiencies

1

Sarah P. Georgiadou and Dimitrios P. Kontoyiannis

Abstract

IFIs are important causes of morbidity and mortality in patients with either primary or acquired immunodeficiency. A wide spectrum of invasive mold and yeast infections are variably implicated depending on the type of immune deficit. A high index of suspicion is needed as prompt diagnosis of IFIs remains a challenge. Establishment of diagnosis is based on host factors, clinical evidence, and microbiological examination. Advancement in molecular diagnostic methods (e.g. serum biomarkers such as 1,3-β-D-glucan or galactomannan) and high-resolution radiological imaging has improved our diagnostic evaluation. The antifungal armamentarium has expanded rapidly in the past few decades.

Abbreviations

CGD	Chronic granulomatous disease
CNS	Central nervous system
HSCT	Hematopoietic stem cell transplantation
IA	Invasive aspergillosis

S.P. Georgiadou
Department of Medicine and Research Laboratory of Internal Medicine, Medical School, University of Thessaly, Larissa, Greece

D.P. Kontoyiannis, MD (✉)
Department of Infectious Diseases, Infectious Diseases, Infection Control, and Employee Health, Unit 402, The University of Texas MD Anderson Cancer Center, 1515 Holcombe Blvd, Houston, TX 77030, USA
e-mail: dkontoyi@mdanderson.org

A. Carvalho (ed.), *Immunogenetics of Fungal Diseases*,
DOI 10.1007/978-3-319-50842-9_1

IC	Invasive candidiasis
IDSA	Infectious Diseases Society of America
IFI	Invasive fungal infection
IPA	Invasive pulmonary aspergillosis
SOT	Solid organ transplantation

1.1 Introduction

IFIs important causes of morbidity and mortality in patients with either primary or acquired immunodeficiency. A wide spectrum of invasive mold and yeast infections are variably implicated depending on the type of immune deficit. A high index of suspicion is needed as prompt diagnosis of IFIs remains a challenge. Establishment of diagnosis is based on host factors, clinical evidence, and microbiological examination. Advancement in molecular diagnostic methods (e.g., serum biomarkers such as 1,3-β-D-glucan or galactomannan) and high-resolution radiological imaging has improved our diagnostic evaluation. The antifungal armamentarium has expanded rapidly in the past few decades. Initiation of antifungal treatment requires careful consideration of several factors such as risk stratification, local fungal epidemiologic patterns, concomitant comorbidities, drug interactions, prior history of antifungal use, and the pharmacologic profile of the antifungal agents. In this chapter, we discuss the most common IFIs in patients with either primary or acquired immunodeficiencies.

1.2 Primary Immunodeficiencies

The term primary immunodeficiency disease represents a group of heterogeneous disorders resulting from inherited defects of the immune system. Depending on which component of the immune system is affected, a number of isolated and pleiotropic immune defects have been described, including humoral immune deficiencies, immunodeficiencies of lymphocytes and natural killer (NK) cells, and disorders resulting from phagocytic and complement defects. Primary immunodeficiencies are usually diagnosed during early life (with more than 80% of cases diagnosed before the third decade of life) and may present with recurrent, protracted, or life-threatening infections caused by common pathogens or with infections caused by opportunistic agents, including fungi. As an effective host immune response against fungal organisms depends on the coordinated contribution of both innate and adaptive immunity [1], IFIs are more common and severe in patients with profound innate defects of the macrophage/monocyte axis with or without defects in T-cell function (Table 1.1).

Table 1.1 Summary of primary immunodeficiencies and associated fungal infections

Disease	Fungal infections
Phagocytic disorders	
Chronic granulomatous disease	*Candida, Aspergillus, Rhizopus, Scedosporium, Trichosporon, Paecilomyces, Acremonium, Exophiala, Penicillium, Absidia, Fusarium, Microascus, Inonotus, Chrysosporium, Cladophialophora, Neosartorya, Alternaria*
Myeloperoxidase deficiency	*Candida*
Leukocyte adhesion deficiency	*Candida, Aspergillus, Fusarium*
Congenital neutropenias	*Candida, Aspergillus, Mucor*
Defects in the IFN-γ/IL-12 axis	Endemic fungi (*Histoplasma, Paracoccidioides*)
Chédiak-Higashi syndrome	NS
Cellular and combined immunodeficiencies	
Severe combined immunodeficiency	*Candida, Aspergillus, Cryptococcus, Acremonium*
DiGeorge syndrome	*Aspergillus*
X-linked hyper-IgM syndrome	*Candida, Cryptococcus, Histoplasma, Paracoccidioides*
Wiskott-Aldrich syndrome	*Candida, Aspergillus*
Humoral immunodeficiencies	
Common variable immunodeficiency (CVID)	*Candida, Aspergillus, Histoplasma, Penicillium, Trichophyton*
X-linked/autosomal recessive agammaglobulinemia	NS
IgA deficiency	NS
IgG subclass deficiency	NS
Complement	
Classic, late or alternative complement defects	NS
Mannose-binding lectin pathway defects	*Candida, Aspergillus*
Other primary immunodeficiencies	
Hyper-IgE syndrome	*Candida, Aspergillus,* Endemic fungi (*Histoplasma, Coccidioides*), *Cryptococcus, Trichosporon, Penicillium, Scedosporium*
Chronic mucocutaneous candidiasis	*Candida, Cryptococcus, Histoplasma*
GATA2 deficiency	*Candida, Aspergillus, Histoplasma*
CARD9 deficiency	*Candida, Trichophyton, Phialophora, Exophiala*

NS not susceptible

1.2.1 Phagocytic Disorders

1.2.1.1 Chronic Granulomatous Disease

Chronic granulomatous disease (CGD) is a genetically heterogeneous condition characterized by recurrent, severe bacterial and fungal infections and excessive inflammatory reactions leading to granuloma formation [2]. CGD is caused by defects (absence or malfunction) in the phagocyte nicotinamide adenine dinucleotide phosphate (NADPH) oxidase. This enzymatic defect results in the inability of phagocytes to destroy certain catalase-producing bacteria (such as *Staphylococcus aureus*, *Nocardia* spp., and Gram-negative bacteria, such as *Serratia marcescens*, *Burkholderia cepacia*, and *Salmonella* spp.) as well as fungi [3–6]. The diagnosis is made by neutrophil function testing, and the exact defect is determined by genotyping [7]. The frequency of CGD has been estimated to range between 1/200,000 and 1/250,000 live births [8]. The disease primarily affects males as most mutations are X-linked; less patients carry an autosomal recessive form [8, 9]. CGD is the primary immunodeficiency with the highest incidence of fungal infections. Most IFIs among CGD patients are caused by *Aspergillus* spp. and, to a lesser extent, by *Candida* spp. and other fungi [10–13]. The frequency of, and mortality from, IFIs has been markedly reduced since the advent of itraconazole prophylaxis and the use of voriconazole and posaconazole for treatment of filamentous fungal infections (e.g., *Aspergillus*) [14]. The prolonged prophylactic use of interferon (IFN)-γ in patients with CGD appears to be safe although significant reduction in the frequency of serious infections and mortality remains controversial [15, 16]. However, IFIs continue to occur, even in the era of routine prophylaxis with triazoles, and remain the leading cause of infectious death in CGD [5, 17].

Aspergillus infections in CGD patients: *Aspergillus* spp. constitute a major pathogen, being responsible for one-third of all deaths. *Aspergillus fumigatus* and *A. nidulans* are the most commonly isolated species [18]. Importantly, *A. nidulans* infections are seldom reported in other immunocompromised patients, indicating a unique interaction between this fungus and the CGD host and leading to more severe implications than that of *A. fumigatus* [19, 20]. The lungs, the liver, and bones are the most commonly affected organs [18, 21]; however, chronic lymphatic and skin involvement have also been described [5]. Most cases of IPA are suggested on routine chest imaging. Of note, the serum biomarkers such as galactomannan and 1,3-β-D-glucan are of limited value in CGD. Radiographic findings of pulmonary disease include segmental and multilobar consolidation, perihilar infiltrates, multiple small nodules, peripheral nodular masses, and pleural effusions. In contrast to neutropenic patients, the incidence of "classic" radiological signs of lung infection such as the halo, air crescent, and other signs of cavitation appears low [22]. Routine use of itraconazole for prophylaxis has been implemented for almost 15 years, although posaconazole may be an alternative. Management of IA typically requires prolonged courses of antifungal therapy. Surgery may be required for complete resolution in selected cases, especially in the setting of osteomyelitis or infections due to *A. nidulans* [21, 23, 24]. In the case of refractory or life-threatening IA, other interventions may be considered as adjunctive therapy. Transfusion of granulocytes from healthy donors may partially restore the patient's impaired phagocytic activity and potentially improve outcome [25]. IFN-γ has also been used as adjunctive therapy of IA in CGD patients in a number of case reports though its effectiveness is controversial [16, 26, 27]. HSCT is the only curative strategy for CGD and may be appropriate in selected patients with refractory IA [28].

Candida infections in CGD patients: *Candida* is considered an uncommon pathogen in the CGD population. In a recent review of 68 cases of non-*Aspergillus* IFIs in 65 CGD patients, only six cases (8.8%) were due to *Candida* infections and the main sites of involvement were the liver, the spleen, skin, and soft tissue [29]. In the US registry of 368 CGD patients, *Candida* spp. were isolated from 20% of meningitis cases (the most common cause), 11% of fungemia cases, 7% of suppurative adenitis cases, 4% of subcutaneous abscesses cases, 2% of liver abscesses, and 2% of pneumonia cases [8]. In the largest European cohort to date of 429 patients with CGD, *Candida* spp. were isolated from 3% of patients with septicemia, 2% of those with pneumonia, <1% of liver abscesses, and 0.5% with lymphadenitis [28]. There are no data on the relative frequency of different *Candida* spp. isolated from CGD patients. A number of antifungal agents, including azoles, echinocandins, and amphotericin B, have been used in the treatment of *Candida* infections in CGD patients. Immunotherapy with IFN-γ has also been proposed for the treatment of IC in CGD patients, either for prevention or adjunctive therapy [29].

Other fungal infections in CGD patients: Data concerning non-*Aspergillus* IFIs in CGD patients are limited in the description of individual cases or small case series. Nevertheless, such infections are far less common than IA in this patient population. Among other IFIs in these patients, *Paecilomyces* spp. have been frequently reported, being the third most common cause of osteomyelitis in the US registry of 368 CGD patients (8% of cases) and the cause in 1% of pneumonia cases [8]. Nonetheless, in a recent review of 68 cases of non-*Aspergillus* IFIs in 65 CGD patients, the most prevalent fungal infections were associated with *Mucorales* spp. and *Trichosporon* spp. found in nine cases each (13.2%), followed by *Scedosporium* spp. in eight cases (11.7%) and *Paecilomyces* spp. in six cases (8.8%). The most commonly affected organs were the lungs, skin and soft tissue, gastrointestinal tract, liver, and central nervous system [29].

A number of other fungal species have also been reported sporadically to cause IFIs in CGD patients, including *Acremonium*, *Exophiala*, *Penicillium*, *Absidia*, *Fusarium*, *Chrysosporium*, *Cladophialophora*, *Neosartorya*, and *Alternaria* [10, 11, 29]. As the literature on non-*Aspergillus* IFIs in patients with CGD is scattered, it is difficult to define the best treatment for each of these rare infections.

1.2.1.2 Myeloperoxidase Deficiency

Myeloperoxidase (MPO) deficiency is an autosomal recessive inherited disorder, with a variable clinical phenotype. It is the most common primary phagocyte disorder as 1 in 4000 individuals has complete MPO deficiency, whereas 1 in 2000 has a partial defect [30, 31]. Myeloperoxidase is the most abundant enzyme in the azurophilic granules and plays a critical role in bacterial killing by neutrophils and monocytes [32].

More than 95% of MPO-deficient patients are entirely asymptomatic. Of the small percentage of MPO-deficient patients with clinical findings, infections due to different *Candida* strains are the most frequently reported [30]. Mucocutaneous, meningeal, and bone infections, as well as sepsis, have been described [33–35]. The susceptibility to invasive *Candida* infections appears to be increased in the presence of other comorbidities, especially diabetes mellitus [36]. Antifungal prophylaxis is not routinely recommended.

1.2.1.3 Leukocyte Adhesion Deficiency

Leukocyte migration to sites of inflammation is a dynamic process, involving multiple steps in an adhesion cascade. Various adhesion molecules are expressed on both resting and stimulated endothelial cells and leukocytes. Defects in a number of these adhesion molecules result in rare, inherited leukocyte adhesion deficiency (LAD) syndromes and are typically diagnosed very early in the neonatal period: LAD I, in which the β-2-integrin family is deficient or defective; LAD II, in which the fucosylated carbohydrate ligands for selectins are absent; LAD III, in which activation of all β-integrins is defective; and LAD IV, with Rac2 (Ras-related C3 botulinum toxin substrate 2) deficiency, which is involved in the regulation of NADPH oxidase and the actin cytoskeleton. Although the infection burden of these newborns might be severe, only a few case reports have shown increased susceptibility of these patients to IFIs caused by *Candida* spp., *Aspergillus* spp., and *Fusarium* spp. [37–39].

1.2.1.4 Congenital Neutropenias

The term "congenital neutropenia" is used to indicate neutropenia starting at or around birth, due to a primary bone marrow failure syndrome. It refers primarily to the following three conditions: severe congenital neutropenia (Kostmann syndrome), cyclic neutropenia, and Shwachman-Diamond syndrome. Interestingly, despite the protracted neutropenia, IFIs are infrequent in these patients whose other immune functions are intact. Nevertheless, a few cases with IFIs due to *Candida* spp., *Aspergillus* spp., and mucormycosis have been published [40–43]. Treatment with recombinant human granulocyte colony-stimulating factor (G-CSF) increases neutrophil count and decreases the incidence of severe infections; in the absence of response to G-CSF, HSCT is indicated [44, 45].

1.2.1.5 Defects in the IFN-γ/IL-12 Axis

This heterogeneous group of immune disorders is caused by defects in components of the IL-12, the IL-12 receptor, or the IFN-γ receptor. IL-12 is the main stimulus for production of IFN-γ by Th1 T cells and NK cells; IFN-γ is a critical cytokine in the development of innate and adaptive immune responses to a variety of infectious agents [46]. Patients with these defects have been reported to develop disseminated infections caused by endemic mycoses (*H. capsulatum* and *Paracoccidioides brasiliensis*) [47, 48].

1.2.1.6 Chédiak-Higashi Syndrome

Chédiak-Higashi syndrome (CHS) is a rare autosomal recessive disorder with severe congenital neutropenia that is characterized by recurrent pyogenic infections, hypopigmentation, progressive neurologic dysfunction, and mild coagulation defects. Eighty percent of these patients develop eventually the "accelerated phase" of the disease characterized by massive lymphohistiocytic infiltration of virtually all organ systems which is frequently lethal. Optimal treatment is HSCT [49]. However, these patients do not exhibit increased susceptibility to IFIs.

1.2.2 Cellular and Combined Immunodeficiencies

1.2.2.1 Severe Combined Immunodeficiency

Severe combined immunodeficiency (SCID) is a syndrome caused by mutations in different genes whose products are essential for the development and function of both T and B cells. In some cases, the molecular defect results in isolated T-cell dysfunction or T-cell lymphopenia, while B-cell numbers are normal. However, since B cells depend on signals from T cells to produce antibodies, serious T-cell dysfunction typically affects humoral immunity. NK cells are present in approximately 50% of patients with SCID and may partially provide protection against bacterial and viral infections in these patients. The incidence of SCID is estimated to be 1:50,000–1:500,000 live births. More than half of SCID cases are X-linked [50, 51]. The classic symptoms of SCID are chronic diarrhea, failure to thrive, and severe recurrent infections that are almost always fatal in the first year of life without treatment [52, 53]. Intracellular pathogens are usually implicated (especially *Pneumocystis jiroveci*), viruses, bacteria, and fungi [54–56].

Regarding IFIs, persistent mucocutaneous *Candida* spp. infection is frequent [57]. Moreover, cases of *C. albicans* meningitis and IPA in patients with SCID have been described [55, 58–60]. Sporadic cases of other rare fungal infections have also been reported: a severe disseminated cryptococcal infection in a 23-month-old boy [61] and an invasive gastrointestinal infection due to *Acremonium falciforme* in an 11-month-old girl with SCID who had received a haploidentical T-cell-depleted bone marrow transplantation [62]. The most common curative strategy for all forms of SCID is HSCT or, alternatively, gene therapy [63].

1.2.2.2 DiGeorge Syndrome (22q11.2 Deletion)

DiGeorge syndrome (DGS) is characterized by signs and symptoms associated with defective development of the pharyngeal pouch system. The classic triad of features of DGS on presentation is congenital cardiovascular abnormalities, hypoplastic thymus, and hypocalcemia (resulting from parathyroid hypoplasia) [64]. Thymic hypoplasia in DGS results in a range of T-cell deficits. Most patients with DGS have mild defects in T-cell numbers and are not overtly immunodeficient. Nonetheless, approximately 1% have a complete absence of thymic tissue and severe immunodeficiency. This form of DGS, called complete DGS, is considered to be a type of SCID with analogous clinical manifestations. A few cases of opportunistic IFIs such as pulmonary and disseminated aspergillosis have been described [65, 66].

1.2.2.3 X-Linked Hyper-IgM Syndrome

The hyperimmunoglobulin M (hyper-IgM or HIGM) syndromes include a heterogeneous group of conditions characterized by normal or increased levels of serum IgM associated with deficiency of IgG, IgA, and IgE and poor antibody function [67]. CD40 ligand (CD40L) deficiency is the most common form of hyper-IgM syndrome. It is inherited as an X-linked condition. The estimated minimal incidence is approximately 1 in 1,000,000 live births. This disease affects the interaction between activated CD4+ T cells and cell types expressing CD40 (B cells, dendritic cells, monocyte/macrophages, platelets, activated endothelial and epithelial cells) and leads to a combined cellular and humoral immunodeficiency [68]. The clinical phenotype of CD40L deficiency is marked not only by recurrent sinopulmonary infections but also by opportunistic infections and liver disease [67]. *Pneumocystis jiroveci* pneumonia is a common clinical feature [69]. Data from the HIGM syndrome registry of the Latin American Society for Immunodeficiencies (LASID) in 58 patients demonstrated several IFIs including *Candida* (n = 6), *Aspergillus* (n = 2), *Paracoccidioides brasiliensis* (n = 1), *Histoplasma capsulatum* (n = 1), and *Cryptococcus neoformans* (n = 1) [70]. In a previous review of 79 patients from the national registry of the USA, the most common fungal pathogens implicated were *Candida*, *Cryptococcus*, and *Histoplasma* [71]. Similarly, in a recent cohort of 11 HIGM patients, nine patients (82%) had IFIs such as *P. jiroveci* and *Candida albicans* and *Paracoccidioides brasiliensis* [72]. Cases of cryptococcal meningoencephalitis or disseminated disease have also been reported [73–76]. Treatment of hyper-IgM syndrome requires regular administration of intravenous immune globulins. However, the only definitive cure for CD40L deficiency is HSCT [77, 78].

1.2.2.4 Wiskott-Aldrich Syndrome

Wiskott-Aldrich syndrome (WAS) is an X-linked disorder caused by mutations in the gene that encodes the Wiskott-Aldrich syndrome protein (WASp). WASp encodes a 502–amino acid protein that is expressed in hematopoietic stem cell lineages and is associated with cell signaling and cytoskeleton reorganization. The main clinical features of WAS include susceptibility to infections related with adaptive and innate immune deficiency, thrombocytopenia, eczema, and increased risk for autoimmunity and malignancy [79]. WAS is a rare disorder with an estimated incidence of approximately 1 in 100,000 live births. Susceptibility to infections in patients with WAS depends largely upon the effect of the type of mutation on the WASp expression and function. Patients with severe WASp deficiency may have recurrent infections during early infancy, but in the majority of cases, the frequency of infections increases with age [80]. IFIs were reported in 12 out of 50 patients

(24%) with WAS, including three cases with aspergillosis and nine patients with candidiasis, all of them having either no detectable WASp or C-terminal-truncated WASp [81].

1.2.3 Humoral Immunodeficiencies

1.2.3.1 Common Variable Immunodeficiency (CVID)

Common variable immunodeficiency (CVID) is a congenital heterogeneous immunodeficiency disorder characterized by impaired B-cell differentiation with defective immunoglobulin production. CVID is defined by the markedly reduced serum concentrations of IgG, in combination with low levels of IgA and/or IgM, and poor or absent response to immunizations. Clinical manifestations of this disorder include recurrent infections, chronic lung disease, autoimmune disorders, gastrointestinal disease, and a raised susceptibility to lymphoma [82, 83]. Its frequency is estimated to affect approximately as many as 1 in 25,000 individuals, being the most common form of humoral immunodeficiency in adults and children [84]. Nonetheless, IFIs consist only of a very small proportion of these infections; in a single-center cohort study including 90 patients with CVID, only 0.9% of total infections were of fungal origin, including one case with IPA [85]. Case reports of various IFIs such as hepatic abscess due to *Aspergillus terreus*, allergic bronchopulmonary aspergillosis, disseminated histoplasmosis, and systemic *Penicillium marneffei* infection have been published [86–90]. Increased susceptibility to superficial infections such as oropharyngeal candidiasis and nail infections with *Candida albicans* and *Trichophyton mentagrophytes* has been also demonstrated [91, 92].

Replacement immunoglobulin is the standard treatment, although there are few consistent data on optimal dosages and target trough IgG levels required for infection prevention [93, 94].

1.2.3.2 X-Linked/Autosomal Recessive Agammaglobulinemia: IgA Deficiency and IgG Subclass Deficiency

X-linked agammaglobulinemia (XLA) is a primary humoral immunodeficiency characterized by severe hypogammaglobulinemia, antibody deficiency, and increased susceptibility to infections due to mutations in the gene encoding Btk (Bruton's tyrosine kinase). Clinical manifestations are generally overt between 3 and 18 months of age [95]. XLA is a rare disorder with estimated frequency of 1 in 190,000 male births [96].

Autosomal recessive agammaglobulinemias (ARAs) are characterized by the same clinical and laboratory features of XLA with variable mutations in the genes contributing to the maturation and function of B cells [97–99].

Selective IgA deficiency (sIgAD) is defined as the isolated deficiency of serum IgA with normal serum levels of IgG and IgM. It is the most common immunologic defect with an estimated frequency of 1 in 100 to 1 in 1000 individuals in Caucasian, Black, and Arab populations [100]. The clinical manifestations of sIgAD are variable, ranging from no symptoms to recurrent infections, most often affecting the sinopulmonary or the gastrointestinal tract, and autoimmune disorders [101].

IgG subclass deficiency is defined as the relative lack of one or more IgG subclasses (there are four IgG subclasses: IgG1, IgG2, IgG3, and IgG4) with a normal concentration of total serum IgG; affected patients have recurrent severe infections [102].

Nevertheless, patients with either of the above disorders do not generally demonstrate increased susceptibility to IFIs.

1.2.4 Complement

1.2.4.1 Classic, Late, or Alternative Complement Defects

Most inherited disorders of the classical pathway components belong to autosomal recessive forms. Defects in components of the alternative pathway, including factor D and properdin, are rare and inherited with an X-linked way. The main clinical manifestations in patients with deficiencies in the components of the classical or alternative complement pathway are autoimmune disorders and recurrent infections with encapsulated bacteria such as *Streptococcus pneumoniae*, *Haemophilus influenzae* type b, and *Neisseria meningitides* [103, 104]. Patients with either of the above disorders do not generally exhibit increased susceptibility to IFIs.

1.2.4.2 Mannose-Binding Lectin Pathway Defects

Mannose-binding lectin (MBL) is a recognition molecule of the lectin pathway of complement and a key component of innate immunity. The MBL pathway defect has been classified as a commonly occurring immune disorder, affecting approximately 30% of the human population [105, 106]. Several studies suggest MBL deficiency is associated with various manifestations of aspergillosis and candidiasis [107–109].

1.2.5 Other Primary Immunodeficiencies

1.2.5.1 Hyper-IgE Syndrome

Hyper-IgE syndrome (HIES) or "Job syndrome" is a rare complex primary immunodeficiency disorder characterized by recurrent skin and sinopulmonary infections; chronic eczematous dermatitis; connective tissue, skeletal, vascular, and dental abnormalities; eosinophilia; and elevated serum IgE levels. In addition to elevated levels of serum IgE, there are also defects in polymorphonuclear leukocyte chemotaxis and associated immune regulatory defects. Dominant-negative mutations in the signal transducer and activator of transcription 3 (STAT3) gene result in the classical multisystem form of HIES with variable penetrance, whereas a null mutation in the tyrosine kinase 2 (TYK2) gene causes an autosomal recessive HIES with abnormalities limited to the immune system. In either case, signal transduction for multiple cytokines, including IL-6 and IL-23, is defective, resulting in impaired Th17 function [110–114].

Sinopulmonary infections are usually of bacterial origin. Notably, pneumonias are frequently complicated by bronchiectasis, bronchopleural fistulae, and pneumatoceles. The latter can become superinfected with *Aspergillus* spp. In general, *Aspergillus* infections are not that rare in patients with HIES, especially when cavitary lesions are present [115]. Cases of allergic bronchopulmonary aspergillosis, skeletal aspergillosis, and disseminated disease with brain lesions have been reported [116–118]. Patients with HIES are also at increased risk for superficial candidiasis such as mucocutaneous infection and *Candida* onychomycosis or severe disseminated and localized invasive infections such as *Candida* endocarditis or endophthalmitis [119–122]. Several other opportunistic yeast infections including endemic mycoses (ileocecal and rectal histoplasmosis and *Coccidioides immitis* meningitis), cryptococcal infections (meningitis, esophageal and colon infection), and *Trichosporon asahii* infection (generalized lymphadenopathy) have been described [123–131]: cases of recurrent pneumonia with lung abscesses caused by *Penicillium marneffei* and disseminated infection with *Scedosporium prolificans* have been reported [116, 132].

Recombinant human IFN-γ has been administered beneficially in a few patients with HIES, although a randomized controlled trial has not been conducted yet. HSCT has also been reported in a small number of cases, with mixed outcomes [70, 133].

1.2.5.2 Chronic Mucocutaneous Candidiasis

Chronic mucocutaneous candidiasis (CMC) is a heterogeneous group of clinical disorders characterized by chronic noninvasive *Candida* infections of the skin, nails, and mucous membranes and associated autoimmune manifestations (mainly of endocrine system). A common immunologic abnormality is the failure of the patient's T lymphocytes to produce cytokines that are essential for expression of cell-mediated immunity to *Candida* [134]. Autoimmune polyendocrinopathy-candidiasis-ectodermal dystrophy disorder (APECED), also known as autoimmune polyendocrine syndrome type 1, is a rare autosomal recessive disease where patients suffer from CMC as well as autoimmune polyendocrinopathy, most commonly hypoparathyroidism and adrenal insufficiency, and skin dystrophy [135].

Apart from *Candida* infections, a case of disseminated histoplasmosis with fulminant hemophagocytic syndrome and cases with cryptococcal infections have been reported in patients with CMC [134, 136].

1.2.5.3 GATA2 Deficiency

GATA2 deficiency is a germline disorder that causes a wide spectrum of phenotypes including viral and bacterial infections, cytopenias (typically monocytopenia, NK cell cytopenia, and B-cell lymphopenia), myelodysplasia, myeloid leukemias, pulmonary alveolar proteinosis, and lymphedema. The age of clinical presentation ranges from early childhood to late adulthood [137]. In a recent review of 54 patients with GATA2 deficiency evaluated at the National Institutes of Health, severe fungal infections were observed in 16% of patients: IA in 9%, disseminated histoplasmosis in 5%, and mucosal candidiasis in 5% [138].

1.2.5.4 CARD9 Deficiency

Caspase recruitment domain-containing protein 9 (CARD9) is an adaptor molecule that mediates intracellular signaling downstream of innate pattern recognition receptors that are involved in antifungal immunity. CARD9 deficiency is a recently reported autosomal recessive primary immunodeficiency characterized by increased susceptibility to fungal infections in otherwise healthy patients with severe forms of disease caused by *Candida*, *Trichophyton*, *Phialophora*, and *Exophiala* species [139–142]. Interestingly, in a recent study, the critical role of CARD9-dependent neutrophil trafficking into the CNS and the susceptibility of CARD9-deficient humans for CNS fungal infections with *Candida* were demonstrated [143].

1.3 Acquired Immunodeficiencies

During the last 30 years, the increasing frequency of organ transplantations, the advent of the human immunodeficiency virus epidemic, and the ever-increasing use of either old or novel immunosuppressive drugs have dramatically increased the population of patients with acquired immunodeficiencies and thus the incidence of IFIs causing potentially lethal disease. Undoubtedly, it has become essential for physicians to increase their awareness and understanding of medically important fungi.

1.3.1 Hematological Malignancies

1.3.1.1 Acute Leukemias/Myelodysplastic Syndrome

IFIs are one of the major causes of morbidity and mortality in patients with acute leukemia (AL) and myelodysplastic syndrome. In a recent study, the cumulative probability of developing IFI was found to be 11.1% at 100 days after the diagnosis of AL [144]. Individuals at increased risk for developing an IFI include those with neutropenia (<500 neutrophils/mm^3 for >10 days) [145]. Among AL, acute myeloid leukemia (AML) might present greater risk than acute lymphoid leukemia (ALL) in acquiring IFIs [146, 147]. The higher rate in AML is believed to be related to either an intrinsic functional defect or to a reduction in the absolute numbers of neutrophils at the start of treatment [148]. Unfortunately, IFIs continue to appear to be underdiagnosed antemortem. A report identified IFIs in 314 of 1017 (31%) autopsies in patients with hematological malignancies, of which only 25% were identified antemortem [146]. Of note, during the past two decades, a significant decrease in the death rate due to IFIs was observed (44% during 1995–2000 vs. 28% during 2001–2004). The decline in mortality could be attributed to the higher suspicion of IFIs and more accurate diagnostic approaches, including non-culture-based serum biomarkers (1,3-B-D-glucan and *Aspergillus* galactomannan) and computed tomography (CT)-guided biopsy, as well as the availability of more potent broad-spectrum and less toxic antifungal agents such as the new triazoles and the lipid formulations of amphotericin B [147].

The vast majority of the IFIs are attributed to *Aspergillus* and *Candida* spp.; nevertheless the spectrum of fungal pathogens has changed in the last few decades. Specifically, these changes include reduction in the frequency of IC, increase in azole-resistant non-*C. albicans* spp. (e.g., *C. krusei* and *C. glabrata*), increase in non-*A. fumigatus* spp., as well as increase in *non-Aspergillus* molds (e.g., fusariosis and mucormycosis). The explanation for these changes is rather multifactorial: increasing use of azole antifungals as prophylaxis, thus creating "selection pressure," and the use of autologous peripheral blood stem cell transplants and novel immunosuppressive agents [149].

IC most frequently affects the bloodstream, whereas lungs and sinuses are the most common sites for IA [144, 150]. The most frequent sites of infection for mucormycosis are the lung and sino-orbital [151, 152]. In one study in neutropenic leukemic patients, bloodstream infections were the site of infection in 93% (25 out of 27) patients with IC. The lungs (73%) were the most common site of infection, followed by the sinuses (17%) and disseminated disease (7%) in 41 patients with IA [153]. Another study found that the most frequent sites for infection of mucormycosis were the lungs (64%) and the orbito-sinus-facial structures (24%), while cerebral involvement and disseminated infection were observed in only 19% and 8% of the cases, respectively [151].

The European Organization for Research and Treatment of Cancer/Mycoses Study Group (EORTC/MSG) has developed standard diagnostic criteria based on host factors, microbiological and clinical evidence for IFI. These criteria categorize the degree of certainty of the diagnosis of IFI in patients with cancer and recipients of HSCT as proven, probable, and possible IFIs. The demonstration of fungal element or positive culture from a site, accompanied by associated pathological, clinical, or radiological evidence of tissue damage, establishes the diagnosis of an IFI. Opposite to IC, blood cultures have a very poor sensitivity for the detection of molds, aspergillosis and mucormycosis. In addition, invasive procedures required to obtain tissue specimen from leukemic patients with multiple comorbidities or coagulopathy are undoubtedly challenging. Lately, serological biomarkers, 1,3-β-D-glucan and galactomannan assays, have been demonstrated as useful diagnostic tools for IFI diagnosis with high sensitivity and specificity, especially with serial sample monitoring [154]. However, false positivity is still a possibility (e.g., use of certain β-lactam antibiotics, bacterial infections), as well as false-negative results (e.g., prior use of antifungal therapy) [155, 156]. Moreover, early use of high-resolution radiological modalities can help in detection of IFI in the early stage, which influences the outcome. Lung CT findings, such as the halo sign, air crescent sign, or cavity within area of consolidation, may help establish the diagnosis of an angioinvasive fungal pneumonia. Especially, the halo sign is considered an early feature of IFI, and initiation of antifungal drugs when the halo sign is still present leads to improved outcome [157]. Similarly, target-like abscesses (bull's-eye lesions) in the liver and/or spleen demonstrated by CT, magnetic resonance imaging, or ultrasound may assist in the diagnosis of chronic disseminated candidiasis [154].

Early initiation of antifungal treatment is essential in this patient population, as delay in antifungal therapy is associated with an increased mortality [158, 159]. Broad-spectrum antifungal therapy in high-risk neutropenic patients with fever for 3 or more days, and nonresponsive to broad-spectrum antibiotics, has been considered to be the standard of care and is characterized as empirical therapy. On the contrary, a treatment approach based on the prompt utilization of diagnostic serological tests in the face of possible IFI, as well as early radiological imaging, tissue sampling, and cytological or histopathological examination, is characterized as preemptive therapy [145]. A recent multicenter randomized non-inferiority trial of preemptive versus empirical antifungal therapy in high-risk febrile neutropenic patients with hematological malignancies showed no difference in mortality, except for patients receiving induction chemotherapy for AML, in which empirical treatment may provide better survival rates [160].

The IDSA recommends the use of echinocandin or lipid formulation of amphotericin B (LFAMB) as the first-line treatment for candidemia in neutropenic patients. Fluconazole is recommended for patients who are not critically ill and without prior azole exposure. Voriconazole is recommended when additional coverage for molds is desired. Of note, echinocandins are preferred for infections due to *C. glabrata*, fluconazole or LFAMB for *C. parapsilosis*, and echinocandin, LFAMB, or voriconazole for *C. krusei*. Candidemia without metastatic complications requires at least a 2-week antifungal treatment after documented clearance of *Candida* from the bloodstream and resolution of neutropenia and symptoms attributable to candidemia. Intravascular catheter removal is recommended, although controversial [161]. In addition, IDSA recommends voriconazole as the primary treatment of IA. LFAMB may be considered as alternative primary therapy [162]. Although frequently used, combination therapy is not routinely recommended based on the lack of convincing clinical data; nevertheless, in a recent phase III prospective, randomized, double blind trial, compared with voriconazole monotherapy, combination treatment with anidulafungin led to higher survival in a subgroup of patients who had an early galactomannan-driven diagnosis of IA [163]. Moreover, addition of another antifungal agent or switch to another drug class for salvage therapy should be individualized. For salvage therapy, agents include LFAMB, caspofungin, micafungin, posaconazole, or itraconazole. Dosage regimens for treatment of IA and major toxicities of antifungal agents are shown in Tables 1.2, 1.3 and 1.4. Surgical resection of *Aspergillus*-infected tissue is recommended in selected patients with lesions that are contiguous with the great vessels. Therapy should be continued throughout the period of immunosuppression and until lesions have resolved [162]. Successful management of mucormycosis is dependent on the reversal of underlying predisposing risk factors, surgical debridement, as well as prompt antifungal therapy. High-risk patients receiving voriconazole prophylaxis should be considered for empirical antifungal therapy with coverage against mucormycosis. High dose of an LFAMB-based regimen is the cornerstone of primary therapy [164]. Susceptibility to amphotericin B and triazoles is variable for *Fusarium* and the echinocandins offer no activity against this pathogen; thus, most experts would consider the use of voriconazole as first-line therapy for fusariosis [165, 166]. *Scedosporium* spp. is intrinsically resistant to polyene antifungals, and third-generation triazoles are also considered first-line therapy for *S. apiospermum*. Notably, S. *prolificans* is intrinsically resistant to all antifungal agents [167]. Regarding cryptococcosis, for CNS or other severe disease, current IDSA guidelines recommend amphotericin B plus flucytosine for 2 weeks, followed by fluconazole orally at 400–800 mg for up to 10 weeks, followed by a decreased dose of fluconazole (200 mg) for 6–12 months [168] (Table 1.4).

Table 1.2 Dosage regimens for treatment of aspergillosis

Drug	Loading dose	Daily dose	Route
D-AMB	–	1–1.5 mg/kg	IV only
Lipid AMB	–	3–5 mg/kg	IV only
Itraconazole IV	200 mg bid × 2 days	200 mg	IV
Itraconazole solution	200 mg bid × 2 days	200 mg	PO
Posaconazole tabs	300 mg bid × 2 doses	300 mg	PO
Posaconazole IV	300 mg bid × 2 doses	300 mg	IV
Posaconazole (susp)	-	200 mg q 6 h	PO
Voriconazole IV	6 mg/kg q 12 h × 2 doses	4 mg/kg q 12 h	IV
Voriconazole tabs	–	200 mg q 12 h (>40 kg)	PO
		100 mg q 12 h (<40 kg)	
Isavuconazole	200 mg tid × 2 days	200 mg	IV
			PO
Caspofungin	70 mg × 1 dose	50 mg	IV
Micafungin	–	100–150 mg	IV
Anidulafungin	200 mg × 1 dose	100 mg	IV

D-AMB amphotericin B deoxycholate, *IV* intravenous, *PO* per os (oral)

Table 1.3 Major toxicities of antifungal agents used for treatment of IFIs

Amphotericin B deoxycholate	Infusion-related reactions (headache, chills, hypotension); nephrotoxicity; hypokalemia; hypomagnesemia; anemia; nausea, vomiting; fever; localized phlebitis
Amphotericin B-lipid formulations	Infusion-related reactions (headache, chills, hypotension) (not common); nephrotoxicity (not common); peripheral edema; nausea, vomiting; hypokalemia; hypomagnesemia; anemia; hepatotoxicity
Flucytosine	Anemia; leukopenia; thrombocytopenia; hepatotoxicity; nephrotoxicity; headache; rash; nausea, vomiting
Fluconazole	Nausea, vomiting; headache; hepatotoxicity (rare); drug interactions
Itraconazole	Nausea, vomiting; headache; hepatotoxicity (rare); pulmonary edema; drug interactions; neuropathy
Posaconazole	Hepatotoxicity (rarely requires discontinuation); neuropathy (rare)
Voriconazole	Visual; rash; nausea, vomiting; headache; hepatotoxicity; drug interactions; bone fluorosis[a]; increased risk for skin cancers[a]; neuropathy
Echinocandins	Fever; nausea; flushing; rash; some drug interactions; phlebitis

[a]Chronic use

1.3.1.2 Chronic Lymphoproliferative Disorders

IFIs seem to be a less frequent cause of morbidity and mortality in patients with chronic lymphoproliferative disorders. In a retrospective, monocentric study of 42 patients with lymphoproliferative diseases, between January 2004 and February 2012, the incidence of probable/proven IFI was 3% (molds 2.3%, yeasts 0.5%, mixed infections 0.2%). The overall rate of response to therapy was 64%. Fungal-attributable mortality rate was 17%, with a significant difference between molds and yeasts (16% vs. 25%). At univariate analysis, the only risk factors

Table 1.4 Therapy of invasive pulmonary aspergillosis (IPA)

Primary	Alternative	Comments
Voriconazole (6 mg/kg IV every 12 h for 1 day, followed by 4 mg/kg IV every 12 h; oral dosage is 200 mg every 12 h) or isavuconazole loading dose of 200 mg three times daily either IV or orally for the first 2 days, then 200 mg/day	Primary: L-AMB (3–5 mg/kg/day IV), isavuconazole 200 mg every 6 h for 6 doses, then 200 mg daily Salvage: ABLC (5 mg/kg/day IV), caspofungin (70 mg/day IV × 1, then 50 mg/day IV thereafter), micafungin (100–150 mg/day IV), posaconazole (dose depends on formulation), itraconazole (dose depends on formulation)	Primary combination therapy is not routinely recommended based on lack of clinical data; addition of another agent or switch to another drug class for salvage therapy may be considered in individual patients
Prophylaxis against invasive aspergillosis		
Posaconazole (200 mg every 8 h)	Itraconazole (200 mg every 12 h IV for 2 days, then 200 mg every 24 h IV) or itraconazole (200 mg PO every 12 h); micafungin (50 mg /day)	Efficacy of posaconazole prophylaxis demonstrated in high-risk patients (patients with GVHD and neutropenic patients with AML or MDS)

related to mortality were severe and prolonged neutropenia and age [169]. In another retrospective cohort study of patients admitted between 1999 and 2003 to 18 hematology wards in Italy, of the 4301 patients with lymphoma (Hodgkin's, 844; non-Hodgkin's, 3457), incidence of IFIs was 1.6% in non-Hodgkin's disease (0.9% mold infections and 0.7% yeast infections) and 0.7% in Hodgkin's disease (0.35% mold infections and 0.35% yeast infections), respectively. Attributable mortality was approximately 52–67% for aspergillosis and 19% for candidemia [170].

1.3.1.3 Multiple Myeloma

Patients with multiple myeloma (MM) are at increased risk for infection. Pyogenic infections especially due to *S. pneumoniae*, *H. influenzae*, and *Escherichia coli* and reactivation of latent viral infections are a leading cause of morbidity and mortality in patients with MM. The rate of infections is highest in the first 3–4 months of induction therapy and in the setting of relapsed disease. Factors that contribute to the increased risk of infection include impaired lymphocyte function, suppression of normal plasma cell function, hypogammaglobulinemia, chemotherapy-induced neutropenia, and novel immunomodulatory drugs [171]. The prevalence of IFIs in this population is low; in a recent study, the overall IFI rate was 2.4% with an invasive mold infection rate of 0.8%. However, the number of lines of therapy was significantly associated with an increased risk of developing an IFI. This finding suggests cumulative exposure to immunosuppressive treatment, and disease burden is a greater determinant of IFI risk than type of individual therapy [172]. In a retrospective cohort study of patients admitted between 1999 and 2003 to 18 hematology wards in Italy, of the 1616 patients with MM, incidence of IFIs was 0.5% (0.3%

mold infections and 0.2% yeast infections). Attributable mortality was approximately 75% for aspergillosis and 33% for candidemia [170].

1.3.2 Solid Tumors

Empirical antifungal therapy for IFIs should be considered for cancer patients with persistent or recurrent fever after 4–7 days of broad-spectrum antibiotics and whose overall duration of neutropenia is expected to be more than 7 days, after intensive cytotoxic chemotherapy. Nonetheless, patients with solid tumors typically have a short duration of neutropenia (less than 7 days) [145, 173]. IC is the most prevalent IFI in this group of patients and different risk factors for IFIs have been reported, compared with patient with hematological malignancies; in a retrospective comparative study, candidemia in patients with hematological malignancies was more likely to occur in the setting of chemotherapy, corticosteroids, neutropenia, mucositis, and tunneled central venous catheters (CVC), whereas surgery, intensive care unit admission, and invasive procedures (mechanical ventilation, parenteral nutrition, and CVC) were more frequent in patients with solid tumors [174]. Likewise, in another study, gastrointestinal surgery and the use of CVC were independently associated with risk for candidemia in non-neutropenic adults with solid tumors [175]. In addition, removal of a CVC at or within 5 days of onset has been associated with decreased mortality [176].

IA has been reported only rarely among patients with solid tumors. In a retrospective study, aspergillosis was found to occur predominantly in patients having brain tumors (primary or metastatic) as their underlying malignancy who were treated with high-dose corticosteroids. Conversely, prolonged and profound neutropenia, a well-known risk factor for aspergillosis in patients with underlying hematologic malignancies, was reported to have occurred only once in this study, most likely because neutropenia is transient and not profound in patients with solid tumors. Response to treatment was better in these patients compared with patients with hematologic malignancies [177].

1.3.3 Transplantation

1.3.3.1 Hematopoietic Cell Transplantation

IFIs in oncology and transplant populations have been associated with significant morbidity and mortality. The Transplant-Associated Infection Surveillance Network (TRANSNET), a network of 23 transplant centers in the USA, prospectively studied the epidemiology of IFIs in HSCT populations over a 5-year period (March 2001 to March 2006) and provided an estimation of the fungal disease burden [178]. The overall incidence of IFIs in the HSCT population was 3.4%: *Aspergillus* accounted for 43% of infections and *Candida* accounted for 28%, followed by other molds including *Fusarium* and *Scedosporium* (16%) and mucormycosis (8%). Mortality was high and 1-year survival was low: 1-year survival for *Fusarium* infections and

IA was 6% and 25%, respectively; moreover, survival among patients with mucormycosis and candidiasis was 28% and 34%, respectively [178]. The timeline for IFIs following HSCT is typically divided into three periods, early onset (≤40 days post HSCT), late onset (41–180 days post HSCT), and very late onset (>180 days post HSCT). In the TRANSNET cohort, 66% of *Candida* infections among autologous HSCT recipients occurred within the first 30 days. On the contrary, *Aspergillus* and other mold infections tend to occur later after HSCT: for example, 22% of cases among allogeneic HSCT recipients were early onset and 47% occurred more than 120 days after transplantation [178]. Notably, IA occurs more frequently and is presented later after allogeneic HSCT compared with autologous HSCT. In addition, the majority (56%) of mucormycosis infections occur after 90 days following HSCT and are usually associated with graft-versus-host disease (GVHD).

Risk factors for IFI include those associated with the host, the transplanted graft, and complications of the procedure. For example, host (e.g., older age) and transplant factors (e.g., human leukocyte antigen mismatch) contribute in early appearance of IFIs, while complications of the transplant procedure (e.g., GVHD and cytomegalovirus [CMV] disease) contribute in late appearance of IFIs [179–181]. Other biological factors such as malnutrition, iron overload, diabetes mellitus, and cytopenias are essential throughout the posttransplant course [179]. Interestingly, host genetic differences may also contribute to the patients' risk of developing IFI; studies in HSCT populations have shown that polymorphisms in Toll-like receptor 4, genetic variations within the plasminogen gene, as well as the genetic deficiency of the soluble pattern recognition receptor known as long pentraxin 3 (PTX3) may influence susceptibility to IA after transplant [182–184].

Treatment of IFIs in this patients' population is based on the same guidelines as in other patients with hematological malignancies. Special attention is given to azoles, especially voriconazole due to its drug interactions with other agents such as calcineurin inhibitors, and drug levels should be monitored during therapy [185, 186].

1.3.3.2 Solid Organ Transplantation

The TRANSNET, a consortium of 23 transplant centers, including 15 that contributed to the organ transplant recipient dataset, prospectively studied the epidemiology of IFIs in solid organ transplant (SOT) recipients over a 5-year period (March 2001 to March 2006) in the USA [187]. Among these patients, *Candida* infections were significantly more common (53%) than *Aspergillus* infections (19%) except for lung transplant recipients. In the latter population, *Aspergillus* was the most common fungal pathogen. Other IFIs included cryptococcosis (8%), non-*Aspergillus* molds (8%), endemic fungi (5%), and mucormycosis (2%). The mortality associated with IFIs in the SOT population was high, but lower than in HSCT patients [187].

The timeline for IFIs following SOT has been divided into three periods: the first month, months 2 through 6, and more than 6 months after the transplant procedure [188]. Historically, infections due to *Candida* occur early post SOT [189]; however, TRANSNET data showed a later appearance of candidiasis, with median time to diagnosis of 103 days posttransplantation [187]. Furthermore, most *Aspergillus* infections historically occur within the first year following SOT; tracheobronchial and/or anastomotic *Aspergillus* infections typically occur early within the first 90 days posttransplant [190, 191]. Thus, the American Society of Transplantation guidelines recommend continuing prophylaxis following lung transplantation at least until bronchial anastomosis remodeling is complete [192]. In addition, *Cryptococcus* and the endemic mycoses tend to occur even later in the posttransplant period [188]. In the TRANSNET cohort, median time to diagnosis of cryptococcosis and endemic mycoses was 575 and 343 days, respectively [187, 193].

Risk factors for IFIs in SOT patients include rejection and exogenous immunosuppressive agents, particularly high-dose steroids and antilymphocyte antibody treatment, prolonged operative time requiring multiple blood transfusions, and infection with certain viruses, especially CMV [194–196]. Treatment of IFIs in this patients' population is based on the same principles as in other patients with hematological malignancies and HSCT.

1.3.4 Human Immunodeficiency Virus (Acquired Immunodeficiency Syndrome)

Acquired immunodeficiency syndrome (AIDS) is defined as a CD4 cell count <200 cells/microL or the presence of any AIDS-defining condition regardless of the CD4 cell count in patients with human immunodeficiency virus infection (HIV) (1993 CDC Revised Classification System). AIDS-defining conditions are opportunistic illnesses that occur more frequently or more severely in immunocompromised hosts. These include mainly opportunistic infections, such as *Pneumocystis jiroveci* pneumonia, toxoplasmosis, disseminated *Mycobacterium avium* infection as well as IFIs such as pulmonary candidiasis, disseminated cryptococcosis, and disseminated endemic mycoses. Survival after first AIDS-defining conditions diagnosis has improved markedly since 1981. Some AIDS-defining conditions such as brain lymphoma and progressive multifocal leukoencephalopathy remain associated with substantially higher mortality risk than others [197]. Following the introduction of highly active anti-retroviral therapy (HAART), there has been a marked reduction of opportunistic IFIs, which represent today 20–25% of the number of infections observed in the mid-1990s. According to a recent study in HIV/AIDS patients, the IFI incidence is 54.3/1000 hospitalization/year, with a lethality of 37.7%. Cryptococcosis represents the main opportunistic IFI in the population, followed by histoplasmosis. Nosocomial pathogenic yeast infections are caused principally by *Candida* spp. [198]. Similarly, in another recent study, of the 320 fungal isolates identified from 303 HIV patients with IFIs, 50% included *Cryptococcus*, 33.1% *Candida*, 9.1% *Histoplasma*, and 4.4% *Aspergillus*. In addition, *Candida* infection occurred mainly as candidemia (86.0%), *Cryptococcus* as central nervous system infection (76.7%), *Histoplasma* as disseminated infection (74.1%), and *Aspergillus* as pulmonary infection (81.8%). The CD4 cell count was ≤200 cells/μL in 91.2% of patients with available data [199]. However, prognosis improved significantly after the introduction of the HAART era [200, 201]. In an autopsy study, in 1630 patients with AIDS who died between 1984 and 2002, IFIs were identified in 297 (18.2%). Their prevalence significantly decreased over time (from 25.0% in 1984–1988 to 15% in 1998–2002; $p = 0.004$), mainly owing to a significant decrease in pneumocystosis ($p = 0.017$) and cryptococcosis ($p = 0.003$), whereas the prevalence of aspergillosis and histoplasmosis remained relatively stable and of candidiasis and mucormycosis tended to increase in the last years ($p = 0.028$ and $p = 0.042$, respectively). IFIs were suspected or confirmed during life in only 46.8% of the cases [202].

1.3.5 Immunosuppressive Agents

Systemic glucocorticoids are extensively used in bone marrow transplantation, solid organ transplantation, and treatment of hematological malignancies, vascular-collagen disorders, and chronic pulmonary conditions. This widespread use of glucocorticoids which have potent, pleiotropic effects on the immune system has expanded the population of profoundly immunocompromised patients susceptible to life-threatening IFIs [203, 204]. IA is the most common invasive mold infection associated with glucocorticoids; there are significant differences between the histopathological features of IPA in glucocorticoid-induced immunosuppression and IA caused by neutropenia with mainly neutrophilic and monocytic infiltrates, inflammatory necrosis, scant intra-alveolar hemorrhaging, and a paucity of hyphae and angioinvasion [205]. The immune dysfunction and hyperglycemic state induced by glucocorticoids account also for the predilection for IFIs caused by *Mucorales* molds [152]. Glucocorticoids have also been recognized as a risk factor for candidemia and IC [206, 207] as well as cryptococcosis [208].

Tumor necrosis factor (TNF)-α inhibitors are being used increasingly in the treatment of inflammatory bowel and rheumatic diseases and can be associated with adverse events, including common infections, and rarely the development of serious life-threatening opportunistic infections. TNF-α inhibitors have the ability to prevent an effective patient granulomatous response, and this may be associated with an increased risk of developing mycobacterial and certain IFIs, including endemic mycoses such as histoplasmosis, blastomycosis, and coccidioidomycosis and other IFIs such as invasive candidiasis, aspergillosis, mucormycosis, and cryptococcosis [209–211].

Therapy with alemtuzumab, an anti-CD52 monoclonal antibody, is associated with profound defects in cell-mediated immunity, as well as neutropenia in patients with chronic lymphocytic leukemia (CLL), GVHD, and allogeneic HSCT (as a conditioning regimen). Alemtuzumab has been implicated in a wide range of infections including IFIs. Severe infections have included aspergillosis, mucormycosis, and candidiasis [212]. Also, with the use of purine analogs (e.g., fludarabine), which results in quantitative and qualitative T-cell abnormalities, a wide spectrum of infectious complications including opportunistic infections caused by organisms such as

Candida, *Aspergillus*, and *Cryptococcus* have been reported in patients with CLL, refractory AML, and non-Hodgkin's lymphoma [213, 214].

References

1. Romani L. Immunity to fungal infections. Nat Rev Immunol. 2004;4(1):1–23. doi:10.1038/nri1255.
2. Holland SM. Chronic granulomatous disease. Hematol Oncol Clin N Am. 2013;27(1):89–99, viii. doi:10.1016/j.hoc.2012.11.002.
3. Ben-Ari J, Wolach O, Gavrieli R, Wolach B. Infections associated with chronic granulomatous disease: linking genetics to phenotypic expression. Expert Rev Anti-Infect Ther. 2012;10(8):881–94. doi:10.1586/eri.12.77.
4. Heyworth PG, Cross AR, Curnutte JT. Chronic granulomatous disease. Curr Opin Immunol. 2003;15(5):578–84.
5. Marciano BE, Spalding C, Fitzgerald A, Mann D, Brown T, Osgood S, Yockey L, Darnell DN, Barnhart L, Daub J, Boris L, Rump AP, Anderson VL, Haney C, Kuhns DB, Rosenzweig SD, Kelly C, Zelazny A, Mason T, DeRavin SS, Kang E, Gallin JI, Malech HL, Olivier KN, Uzel G, Freeman AF, Heller T, Zerbe CS, Holland SM. Common severe infections in chronic granulomatous disease. Clin Infect Dis: Off Publ Infect Dis Soc Am. 2015;60(8):1176–83. doi:10.1093/cid/ciu1154.
6. Liese J, Kloos S, Jendrossek V, Petropoulou T, Wintergerst U, Notheis G, Gahr M, Belohradsky BH. Long-term follow-up and outcome of 39 patients with chronic granulomatous disease. J Pediatr. 2000;137(5):687–93. doi:10.1067/mpd.2000.109112.
7. Roos D, de Boer M. Molecular diagnosis of chronic granulomatous disease. Clin Exp Immunol. 2014;175(2):139–49. doi:10.1111/cei.12202.
8. Winkelstein JA, Marino MC, Johnston Jr RB, Boyle J, Curnutte J, Gallin JI, Malech HL, Holland SM, Ochs H, Quie P, Buckley RH, Foster CB, Chanock SJ, Dickler H. Chronic granulomatous disease. Report on a national registry of 368 patients. Medicine. 2000;79(3):155–69.
9. Segal BH, Leto TL, Gallin JI, Malech HL, Holland SM. Genetic, biochemical, and clinical features of chronic granulomatous disease. Medicine. 2000;79(3):170–200.
10. Antachopoulos C, Walsh TJ, Roilides E. Fungal infections in primary immunodeficiencies. Eur J Pediatr. 2007;166(11):1099–117. doi:10.1007/s00431-007-0527-7.
11. Antachopoulos C. Invasive fungal infections in congenital immunodeficiencies. Clin Microbiol Infect: Off Publ Eur Soc Clin Microbiol Infect Dis. 2010;16(9):1335–42. doi:10.1111/j.1469-0691.2010.03289.x.
12. Lanternier F, Cypowyj S, Picard C, Bustamante J, Lortholary O, Casanova JL, Puel A. Primary immunodeficiencies underlying fungal infections. Curr Opin Pediatr. 2013;25(6):736–47. doi:10.1097/MOP.0000000000000031.
13. Beaute J, Obenga G, Le Mignot L, Mahlaoui N, Bougnoux ME, Mouy R, Gougerot-Pocidalo MA, Barlogis V, Suarez F, Lanternier F, Hermine O, Lecuit M, Blanche S, Fischer A, Lortholary O, French PIDSGC. Epidemiology and outcome of invasive fungal diseases in patients with chronic granulomatous disease: a multicenter study in France. Pediatr Infect Dis J. 2011;30(1):57–62. doi:10.1097/INF.0b013e3181f13b23.
14. Bortoletto P, Lyman K, Camacho A, Fricchione M, Khanolkar A, Katz BZ. Chronic granulomatous disease: a large, single-center U.S. experience. Pediatr Infect Dis J. 2015;34:1110. doi:10.1097/inf.0000000000000840.
15. Marciano BE, Wesley R, De Carlo ES, Anderson VL, Barnhart LA, Darnell D, Malech HL, Gallin JI, Holland SM. Long-term interferon-gamma therapy for patients with chronic granulomatous disease. Clin Infect Dis: Off Publ Infect Dis Soc Am. 2004;39(5):692–9. doi:10.1086/422993.

16. Kobayashi S, Murayama S, Takanashi S, Takahashi K, Miyatsuka S, Fujita T, Ichinohe S, Koike Y, Kohagizawa T, Mori H, Deguchi Y, Higuchi K, Wakasugi H, Sato T, Wada Y, Nagata M, Okabe N, Tatsuzawa O. Clinical features and prognoses of 23 patients with chronic granulomatous disease followed for 21 years by a single hospital in Japan. Eur J Pediatr. 2008;167(12):1389–94. doi:10.1007/s00431-008-0680-7.
17. Salvator H, Mahlaoui N, Catherinot E, Rivaud E, Pilmis B, Borie R, Crestani B, Tcherakian C, Suarez F, Dunogue B, Gougerot-Pocidalo MA, Hurtado-Nedelec M, Dreyfus JF, Durieu I, Fouyssac F, Hermine O, Lortholary O, Fischer A, Couderc LJ. Pulmonary manifestations in adult patients with chronic granulomatous disease. Eur Respir J. 2015;45(6):1613–23. doi:10.1183/09031936.00118414.
18. Blumental S, Mouy R, Mahlaoui N, Bougnoux ME, Debre M, Beaute J, Lortholary O, Blanche S, Fischer A. Invasive mold infections in chronic granulomatous disease: a 25-year retrospective survey. Clin Infect Dis: Off Pub Infect Dis Soc Am. 2011;53(12):e159–69. doi:10.1093/cid/cir731.
19. Henriet SS, Verweij PE, Warris A. Aspergillus nidulans and chronic granulomatous disease: a unique host-pathogen interaction. J Infect Dis. 2012;206(7):1128–37. doi:10.1093/infdis/jis473.
20. Segal BH, DeCarlo ES, Kwon-Chung KJ, Malech HL, Gallin JI, Holland SM. Aspergillus nidulans infection in chronic granulomatous disease. Medicine. 1998;77(5):345–54.
21. Dotis J, Roilides E. Osteomyelitis due to Aspergillus species in chronic granulomatous disease: anupdateoftheliterature.Mycoses.2011;54(6):e686–96.doi:10.1111/j.1439-0507.2010.02001.x.
22. Thomas KE, Owens CM, Veys PA, Novelli V, Costoli V. The radiological spectrum of invasive aspergillosis in children: a 10-year review. Pediatr Radiol. 2003;33(7):453–60. doi:10.1007/s00247-003-0919-4.
23. Falcone EL, Holland SM. Invasive fungal infection in chronic granulomatous disease: insights into pathogenesis and management. Curr Opin Infect Dis. 2012;25(6):658–69. doi:10.1097/QCO.0b013e328358b0a4.
24. Hodiamont CJ, Dolman KM, Ten Berge IJ, Melchers WJ, Verweij PE, Pajkrt D. Multiple-azole-resistant Aspergillus fumigatus osteomyelitis in a patient with chronic granulomatous disease successfully treated with long-term oral posaconazole and surgery. Med Mycol. 2009;47(2):217–20. doi:10.1080/13693780802545600.
25. Shigemura T, Nakazawa Y, Yoshikawa K, Hirabayashi K, Saito S, Kobayashi N, Sakashita K, Shiohara M, Wada T, Shimodaira S, Agematsu K, Koike K. Successful cord blood transplantation after repeated transfusions of unmobilized neutrophils in addition to antifungal treatment in an infant with chronic granulomatous disease complicated by invasive pulmonary aspergillosis. Transfusion. 2014;54(3):516–21. doi:10.1111/trf.12325.
26. Al-Tawfiq JA, Al-Abdely HM. Vertebral osteomyelitis due to Aspergillus fumigatus in a patient with chronic granulomatous disease successfully treated with antifungal agents and interferon-gamma. Med Mycol. 2010;48(3):537–41. doi:10.3109/13693780903325290.
27. Martire B, Rondelli R, Soresina A, Pignata C, Broccoletti T, Finocchi A, Rossi P, Gattorno M, Rabusin M, Azzari C, Dellepiane RM, Pietrogrande MC, Trizzino A, Di Bartolomeo P, Martino S, Carpino L, Cossu F, Locatelli F, Maccario R, Pierani P, Putti MC, Stabile A, Notarangelo LD, Ugazio AG, Plebani A, De Mattia D, Ipinet. Clinical features, long-term follow-up and outcome of a large cohort of patients with chronic granulomatous disease: an Italian multicenter study. Clin Immunol. 2008;126(2):155–64. doi:10.1016/j.clim.2007.09.008.
28. van den Berg JM, van Koppen E, Ahlin A, Belohradsky BH, Bernatowska E, Corbeel L, Espanol T, Fischer A, Kurenko-Deptuch M, Mouy R, Petropoulou T, Roesler J, Seger R, Stasia MJ, Valerius NH, Weening RS, Wolach B, Roos D, Kuijpers TW. Chronic granulomatous disease: the European experience. PLoS One. 2009;4(4):e5234. doi:10.1371/journal.pone.0005234.
29. Dotis J, Pana ZD, Roilides E. Non-Aspergillus fungal infections in chronic granulomatous disease. Mycoses. 2013;56(4):449–62. doi:10.1111/myc.12049.

30. Parry MF, Root RK, Metcalf JA, Delaney KK, Kaplow LS, Richar WJ. Myeloperoxidase deficiency: prevalence and clinical significance. Ann Intern Med. 1981;95(3):293–301.
31. Kitahara M, Eyre HJ, Simonian Y, Atkin CL, Hasstedt SJ. Hereditary myeloperoxidase deficiency. Blood. 1981;57(5):888–93.
32. Hampton MB, Kettle AJ, Winterbourn CC. Inside the neutrophil phagosome: oxidants, myeloperoxidase, and bacterial killing. Blood. 1998;92(9):3007–17.
33. Weber ML, Abela A, de Repentigny L, Garel L, Lapointe N. Myeloperoxidase deficiency with extensive candidal osteomyelitis of the base of the skull. Pediatrics. 1987;80(6):876–9.
34. Nguyen C, Katner HP. Myeloperoxidase deficiency manifesting as pustular candidal dermatitis. Clin Infect Dis: Off Publ Infect Dis Soc Am. 1997;24(2):258–60.
35. Chiang AK, Chan GC, Ma SK, Ng YK, Ha SY, Lau YL. Disseminated fungal infection associated with myeloperoxidase deficiency in a premature neonate. Pediatr Infect Dis J. 2000;19(10):1027–9.
36. Cech P, Stalder H, Widmann JJ, Rohner A, Miescher PA. Leukocyte myeloperoxidase deficiency and diabetes mellitus associated with *Candida albicans* liver abscess. Am J Med. 1979;66(1):149–53.
37. Valentini P, De Sole P, De Luca D, Plaisant P, Puggioni P, Rossi MC, Rumi C, Ranno O. Decreased chemiluminescence in leukocyte adhesion deficiency presenting with recurrent sepsis, amoebiasis and *Candida albicans* urinary tract infection. Minerva Med. 2006;97(5):437–42.
38. Mellouli F, Ksouri H, Barbouche R, Maamer M, Hamed LB, Hmida S, Hassen AB, Bejaoui M. Successful treatment of Fusarium solani ecthyma gangrenosum in a patient affected by leukocyte adhesion deficiency type 1 with granulocytes transfusions. BMC Dermatol. 2010;10:10. doi:10.1186/1471-5945-10-10.
39. Kuijpers TW, van Bruggen R, Kamerbeek N, Tool AT, Hicsonmez G, Gurgey A, Karow A, Verhoeven AJ, Seeger K, Sanal O, Niemeyer C, Roos D. Natural history and early diagnosis of LAD-1/variant syndrome. Blood. 2007;109(8):3529–37. doi:10.1182/blood-2006-05-021402.
40. Mamishi S, Esfahani SA, Parvaneh N, Diestelhorst J, Rezaei N. Severe congenital neutropenia in 2 siblings of consanguineous parents. The role of HAX1 deficiency. J Investig Allergol Clin Immunol. 2009;19(6):500–3.
41. Fahimzad A, Chavoshzadeh Z, Abdollahpour H, Klein C, Rezaei N. Necrosis of nasal cartilage due to mucormycosis in a patient with severe congenital neutropenia due to HAX1 deficiency. J Investig Allergol Clin Immunol. 2008;18(6):469–72.
42. Dallorso S, Manzitti C, Dodero P, Faraci M, Rosanda C, Castagnola E. Uneventful outcome of unrelated hematopoietic stem cell transplantation in a patient with leukemic transformation of Kostmann syndrome and long-lasting invasive pulmonary mycosis. Eur J Haematol. 2003;70(5):322–5.
43. Al-Kindi H, Abdoon H, Alkhabori M, Daar S, Beshlawi I, Wali YA. Invasive candidal laryngitis as a manifestation of cyclic neutropenia in an Omani infant. Pediatr Hematol Oncol. 2008;25(4):339–44. doi:10.1080/08880010802016144.
44. Ferry C, Ouachee M, Leblanc T, Michel G, Notz-Carrere A, Tabrizi R, Flood T, Lutz P, Fischer A, Gluckman E, Donadieu J. Hematopoietic stem cell transplantation in severe congenital neutropenia: experience of the French SCN register. Bone Marrow Transplant. 2005;35(1):45–50. doi:10.1038/sj.bmt.1704718.
45. Carlsson G, Winiarski J, Ljungman P, Ringden O, Mattsson J, Nordenskjold M, Touw I, Henter JI, Palmblad J, Fadeel B, Hagglund H. Hematopoietic stem cell transplantation in severe congenital neutropenia. Pediatr Blood Cancer. 2011;56(3):444–51. doi:10.1002/pbc.22836.
46. Rosenzweig SD, Holland SM. Phagocyte immunodeficiencies and their infections. J Allergy Clin Immunol. 2004;113(4):620–6. doi:10.1016/j.jaci.2004.02.001.
47. Zerbe CS, Holland SM. Disseminated histoplasmosis in persons with interferon-gamma receptor 1 deficiency. Clin Infect Dis: Off Publ Infect Dis Soc Am. 2005;41(4):e38–41. doi:10.1086/432120.

48. Moraes-Vasconcelos D, Grumach AS, Yamaguti A, Andrade ME, Fieschi C, de Beaucoudrey L, Casanova JL, Duarte AJ. Paracoccidioides brasiliensis disseminated disease in a patient with inherited deficiency in the beta1 subunit of the interleukin (IL)-12/IL-23 receptor. Clin Infect Dis: Off Publ Infect Dis Soc Am. 2005;41(4):e31–7. doi:10.1086/432119.
49. Kaplan J, De Domenico I, Ward DM. Chediak-Higashi syndrome. Curr Opin Hematol. 2008;15(1):22–9. doi:10.1097/MOH.0b013e3282f2bcce.
50. Geha RS, Notarangelo LD, Casanova JL, Chapel H, Conley ME, Fischer A, Hammarstrom L, Nonoyama S, Ochs HD, Puck JM, Roifman C, Seger R, Wedgwood J, International Union of Immunological Societies Primary Immunodeficiency Diseases Classification C. Primary immunodeficiency diseases: an update from the International Union of Immunological Societies Primary Immunodeficiency Diseases Classification Committee. J Allergy Clin Immunol. 2007;120(4):776–94.
51. Kumar A, Teuber SS, Gershwin ME. Current perspectives on primary immunodeficiency diseases. Clin Dev Immunol. 2006;13(2–4):223–59. doi:10.1080/17402520600800705.
52. Lahood NN, Hershfield MS, Leiva LE, Sorensen RU. Recurrent infection, chronic diarrhea, and failure to thrive in a seven-month-old infant. Ann Allergy. 1991;67(4):389–93.
53. Walcott DW, Linehan T, Hilman BC, Hershfield MS, el Dahr J. Failure to thrive, diarrhea, cough, and oral candidiasis in a three-month-old boy. Ann Allergy. 1994;72(5):408–14.
54. Dominguez-Pinilla N, Allende-Martinez L, Corral Sanchez MD, Arocena Jde I, Gonzalez-Granado LI. Presentation of severe combined immunodeficiency with respiratory syncytial virus and pneumocystis co-infection. Pediatr Infect Dis J. 2015;34(4):433–4. doi:10.1097/INF.0000000000000569.
55. Lauzon D, Delage G, Brochu P, Michaud J, Jasmin G, Joncas JH, Lapointe N. Pathogens in children with severe combined immune deficiency disease or AIDS. CMAJ: Can Med Assoc J = J de l'Assoc Med Can. 1986;135(1):33–8.
56. Lundgren IS, Englund JA, Burroughs LM, Torgerson TR, Skoda-Smith S. Outcomes and duration of Pneumocystis jiroveci pneumonia therapy in infants with severe combined immunodeficiency. Pediatr Infect Dis J. 2012;31(1):95–7. doi:10.1097/INF.0b013e31822db772.
57. Fogarty L. Thrush and septic shock in a two-month-old. Pediatr Infect Dis J. 1996;15(6):553–4. 559–560.
58. Smego Jr RA, Devoe PW, Sampson HA, Perfect JR, Wilfert CM, Buckley RH. Candida meningitis in two children with severe combined immunodeficiency. J Pediatr. 1984;104(6):902–4.
59. Kobayashi S, Murayama S, Tatsuzawa O, Koinuma G, Kawasaki K, Kiyotani C, Kumagai M. X-linked severe combined immunodeficiency (X-SCID) with high blood levels of immunoglobulins and Aspergillus pneumonia successfully treated with micafangin followed by unrelated cord blood stem cell transplantation. Eur J Pediatr. 2007;166(3):207–10. doi:10.1007/s00431-006-0224-y.
60. Yoshihara T, Morimoto A, Nakauchi S, Fujii N, Tsunamoto K, Misawa A, Hibi S, Imashuku S. Successful transplantation of haploidentical CD34+ selected bone marrow cells for an infantile case of severe combined immunodeficiency with aspergillus pneumonia. Pediatr Hematol Oncol. 2002;19(6):439–43. doi:10.1080/08880010290097215.
61. Alsum Z, Al-Saud B, Al-Ghonaium A, Bin Hussain I, Alsmadi O, Al-Mousa H, Ayas M, Al-Dhekri H, Arnaout R, Al-Muhsen S. Disseminated cryptococcal infection in patient with novel JAK3 mutation severe combined immunodeficiency, with resolution after stem cell transplantation. Pediatr Infect Dis J. 2012;31(2):204–6. doi:10.1097/INF.0b013e318239c3b3.
62. Lau YL, Yuen KY, Lee CW, Chan CF. Invasive Acremonium falciforme infection in a patient with severe combined immunodeficiency. Clin Infect Dis: Off Publ Infect Dis Soc Am. 1995;20(1):197–8.
63. Rivers L, Gaspar HB. Severe combined immunodeficiency: recent developments and guidance on clinical management. Arch Dis Child. 2015;100(7):667–72. doi:10.1136/archdischild-2014-306425.
64. McDonald-McGinn DM, Sullivan KE. Chromosome 22q11.2 deletion syndrome (DiGeorge syndrome/velocardiofacial syndrome). Medicine. 2011;90(1):1–18. doi:10.1097/MD.0b013e3182060469.

65. Marcinkowski M, Bauer K, Stoltenburg-Didinger G, Vogel M, Versmold H. Fatal aspergillosis with brain abscesses in a neonate with DiGeorge syndrome. Pediatr Infect Dis J. 2000;19(12):1214–6.
66. Sergi C, Serpi M, Muller-Navia J, Schnabel PA, Hagl S, Otto HF, Ulmer HE. CATCH 22 syndrome: report of 7 infants with follow-up data and review of the recent advancements in the genetic knowledge of the locus 22q11. Pathologica. 1999;91(3):166–72.
67. Davies EG, Thrasher AJ. Update on the hyper immunoglobulin M syndromes. Br J Haematol. 2010;149(2):167–80. doi:10.1111/j.1365-2141.2010.08077.x.
68. Allenspach E, Rawlings DJ, Scharenberg AM. X-linked severe combined immunodeficiency. In: Pagon RA, Adam MP, Ardinger HH et al., editors. GeneReviews(R). Seattle: University of Washington; 1993
69. Levy J, Espanol-Boren T, Thomas C, Fischer A, Tovo P, Bordigoni P, Resnick I, Fasth A, Baer M, Gomez L, Sanders EA, Tabone MD, Plantaz D, Etzioni A, Monafo V, Abinun M, Hammarstrom L, Abrahamsen T, Jones A, Finn A, Klemola T, DeVries E, Sanal O, Peitsch MC, Notarangelo LD. Clinical spectrum of X-linked hyper-IgM syndrome. J Pediatr. 1997;131(1 Pt 1):47–54.
70. Cabral-Marques O, Klaver S, Schimke LF, Ascendino EH, Khan TA, Pereira PV, Falcai A, Vargas-Hernandez A, Santos-Argumedo L, Bezrodnik L, Moreira I, Seminario G, Di Giovanni D, Raccio AG, Porras O, Weber CW, Ferreira JF, Tavares FS, de Carvalho E, Valente CF, Kuntze G, Galicchio M, King A, Rosario-Filho NA, Grota MB, dos Santos Vilela MM, Di Gesu RS, Lima S, de Souza ML, Talesnik E, Mansour E, Roxo-Junior P, Aldave JC, Goudouris E, Pinto-Mariz F, Berron-Ruiz L, Staines-Boone T, Calderon WO, del Carmen Zarate-Hernandez M, Grumach AS, Sorensen R, Durandy A, Torgerson TR, Carvalho BT, Espinosa-Rosales F, Ochs HD, Condino-Neto A. First report of the Hyper-IgM syndrome Registry of the Latin American Society for Immunodeficiencies: novel mutations, unique infections, and outcomes. J Clin Immunol. 2014;34(2):146–56. doi:10.1007/s10875-013-9980-4.
71. Winkelstein JA, Marino MC, Ochs H, Fuleihan R, Scholl PR, Geha R, Stiehm ER, Conley ME. The X-linked hyper-IgM syndrome: clinical and immunologic features of 79 patients. Medicine. 2003;82(6):373–84. doi:10.1097/01.md.0000100046.06009.b0.
72. Cabral-Marques O, Schimke LF, Pereira PV, Falcai A, de Oliveira JB, Hackett MJ, Errante PR, Weber CW, Ferreira JF, Kuntze G, Rosario-Filho NA, Ochs HD, Torgerson TR, Carvalho BT, Condino-Neto A. Expanding the clinical and genetic spectrum of human CD40L deficiency: the occurrence of paracoccidioidomycosis and other unusual infections in Brazilian patients. J Clin Immunol. 2012;32(2):212–20. doi:10.1007/s10875-011-9623-6.
73. Malheiro L, Lazzara D, Xerinda S, Pinheiro MD, Sarmento A. Cryptococcal meningoencephalitis in a patient with hyper immunoglobulin M (IgM) syndrome: a case report. BMC Res Notes. 2014;7:566. doi:10.1186/1756-0500-7-566.
74. Simon G, Simon G, Erdos M, Marodi L. Invasive *Cryptococcus laurentii* disease in a nine-year-old boy with X-linked hyper-immunoglobulin M syndrome. Pediatr Infect Dis J. 2005;24(10):935–7.
75. de Gorgolas M, Erice A, Gil A, Gutierrez J, Rivas P, Hernando C, Rodriguez MC. Cryptococcal meningitis in a patient with X-linked hyper-IgM1 syndrome. Scand J Infect Dis. 2005;37(6–7):526–8. doi:10.1080/00365540510036570.
76. Iseki M, Anzo M, Yamashita N, Matsuo N. Hyper-IgM immunodeficiency with disseminated cryptococcosis. Acta Paediatr (Oslo, Norway: 1992). 1994;83(7):780–2.
77. Allewelt H, Martin PL, Szabolcs P, Chao N, Buckley R, Parikh S. Hematopoietic stem cell transplantation for CD40 ligand deficiency: single institution experience. Pediatr Blood Cancer. 2015; doi:10.1002/pbc.25711.
78. Mitsui-Sekinaka K, Imai K, Sato H, Tomizawa D, Kajiwara M, Nagasawa M, Morio T, Nonoyama S. Clinical features and hematopoietic stem cell transplantations for CD40 ligand deficiency in Japan. J Allergy Clin Immunol. 2015; doi:10.1016/j.jaci.2015.02.020.
79. Aldrich RA, Steinberg AG, Campbell DC. Pedigree demonstrating a sex-linked recessive condition characterized by draining ears, eczematoid dermatitis and bloody diarrhea. Pediatrics. 1954;13(2):133–9.

80. Blundell MP, Worth A, Bouma G, Thrasher AJ. The Wiskott-Aldrich syndrome: the actin cytoskeleton and immune cell function. Dis Markers. 2010;29(3–4):157–75. doi:10.3233/dma-2010-0735.
81. Imai K, Morio T, Zhu Y, Jin Y, Itoh S, Kajiwara M, Yata J, Mizutani S, Ochs HD, Nonoyama S. Clinical course of patients with WASP gene mutations. Blood. 2004;103(2):456–64. doi:10.1182/blood-2003-05-1480.
82. Cunningham-Rundles C, Bodian C. Common variable immunodeficiency: clinical and immunological features of 248 patients. Clin Immunol. 1999;92(1):34–48. doi:10.1006/clim.1999.4725.
83. Cunningham-Rundles C. Clinical and immunologic analyses of 103 patients with common variable immunodeficiency. J Clin Immunol. 1989;9(1):22–33.
84. Hermaszewski RA, Webster AD. Primary hypogammaglobulinaemia: a survey of clinical manifestations and complications. Q J Med. 1993;86(1):31–42.
85. Lucas M, Lee M, Lortan J, Lopez-Granados E, Misbah S, Chapel H. Infection outcomes in patients with common variable immunodeficiency disorders: relationship to immunoglobulin therapy over 22 years. J Allergy Clin Immunol. 2010;125(6):1354–60. e1354 doi:10.1016/j.jaci.2010.02.040.
86. Kane S, Brasitus T. Histoplasmosis capsulatum as a cause of lower gastrointestinal bleeding in common variable immunodeficiency. Dig Dis Sci. 2000;45(11):2133–5.
87. Lin WC, Dai YS, Tsai MJ, Huang LM, Chiang BL. Systemic Penicillium marneffei infection in a child with common variable immunodeficiency. J Formos Med Assoc = Taiwan yi zhi. 1998;97(11):780–3.
88. Tinelli M, Zambelli A, Cavanna C, Michelone G. Pulmonary aspergillosis in a case of humoral immunodeficiency. Microbiologica. 1987;10(2):235–40.
89. Trachana M, Roilides E, Gompakis N, Kanellopoulou K, Mpantouraki M, Kanakoudi-Tsakalidou F. Case report. Hepatic abscesses due to Aspergillus terreus in an immunodeficient child. Mycoses. 2001;44(9–10):415–8.
90. Schwartz HJ, Berger M, Hostoffer R. Allergic bronchopulmonary aspergillosis and common variable hypogammaglobulinemia in an adult male patient: case report. J Allergy Clin Immunol. 1996;98(3):708–10.
91. Macura AB, Macura-Biegun A, Pawlik B. Susceptibility to fungal infections of nails in patients with primary antibody deficiency. Comp Immunol Microbiol Infect Dis. 2003;26(4):223–32. doi:10.1016/s0147-9571(02)00051-6.
92. Porter SR, Scully C. Orofacial manifestations in primary immunodeficiencies: common variable immunodeficiencies. J Oral Pathol Med: Off Publ Int Assoc Oral Pathol Am Acad Oral Pathol. 1993;22(4):157–8.
93. Quinti I, Soresina A, Spadaro G, Martino S, Donnanno S, Agostini C, Claudio P, Franco D, Maria Pesce A, Borghese F, Guerra A, Rondelli R, Plebani A. Long-term follow-up and outcome of a large cohort of patients with common variable immunodeficiency. J Clin Immunol. 2007;27(3):308–16. doi:10.1007/s10875-007-9075-1.
94. Quinti I, Soresina A, Guerra A, Rondelli R, Spadaro G, Agostini C, Milito C, Trombetta AC, Visentini M, Martini H, Plebani A, Fiorilli M. Effectiveness of immunoglobulin replacement therapy on clinical outcome in patients with primary antibody deficiencies: results from a multicenter prospective cohort study. J Clin Immunol. 2011;31(3):315–22. doi:10.1007/s10875-011-9511-0.
95. Ochs HD, Smith CI. X-linked agammaglobulinemia. A clinical and molecular analysis. Medicine. 1996;75(6):287–99.
96. Winkelstein JA, Marino MC, Lederman HM, Jones SM, Sullivan K, Burks AW, Conley ME, Cunningham-Rundles C, Ochs HD. X-linked agammaglobulinemia: report on a United States registry of 201 patients. Medicine. 2006;85(4):193–202. doi:10.1097/01.md.0000229482.27398.ad.
97. Khalili A, Plebani A, Vitali M, Abolhassani H, Lougaris V, Mirminachi B, Rezaei N, Aghamohammadi A. Autosomal recessive agammaglobulinemia: a novel non-sense mutation in CD79a. J Clin Immunol. 2014;34(2):138–41. doi:10.1007/s10875-014-9989-3.

98. Lougaris V, Ferrari S, Cattalini M, Soresina A, Plebani A. Autosomal recessive agammaglobulinemia: novel insights from mutations in Ig-beta. Curr Allergy Asthma Rep. 2008;8(5):404–8.
99. Lougaris V, Vitali M, Baronio M, Moratto D, Tampella G, Biasini A, Badolato R, Plebani A. Autosomal recessive agammaglobulinemia: the third case of Igbeta deficiency due to a novel non-sense mutation. J Clin Immunol. 2014;34(4):425–7. doi:10.1007/s10875-014-0033-4.
100. Stiehm ER. The four most common pediatric immunodeficiencies. J Immunotoxicol. 2008;5(2):227–34. doi:10.1080/15476910802129646.
101. Woof JM, Kerr MA. The function of immunoglobulin A in immunity. J Pathol. 2006;208(2):270–82. doi:10.1002/path.1877.
102. Herrod HG. Clinical significance of IgG subclasses. Curr Opin Pediatr. 1993;5(6):696–9.
103. Botto M, Kirschfink M, Macor P, Pickering MC, Wurzner R, Tedesco F. Complement in human diseases: lessons from complement deficiencies. Mol Immunol. 2009;46(14):2774–83. doi:10.1016/j.molimm.2009.04.029.
104. Figueroa JE, Densen P. Infectious diseases associated with complement deficiencies. Clin Microbiol Rev. 1991;4(3):359–95.
105. Bouwman LH, Roep BO, Roos A. Mannose-binding lectin: clinical implications for infection, transplantation, and autoimmunity. Hum Immunol. 2006;67(4–5):247–56. doi:10.1016/j.humimm.2006.02.030.
106. Heitzeneder S, Seidel M, Forster-Waldl E, Heitger A. Mannan-binding lectin deficiency – good news, bad news, doesn't matter? Clin Immunol. 2012;143(1):22–38. doi:10.1016/j.clim.2011.11.002.
107. Harrison E, Singh A, Morris J, Smith NL, Fraczek MG, Moore CB, Denning DW. Mannose-binding lectin genotype and serum levels in patients with chronic and allergic pulmonary aspergillosis. Int J Immunogenet. 2012;39(3):224–32. doi:10.1111/j.1744-313X.2011.01078.x.
108. Vaid M, Kaur S, Sambatakou H, Madan T, Denning DW, Sarma PU. Distinct alleles of mannose-binding lectin (MBL) and surfactant proteins A (SP-A) in patients with chronic cavitary pulmonary aspergillosis and allergic bronchopulmonary aspergillosis. Clin Chem Lab Med. 2007;45(2):183–6. doi:10.1515/cclm.2007.033.
109. van Till JW, Modderman PW, de Boer M, Hart MH, Beld MG, Boermeester MA. Mannose-binding lectin deficiency facilitates abdominal Candida infections in patients with secondary peritonitis. Clin Vaccine Immunol: CVI. 2008;15(1):65–70. doi:10.1128/cvi.00297-07.
110. Farmand S, Sundin M. Hyper-IgE syndromes: recent advances in pathogenesis, diagnostics and clinical care. Curr Opin Hematol. 2015;22(1):12–22. doi:10.1097/moh.0000000000000104.
111. Freeman AF, Holland SM. Clinical manifestations, etiology, and pathogenesis of the hyper-IgE syndromes. Pediatr Res. 2009;65(5 Pt 2):32R–7R. doi:10.1203/PDR.0b013e31819dc8c5.
112. Minegishi Y. Hyper-IgE syndrome. Curr Opin Immunol. 2009;21(5):487–92. doi:10.1016/j.coi.2009.07.013.
113. Sowerwine KJ, Holland SM, Freeman AF. Hyper-IgE syndrome update. Ann N Y Acad Sci. 2012;1250:25–32. doi:10.1111/j.1749-6632.2011.06387.x.
114. Yong PF, Freeman AF, Engelhardt KR, Holland S, Puck JM, Grimbacher B. An update on the hyper-IgE syndromes. Arthritis Res Ther. 2012;14(6):228. doi:10.1186/ar4069.
115. van der Meer JW, Bont L, Verhage J. Aspergillus infection in patients with hyperimmunoglobulin E syndrome. Clin Infect Dis: Off Publ Infect Dis Soc Am. 1998;27(5):1337.
116. Freeman AF, Kleiner DE, Nadiminti H, Davis J, Quezado M, Anderson V, Puck JM, Holland SM. Causes of death in hyper-IgE syndrome. J Allergy Clin Immunol. 2007;119(5):1234–40. doi:10.1016/j.jaci.2006.12.666.
117. Ma H, Kuang L, Lv G, Wang B, Lian Z. Vertebral aspergillosis in a patient with autosomal-dominant hyper-IgE syndrome. Clin Vaccine Immunol: CVI. 2014;21(1):107–9. doi:10.1128/cvi.00529-13.
118. McCallum BJ, Amrol D, Horvath J, Inayat N, Talwani R. A case of allergic bronchopulmonary aspergillosis leading to pneumonia with unusual organisms. South Med J. 2005;98(11):1135–8. doi:10.1097/01.smj.0000184788.50353.83.

119. Huppler AR, Bishu S, Gaffen SL. Mucocutaneous candidiasis: the IL-17 pathway and implications for targeted immunotherapy. Arthritis Res Ther. 2012;14(4):217. doi:10.1186/ar3893.
120. Yates AB, Mehrotra D, Moffitt JE. Candida endocarditis in a child with hyperimmunoglobulinemia E syndrome. J Allergy Clin Immunol. 1997;99(6 Pt 1):770–2.
121. Cobos G, Rubin AI, Gober LM, Treat JR. A case of exuberant candidal onychomycosis in a child with hyper IgE syndrome. J Allergy Clin Immunol Pract. 2014;2(1):99–100. doi:10.1016/j.jaip.2013.10.004.
122. Haslett RS, Moriarty AP, Vijayadurai P, McGalliard JN, Chandna A. Candida endophthalmitis in Job syndrome. Arch Ophthalmol (Chicago, Ill: 1960). 1996;114(5):617–8.
123. Jacobs DH, Macher AM, Handler R, Bennett JE, Collen MJ, Gallin JI. Esophageal cryptococcosis in a patient with the hyperimmunoglobulin E-recurrent infection (Job's) syndrome. Gastroenterology. 1984;87(1):201–3.
124. Hutto JO, Bryan CS, Greene FL, White CJ, Gallin JI. Cryptococcosis of the colon resembling Crohn's disease in a patient with the hyperimmunoglobulinemia E-recurrent infection (Job's) syndrome. Gastroenterology. 1988;94(3):808–12.
125. Garty BZ, Wolach B, Ashkenazi S, Weismart Y, Rachmel A, Nitzan M. Cryptococcal meningitis in a child with hyperimmunoglobulin E syndrome. Pediatr Allergy Immunol: Off Publication Eur Soc Pediatr Allergy Immunol. 1995;6(3):175–7.
126. Odio CD, Lee Milligan K, McGowan K, Rudman Spergel AK, Bishop R, Boris L, Urban A, Welch P, Heller T, Kleiner D, Jackson MA, Holland SM, Freeman AF. Endemic mycoses in patients with STAT3-mutated hyper-IgE (Job) syndrome. J Allergy Clin Immunol. 2015;136:1411. doi:10.1016/j.jaci.2015.07.003.
127. Rana C, Krishnani N, Kumari N, Shastri C, Poddar U. Rectal histoplasmosis in Job's syndrome. Indian J Gastroenterol: Off J Indian Soc Gastroenterol. 2013;32(1):64–5. doi:10.1007/s12664-012-0275-0.
128. Hsu AP, Davis J, Puck JM, Holland SM, Freeman AF. Autosomal dominant hyper IgE syndrome. In: Pagon RA, Adam MP, Ardinger HH, et al., editors. GeneReviews(R). Seattle: University of Washington; 1993.
129. Steiner SJ, Kleiman MB, Corkins MR, Christenson JC, Wheat LJ. Ileocecal histoplasmosis simulating Crohn disease in a patient with hyperimmunoglobulin E syndrome. Pediatr Infect Dis J. 2009;28(8):744–6. doi:10.1097/INF.0b013e31819b65e0.
130. Chakrabarti A, Marhawa RK, Mondal R, Trehan A, Gupta S, Rao Raman DS, Sethi S, Padhyet AA. Generalized lymphadenopathy caused by Trichosporon asahii in a patient with Job's syndrome. Med Mycol. 2002;40(1):83–6.
131. Powers AE, Bender JM, Kumanovics A, Ampofo K, Augustine N, Pavia AT, Hill HR. Coccidioides immitis meningitis in a patient with hyperimmunoglobulin E syndrome due to a novel mutation in signal transducer and activator of transcription. Pediatr Infect Dis J. 2009;28(7):664–6. doi:10.1097/INF.0b013e31819866ec.
132. Ma BH, Ng CS, Lam R, Wan S, Wan IY, Lee TW, Yim AP. Recurrent hemoptysis with Penicillium marneffei and Stenotrophomonas maltophilia in Job's syndrome. Can Respir J: J Can Thorac Soc. 2009;16(4):e50–2.
133. Patel NC, Gallagher JL, Torgerson TR, Gilman AL. Successful haploidentical donor hematopoietic stem cell transplant and restoration of STAT3 function in an adolescent with autosomal dominant hyper-IgE syndrome. J Clin Immunol. 2015;35(5):479–85. doi:10.1007/s10875-015-0167-z.
134. Kirkpatrick CH. Chronic mucocutaneous candidiasis. Pediatr Infect Dis J. 2001;20(2):197–206.
135. Kisand K, Peterson P. Autoimmune polyendocrinopathy candidiasis ectodermal dystrophy: known and novel aspects of the syndrome. Ann N Y Acad Sci. 2011;1246:77–91. doi:10.1111/j.1749-6632.2011.06308.x.
136. Keller FG, Kurtzberg J. Disseminated histoplasmosis: a cause of infection-associated hemophagocytic syndrome. Am J Pediatr Hematol Oncol. 1994;16(4):368–71.

137. Hsu AP, McReynolds LJ, Holland SM. GATA2 deficiency. Curr Opin Allergy Clin Immunol. 2015;15(1):104–9. doi:10.1097/aci.0000000000000126.
138. Spinner MA, Sanchez LA, Hsu AP, Shaw PA, Zerbe CS, Calvo KR, Arthur DC, Gu W, Gould CM, Brewer CC, Cowen EW, Freeman AF, Olivier KN, Uzel G, Zelazny AM, Daub JR, Spalding CD, Claypool RJ, Giri NK, Alter BP, Mace EM, Orange JS, Cuellar-Rodriguez J, Hickstein DD, Holland SM. GATA2 deficiency: a protean disorder of hematopoiesis, lymphatics, and immunity. Blood. 2014;123(6):809–21. doi:10.1182/blood-2013-07-515528.
139. Lanternier F, Mahdaviani SA, Barbati E, Chaussade H, Koumar Y, Levy R, Denis B, Brunel AS, Martin S, Loop M, Peeters J, de Selys A, Vanclaire J, Vermylen C, Nassogne MC, Chatzis O, Liu L, Migaud M, Pedergnana V, Desoubeaux G, Jouvion G, Chretien F, Darazam IA, Schaffer AA, Netea MG, De Bruycker JJ, Bernard L, Reynes J, Amazrine N, Abel L, Van der Linden D, Harrison T, Picard C, Lortholary O, Mansouri D, Casanova JL, Puel A. Inherited CARD9 deficiency in otherwise healthy children and adults with Candida species-induced meningoencephalitis, colitis, or both. J Allergy Clin Immunol. 2015;135(6):1558–68. e1552 doi:10.1016/j.jaci.2014.12.1930.
140. Lanternier F, Barbati E, Meinzer U, Liu L, Pedergnana V, Migaud M, Heritier S, Chomton M, Fremond ML, Gonzales E, Galeotti C, Romana S, Jacquemin E, Angoulvant A, Bidault V, Canioni D, Lachenaud J, Mansouri D, Mahdaviani SA, Adimi P, Mansouri N, Jamshidi M, Bougnoux ME, Abel L, Lortholary O, Blanche S, Casanova JL, Picard C, Puel A. Inherited CARD9 deficiency in 2 unrelated patients with invasive Exophiala infection. J Infect Dis. 2015;211(8):1241–50. doi:10.1093/infdis/jiu412.
141. Gavino C, Cotter A, Lichtenstein D, Lejtenyi D, Fortin C, Legault C, Alirezaie N, Majewski J, Sheppard DC, Behr MA, Foulkes WD, Vinh DC. CARD9 deficiency and spontaneous central nervous system candidiasis: complete clinical remission with GM-CSF therapy. Clin Infect Dis: Off Publ Infect Dis Soc Am. 2014;59(1):81–4. doi:10.1093/cid/ciu215.
142. Lanternier F, Pathan S, Vincent QB, Liu L, Cypowyj S, Prando C, Migaud M, Taibi L, Ammar-Khodja A, Boudghene Stambouli O, Guellil B, Jacobs F, Goffard JC, Schepers K, del Marmol V, Boussofara L, Denguezli M, Larif M, Bachelez H, Michel L, Lefranc G, Hay R, Jouvion G, Chretien F, Fraitag S, Bougnoux ME, Boudia M, Abel L, Lortholary O, Casanova JL, Picard C, Grimbacher B, Puel A. Deep dermatophytosis and inherited CARD9 deficiency. N Engl J Med. 2013;369(18):1704–14. doi:10.1056/NEJMoa1208487.
143. Drummond RA, Collar AL, Swamydas M, Rodriguez CA, Lim JK, Mendez LM, Fink DL, Hsu AP, Zhai B, Karauzum H, Mikelis CM, Rose SR, Ferre EM, Yockey L, Lemberg K, Kuehn HS, Rosenzweig SD, Lin X, Chittiboina P, Datta SK, Belhorn TH, Weimer ET, Hernandez ML, Hohl TM, Kuhns DB, Lionakis MS. CARD9-dependent neutrophil recruitment protects against fungal invasion of the central nervous system. PLoS Pathog. 2015;11(12):e1005293. doi:10.1371/journal.ppat.1005293.
144. Hammond SP, Marty FM, Bryar JM, DeAngelo DJ, Baden LR. Invasive fungal disease in patients treated for newly diagnosed acute leukemia. Am J Hematol. 2010;85(9):695–9. doi:10.1002/ajh.21776.
145. Freifeld AG, Bow EJ, Sepkowitz KA, Boeckh MJ, Ito JI, Mullen CA, Raad II, Rolston KV, Young JA, Wingard JR, Infectious Diseases Society of A. Clinical practice guideline for the use of antimicrobial agents in neutropenic patients with cancer: 2010 update by the infectious diseases society of america. Clin Infect Dis: Off Publ Infect Dis Soc Am. 2011;52(4):e56–93. doi:10.1093/cid/cir073.
146. Chamilos G, Luna M, Lewis RE, Bodey GP, Chemaly R, Tarrand JJ, Safdar A, Raad II, Kontoyiannis DP. Invasive fungal infections in patients with hematologic malignancies in a tertiary care cancer center: an autopsy study over a 15-year period (1989–2003). Haematologica. 2006;91(7):986–9.
147. Auberger J, Lass-Florl C, Ulmer H, Nogler-Semenitz E, Clausen J, Gunsilius E, Einsele H, Gastl G, Nachbaur D. Significant alterations in the epidemiology and treatment outcome of invasive fungal infections in patients with hematological malignancies. Int J Hematol. 2008;88(5):508–15. doi:10.1007/s12185-008-0184-2.

148. Prentice HG, Kibbler CC, Prentice AG. Towards a targeted, risk-based, antifungal strategy in neutropenic patients. Br J Haematol. 2000;110(2):273–84.
149. Singh N. Trends in the epidemiology of opportunistic fungal infections: predisposing factors and the impact of antimicrobial use practices. Clin Infect Dis: Off Publ Infect Dis Soc Am. 2001;33(10):1692–6. doi:10.1086/323895.
150. Pagano L, Caira M, Candoni A, Offidani M, Martino B, Specchia G, Pastore D, Stanzani M, Cattaneo C, Fanci R, Caramatti C, Rossini F, Luppi M, Potenza L, Ferrara F, Mitra ME, Fadda RM, Invernizzi R, Aloisi T, Picardi M, Bonini A, Vacca A, Chierichini A, Melillo L, de Waure C, Fianchi L, Riva M, Leone G, Aversa F, Nosari A. Invasive aspergillosis in patients with acute myeloid leukemia: a SEIFEM-2008 registry study. Haematologica. 2010;95(4):644–50. doi:10.3324/haematol.2009.012054.
151. Pagano L, Offidani M, Fianchi L, Nosari A, Candoni A, Piccardi M, Corvatta L, D'Antonio D, Girmenia C, Martino P, Del Favero A. Mucormycosis in hematologic patients. Haematologica. 2004;89(2):207–14.
152. Petrikkos G, Skiada A, Lortholary O, Roilides E, Walsh TJ, Kontoyiannis DP. Epidemiology and clinical manifestations of mucormycosis. Clin Infect Dis: Off Publ Infect Dis Soc Am. 2012;54(Suppl 1):S23–34. doi:10.1093/cid/cir866.
153. Betts R, Glasmacher A, Maertens J, Maschmeyer G, Vazquez JA, Teppler H, Taylor A, Lupinacci R, Sable C, Kartsonis N. Efficacy of caspofungin against invasive Candida or invasive Aspergillus infections in neutropenic patients. Cancer. 2006;106(2):466–73. doi:10.1002/cncr.21615.
154. De Pauw B, Walsh TJ, Donnelly JP, Stevens DA, Edwards JE, Calandra T, Pappas PG, Maertens J, Lortholary O, Kauffman CA, Denning DW, Patterson TF, Maschmeyer G, Bille J, Dismukes WE, Herbrecht R, Hope WW, Kibbler CC, Kullberg BJ, Marr KA, Munoz P, Odds FC, Perfect JR, Restrepo A, Ruhnke M, Segal BH, Sobel JD, Sorrell TC, Viscoli C, Wingard JR, Zaoutis T, Bennett JE. Revised definitions of invasive fungal disease from the European Organization for Research and Treatment of Cancer/Invasive Fungal Infections Cooperative Group and the National Institute of Allergy and Infectious Diseases Mycoses Study Group (EORTC/MSG) Consensus Group. Clin Infect Dis: Off Publ Infect Dis Soc Am. 2008;46(12):1813–21. doi:10.1086/588660.
155. Marr KA, Balajee SA, McLaughlin L, Tabouret M, Bentsen C, Walsh TJ. Detection of galactomannan antigenemia by enzyme immunoassay for the diagnosis of invasive aspergillosis: variables that affect performance. J Infect Dis. 2004;190(3):641–9. doi:10.1086/422009.
156. Marr KA, Laverdiere M, Gugel A, Leisenring W. Antifungal therapy decreases sensitivity of the Aspergillus galactomannan enzyme immunoassay. Clin Infect Dis: Off Publ Infect Dis Soc Am. 2005;40(12):1762–9. doi:10.1086/429921.
157. Georgiadou SP, Sipsas NV, Marom EM, Kontoyiannis DP. The diagnostic value of halo and reversed halo signs for invasive mold infections in compromised hosts. Clin Infect Dis: Off Publ Infect Dis Soc Am. 2011;52(9):1144–55. doi:10.1093/cid/cir122.
158. Chamilos G, Lewis RE, Kontoyiannis DP. Delaying amphotericin B-based frontline therapy significantly increases mortality among patients with hematologic malignancy who have zygomycosis. Clin Infect Dis: Off Publ Infect Dis Soc Am. 2008;47(4):503–9. doi:10.1086/590004.
159. Taur Y, Cohen N, Dubnow S, Paskovaty A, Seo SK. Effect of antifungal therapy timing on mortality in cancer patients with candidemia. Antimicrob Agents Chemother. 2010;54(1):184–90. doi:10.1128/aac.00945-09.
160. Cordonnier C, Pautas C, Maury S, Vekhoff A, Farhat H, Suarez F, Dhedin N, Isnard F, Ades L, Kuhnowski F, Foulet F, Kuentz M, Maison P, Bretagne S, Schwarzinger M. Empirical versus preemptive antifungal therapy for high-risk, febrile, neutropenic patients: a randomized, controlled trial. Clin Infect Dis: Off Publ Infect Dis Soc Am. 2009;48(8):1042–51. doi:10.1086/597395.
161. Pappas PG, Kauffman CA, Andes D, Benjamin Jr DK, Calandra TF, Edwards Jr JE, Filler SG, Fisher JF, Kullberg BJ, Ostrosky-Zeichner L, Reboli AC, Rex JH, Walsh TJ, Sobel JD. Clinical

practice guidelines for the management of candidiasis: 2009 update by the Infectious Diseases Society of America. Clin Infect Dis: Off Publ Infect Dis Soc Am. 2009;48(5):503–35. doi:10.1086/596757.

162. Walsh TJ, Anaissie EJ, Denning DW, Herbrecht R, Kontoyiannis DP, Marr KA, Morrison VA, Segal BH, Steinbach WJ, Stevens DA, van Burik JA, Wingard JR, Patterson TF. Treatment of aspergillosis: clinical practice guidelines of the Infectious Diseases Society of America. Clin Infect Dis: Off Publ Infect Dis Soc Am. 2008;46(3):327–60. doi:10.1086/525258.
163. Marr KA, Schlamm HT, Herbrecht R, Rottinghaus ST, Bow EJ, Cornely OA, Heinz WJ, Jagannatha S, Koh LP, Kontoyiannis DP, Lee DG, Nucci M, Pappas PG, Slavin MA, Queiroz-Telles F, Selleslag D, Walsh TJ, Wingard JR, Maertens JA. Combination antifungal therapy for invasive aspergillosis: a randomized trial. Ann Intern Med. 2015;162(2):81–9. doi:10.7326/m13-2508.
164. Cornely OA, Arikan-Akdagli S, Dannaoui E, Groll AH, Lagrou K, Chakrabarti A, Lanternier F, Pagano L, Skiada A, Akova M, Arendrup MC, Boekhout T, Chowdhary A, Cuenca-Estrella M, Freiberger T, Guinea J, Guarro J, de Hoog S, Hope W, Johnson E, Kathuria S, Lackner M, Lass-Florl C, Lortholary O, Meis JF, Meletiadis J, Munoz P, Richardson M, Roilides E, Tortorano AM, Ullmann AJ, van Diepeningen A, Verweij P, Petrikkos G. ESCMID and ECMM joint clinical guidelines for the diagnosis and management of mucormycosis 2013. Clin Microbiol Infect: Off Publ Eur Soc Clin Microbiol Infect Dis. 2014;20(Suppl 3):5–26. doi:10.1111/1469-0691.12371.
165. Horn DL, Freifeld AG, Schuster MG, Azie NE, Franks B, Kauffman CA. Treatment and outcomes of invasive fusariosis: review of 65 cases from the PATH Alliance((R)) registry. Mycoses. 2014;57(11):652–8. doi:10.1111/myc.12212.
166. Campo M, Lewis RE, Kontoyiannis DP. Invasive fusariosis in patients with hematologic malignancies at a cancer center: 1998-2009. J Infect. 2010;60(5):331–7. doi:10.1016/j.jinf.2010.01.010.
167. Perfect JR, Marr KA, Walsh TJ, Greenberg RN, DuPont B, de la Torre-Cisneros J, Just-Nubling G, Schlamm HT, Lutsar I, Espinel-Ingroff A, Johnson E. Voriconazole treatment for less-common, emerging, or refractory fungal infections. Clin Infect Dis: Off Publ Infect Dis Soc Am. 2003;36(9):1122–31. doi:10.1086/374557.
168. Perfect JR, Dismukes WE, Dromer F, Goldman DL, Graybill JR, Hamill RJ, Harrison TS, Larsen RA, Lortholary O, Nguyen MH, Pappas PG, Powderly WG, Singh N, Sobel JD, Sorrell TC. Clinical practice guidelines for the management of cryptococcal disease: 2010 update by the infectious diseases society of america. Clin Infect Dis: Off Publ Infect Dis Soc Am. 2010;50(3):291–322. doi:10.1086/649858.
169. Nosari AM, Pioltelli ML, Riva M, Marbello L, Nichelatti M, Greco A, Molteni A, Vismara E, Gabutti C, Volonterio A, Lombardi P, Morra E. Invasive fungal infections in lymphoproliferative disorders: a monocentric retrospective experience. Leuk Lymphoma. 2014;55(8):1844–8. doi:10.3109/10428194.2013.853299.
170. Pagano L, Caira M, Candoni A, Offidani M, Fianchi L, Martino B, Pastore D, Picardi M, Bonini A, Chierichini A, Fanci R, Caramatti C, Invernizzi R, Mattei D, Mitra ME, Melillo L, Aversa F, Van Lint MT, Falcucci P, Valentini CG, Girmenia C, Nosari A. The epidemiology of fungal infections in patients with hematologic malignancies: the SEIFEM-2004 study. Haematologica. 2006;91(8):1068–75.
171. Nucci M, Anaissie E. Infections in patients with multiple myeloma in the era of high-dose therapy and novel agents. Clin Infect Dis: Off Publ Infect Dis Soc Am. 2009;49(8):1211–25. doi:10.1086/605664.
172. Teh BW, Teng JC, Urbancic K, Grigg A, Harrison SJ, Worth LJ, Slavin MA, Thursky KA. Invasive fungal infections in patients with multiple myeloma: a multi-center study in the era of novel myeloma therapies. Haematologica. 2015;100(1):e28–31. doi:10.3324/haematol.2014.114025.
173. Nesher L, Rolston KV. The current spectrum of infection in cancer patients with chemotherapy related neutropenia. Infection. 2014;42(1):5–13. doi:10.1007/s15010-013-0525-9.

174. Bergamasco MD, Garnica M, Colombo AL, Nucci M. Epidemiology of candidemia in patients with hematologic malignancies and solid tumours in Brazil. Mycoses. 2013;56(3):256–63. doi:10.1111/myc.12013.
175. Pasqualotto AC, Rosa DD, Medeiros LR, Severo LC. Candidaemia and cancer: patients are not all the same. BMC Infect Dis. 2006;6:50. doi:10.1186/1471-2334-6-50.
176. Slavin MA, Sorrell TC, Marriott D, Thursky KA, Nguyen Q, Ellis DH, Morrissey CO, Chen SC. Candidaemia in adult cancer patients: risks for fluconazole-resistant isolates and death. J Antimicrob Chemother. 2010;65(5):1042–51. doi:10.1093/jac/dkq053.
177. Ohmagari N, Raad II, Hachem R, Kontoyiannis DP. Invasive aspergillosis in patients with solid tumors. Cancer. 2004;101(10):2300–2. doi:10.1002/cncr.20647.
178. Kontoyiannis DP, Marr KA, Park BJ, Alexander BD, Anaissie EJ, Walsh TJ, Ito J, Andes DR, Baddley JW, Brown JM, Brumble LM, Freifeld AG, Hadley S, Herwaldt LA, Kauffman CA, Knapp K, Lyon GM, Morrison VA, Papanicolaou G, Patterson TF, Perl TM, Schuster MG, Walker R, Wannemuehler KA, Wingard JR, Chiller TM, Pappas PG. Prospective surveillance for invasive fungal infections in hematopoietic stem cell transplant recipients, 2001–2006: overview of the Transplant-Associated Infection Surveillance Network (TRANSNET) Database. Clin Infect Dis: Off Publ Infect Dis Soc Am. 2010;50(8):1091–100. doi:10.1086/651263.
179. Garcia-Vidal C, Upton A, Kirby KA, Marr KA. Epidemiology of invasive mold infections in allogeneic stem cell transplant recipients: biological risk factors for infection according to time after transplantation. Clin Infect Dis: Off Publ Infect Dis Soc Am. 2008;47(8):1041–50. doi:10.1086/591969.
180. Marr KA, Carter RA, Boeckh M, Martin P, Corey L. Invasive aspergillosis in allogeneic stem cell transplant recipients: changes in epidemiology and risk factors. Blood. 2002;100(13):4358–66. doi:10.1182/blood-2002-05-1496.
181. Marr KA, Carter RA, Crippa F, Wald A, Corey L. Epidemiology and outcome of mould infections in hematopoietic stem cell transplant recipients. Clin Infect Dis: Off Publ Infect Dis Soc Am. 2002;34(7):909–17. doi:10.1086/339202.
182. Bochud PY, Chien JW, Marr KA, Leisenring WM, Upton A, Janer M, Rodrigues SD, Li S, Hansen JA, Zhao LP, Aderem A, Boeckh M. Toll-like receptor 4 polymorphisms and aspergillosis in stem-cell transplantation. N Engl J Med. 2008;359(17):1766–77. doi:10.1056/NEJMoa0802629.
183. Zaas AK, Liao G, Chien JW, Weinberg C, Shore D, Giles SS, Marr KA, Usuka J, Burch LH, Perera L, Perfect JR, Peltz G, Schwartz DA. Plasminogen alleles influence susceptibility to invasive aspergillosis. PLoS Genet. 2008;4(6):e1000101. doi:10.1371/journal.pgen.1000101.
184. Cunha C, Aversa F, Lacerda JF, Busca A, Kurzai O, Grube M, Loffler J, Maertens JA, Bell AS, Inforzato A, Barbati E, Almeida B, Santos e Sousa P, Barbui A, Potenza L, Caira M, Rodrigues F, Salvatori G, Pagano L, Luppi M, Mantovani A, Velardi A, Romani L, Carvalho A. Genetic PTX3 deficiency and aspergillosis in stem-cell transplantation. N Engl J Med. 2014;370(5):421–32. doi:10.1056/NEJMoa1211161.
185. Denning DW, Ribaud P, Milpied N, Caillot D, Herbrecht R, Thiel E, Haas A, Ruhnke M, Lode H. Efficacy and safety of voriconazole in the treatment of acute invasive aspergillosis. Clin Infect Dis: Off Publ Infect Dis Soc Am. 2002;34(5):563–71. doi:10.1086/324620.
186. Weiss J, Ten Hoevel MM, Burhenne J, Walter-Sack I, Hoffmann MM, Rengelshausen J, Haefeli WE, Mikus G. CYP2C19 genotype is a major factor contributing to the highly variable pharmacokinetics of voriconazole. J Clin Pharmacol. 2009;49(2):196–204. doi:10.1177/0091270008327537.
187. Pappas PG, Alexander BD, Andes DR, Hadley S, Kauffman CA, Freifeld A, Anaissie EJ, Brumble LM, Herwaldt L, Ito J, Kontoyiannis DP, Lyon GM, Marr KA, Morrison VA, Park BJ, Patterson TF, Perl TM, Oster RA, Schuster MG, Walker R, Walsh TJ, Wannemuehler KA, Chiller TM. Invasive fungal infections among organ transplant recipients: results of the Transplant-Associated Infection Surveillance Network (TRANSNET). Clin Infect Dis: Off Publ Infect Dis Soc Am. 2010;50(8):1101–11. doi:10.1086/651262.

188. Fishman JA, Rubin RH. Infection in organ-transplant recipients. N Engl J Med. 1998;338(24):1741–51. doi:10.1056/nejm199806113382407.
189. Grossi P, Farina C, Fiocchi R, Dalla Gasperina D. Prevalence and outcome of invasive fungal infections in 1,963 thoracic organ transplant recipients: a multicenter retrospective study. Italian Study Group of Fungal Infections in Thoracic Organ Transplant Recipients. Transplantation. 2000;70(1):112–6.
190. Singh N, Husain S. Aspergillus infections after lung transplantation: clinical differences in type of transplant and implications for management. J Heart Lung Transplant: Off Publi Int Soc Heart Transplant. 2003;22(3):258–66.
191. Sole A, Morant P, Salavert M, Peman J, Morales P. Aspergillus infections in lung transplant recipients: risk factors and outcome. Clin Microbiol Infect: Off Publ Eur Soc Clin Microbiol Infect Dis. 2005;11(5):359–65. doi:10.1111/j.1469-0691.2005.01128.x.
192. Fungal infections. Am J Transplant off J Am Soc Transplant Am Soc of Transplant Surg. 2004;4 Suppl 10:110–34. doi:10.1111/j.1600-6135.2004.00735.x.
193. Kauffman CA, Freifeld AG, Andes DR, Baddley JW, Herwaldt L, Walker RC, Alexander BD, Anaissie EJ, Benedict K, Ito JI, Knapp KM, Lyon GM, Marr KA, Morrison VA, Park BJ, Patterson TF, Schuster MG, Chiller TM, Pappas PG. Endemic fungal infections in solid organ and hematopoietic cell transplant recipients enrolled in the Transplant-Associated Infection Surveillance Network (TRANSNET). Transpl Infect Dis:Off J Transplant Soc. 2014;16(2):213–24. doi:10.1111/tid.12186.
194. Issa NC, Fishman JA. Infectious complications of antilymphocyte therapies in solid organ transplantation. Clin Infect Dis Off Publ Infect Dis Soc Am. 2009;48(6):772–86. doi:10.1086/597089.
195. Gabardi S, Kubiak DW, Chandraker AK, Tullius SG. Invasive fungal infections and antifungal therapies in solid organ transplant recipients. Transpl Int: Off J Eur Soc Organ Transplant. 2007;20(12):993–1015. doi:10.1111/j.1432-2277.2007.00511.x.
196. George MJ, Snydman DR, Werner BG, Griffith J, Falagas ME, Dougherty NN, Rubin RH. The independent role of cytomegalovirus as a risk factor for invasive fungal disease in orthotopic liver transplant recipients. Boston Center for Liver Transplantation CMVIG-Study Group. Cytogam, MedImmune, Inc. Gaithersburg, Maryland. Am J Med. 1997;103(2):106–13.
197. Djawe K, Buchacz K, Hsu L, Chen MJ, Selik RM, Rose C, Williams T, Brooks JT, Schwarcz S. Mortality risk after AIDS-defining opportunistic illness among HIV-infected persons – San Francisco, 1981–2012. J Infect Dis. 2015;212(9):1366–75. doi:10.1093/infdis/jiv235.
198. de Oliveira RB, Atobe JH, Souza SA, de Castro Lima Santos DW. Epidemiology of invasive fungal infections in patients with acquired immunodeficiency syndrome at a reference hospital for infectious diseases in Brazil. Mycopathologia. 2014;178(1–2):71–8. doi:10.1007/s11046-014-9755-3.
199. Marukutira T, Huprikar S, Azie N, Quan SP, Meier-Kriesche HU, Horn DL. Clinical characteristics and outcomes in 303 HIV-infected patients with invasive fungal infections: data from the Prospective Antifungal Therapy Alliance registry, a multicenter, observational study. HIV/AIDS (Auckland, NZ). 2014;6:39–47. doi:10.2147/hiv.s53910.
200. Peigne V, Dromer F, Elie C, Lidove O, Lortholary O. Imported acquired immunodeficiency syndrome-related histoplasmosis in metropolitan France: a comparison of pre-highly active anti-retroviral therapy and highly active anti-retroviral therapy eras. AmJTrop Med Hyg. 2011;85(5):934–41. doi:10.4269/ajtmh.2011.11-0224.
201. Moreno A, Perez-Elias M, Casado J, Navas E, Pintado V, Fortun J, Quereda C, Guerrero A. Role of antiretroviral therapy in long-term survival of patients with AIDS-related pulmonary aspergillosis. Eur J Clin Microbiol Infect Dis: Off Publ Eur Soc Clin Microbiol. 2000;19(9):688–93.
202. Antinori S, Nebuloni M, Magni C, Fasan M, Adorni F, Viola A, Corbellino M, Galli M, Vago G, Parravicini C, Ridolfo AL. Trends in the postmortem diagnosis of opportunistic invasive fungal infections in patients with AIDS: a retrospective study of 1,630 autopsies performed between 1984 and 2002. Am J Clin Pathol. 2009;132(2):221–7. doi:10.1309/ajcpraae8lz7dtne.

203. Lionakis MS, Kontoyiannis DP. Glucocorticoids and invasive fungal infections. Lancet (London, England). 2003;362(9398):1828–38. doi:10.1016/s0140-6736(03)14904-5.
204. Lewis RE, Kontoyiannis DP. Invasive aspergillosis in glucocorticoid-treated patients. Med Mycol. 2009;47(Suppl 1):S271–81. doi:10.1080/13693780802227159.
205. Berenguer J, Allende MC, Lee JW, Garrett K, Lyman C, Ali NM, Bacher J, Pizzo PA, Walsh TJ. Pathogenesis of pulmonary aspergillosis. Granulocytopenia versus cyclosporine and methylprednisolone-induced immunosuppression. Am J Respir Crit Care Med. 1995;152(3):1079–86. doi:10.1164/ajrccm.152.3.7663787.
206. Delaloye J, Calandra T. Invasive candidiasis as a cause of sepsis in the critically ill patient. Virulence. 2014;5(1):161–9. doi:10.4161/viru.26187.
207. Nucci M, Colombo AL. Risk factors for breakthrough candidemia. Eur. J Clin Microbiol Infect Dis: Off Publ Eur Soc Clin Microbiol. 2002;21(3):209–11. doi:10.1007/s10096-002-0697-1.
208. Dromer F, Mathoulin S, Dupont B, Laporte A. Epidemiology of cryptococcosis in France: a 9-year survey (1985–1993). French Cryptococcosis Study Group. Clin Infect Dis: Off Publ Infect Dis Soc Am. 1996;23(1):82–90.
209. Salmon-Ceron D, Tubach F, Lortholary O, Chosidow O, Bretagne S, Nicolas N, Cuillerier E, Fautrel B, Michelet C, Morel J, Puechal X, Wendling D, Lemann M, Ravaud P, Mariette X. Drug-specific risk of non-tuberculosis opportunistic infections in patients receiving anti-TNF therapy reported to the 3-year prospective French RATIO registry. Ann Rheum Dis. 2011;70(4):616–23. doi:10.1136/ard.2010.137422.
210. Tsiodras S, Samonis G, Boumpas DT, Kontoyiannis DP. Fungal infections complicating tumor necrosis factor alpha blockade therapy. Mayo Clin Proc. 2008;83(2):181–94.
211. Ford AC, Peyrin-Biroulet L. Opportunistic infections with anti-tumor necrosis factor-alpha therapy in inflammatory bowel disease: meta-analysis of randomized controlled trials. Am J Gastroenterol. 2013;108(8):1268–76. doi:10.1038/ajg.2013.138.
212. Maschmeyer G, Patterson TF. New immunosuppressive agents and risk for invasive fungal infections. Curr Infect Dis Rep. 2009;11(6):435–8.
213. Todd T, Besser M, Gudgin E, Crawley C, Craig JI, Follows G, Marcus RE, Enoch DA, Cargill JS, Ludlam HA, Min SY, Sartori P. Invasive fungal sinusitis in patients treated with fludarabine. J Infect. 2008;56(2):156–8. doi:10.1016/j.jinf.2007.11.002.
214. Henn A, Mellon G, Benoit H, Roos-Weil D, Jaureguiberry S, Mordant P, Fekkar A, Caumes E. Disseminated cryptococcosis, invasive aspergillosis, and mucormycosis in a patient treated with alemtuzumab for chronic lymphocytic leukaemia. Scand J Infect Dis. 2014;46(3):231–4. doi:10.3109/00365548.2013.866269.

Immunity to Fungal Infections

2

Simon Altmeier and Salomé LeibundGut-Landmann

Abstract

Most fungi to which we are regularly exposed through the air or because they are part of our normal microbiota do not usually cause disease in immunocompetent individuals. However, some fungi can become pathogenic if host defenses are breached with symptoms ranging from mild superficial infections to severe systemic diseases that are associated with a high degree of morbidity and mortality. Understanding the immune response against fungal infections is of key importance for the development of better preventive and therapeutic options. However, the host response against different fungal infections are as diverse and distinct as the different fungal diseases themselves. Clinical and basic research during the last decade has brought exciting new insights into the pathogenesis of fungi and revealed important molecular and cellular players in host-fungal interactions and host defense. This chapter summarizes and reviews recent advances in the field that have shaped the current understanding of antifungal immunity.

2.1 Introduction

Most fungal infections are caused by organisms to which we are regularly exposed through the air or because they are part of our normal microbiota. They do not usually cause disease in immunocompetent individuals. However, some fungi can become pathogenic if host defenses are breached with symptoms ranging from mild superficial infections to severe systemic diseases that are associated with a high

S. Altmeier • S. LeibundGut-Landmann (✉)
Section of Immunology, Vetsuisse Faculty, University of Zurich,
Winterthurerstrasse 266a, 8057 Zurich, Switzerland
e-mail: salome.leibundgut-landmann@uzh.ch

A. Carvalho (ed.), *Immunogenetics of Fungal Diseases*,
DOI 10.1007/978-3-319-50842-9_2

degree of morbidity and mortality. Predisposing conditions include immunosuppression by corticosteroids or chemotherapy in transplant recipients and tumor patients, acquired immunodeficiencies such as those occurring as a consequence of HIV infection, antibiotic treatment, or the application of medical devices (e.g., dentures and catheters that promote the formation of biofilms, e.g., by *Candida* spp.). Hereditary immunodeficiencies have recently gained attention as rare but important predisposing factor for fungal infections. The clinical relevance of fungal infections often remains undervalued despite the fact that ~25% of the overall population is affected. While the majority of cases can be treated with available drugs, recurrent, chronic, and invasive forms of disease are more severe and often difficult to treat. They cause far over one million deaths per year worldwide [39]. There is thus an unmet clinical need for more rapid and better diagnostics, safer and more effective antifungal drugs, and preventative vaccines. Clinical and basic research during the last decade has brought exciting new insights into the pathogenesis of fungi and revealed important molecular and cellular players in host-fungal interactions and host defense. In this chapter, we will summarize and review recent advances in the field that have shaped the current understanding of antifungal immunity.

2.2 Human Fungal Pathogens Cause a Diverse Spectrum of Diseases

Fungal pathogens cause a broad spectrum of diseases that manifests as superficial, tissue-invasive, and allergenic syndromes. They can be grouped by the causative fungal agents and by the tissue tropism. The host responses raised against these different types of infections vary greatly and depend on the causative fungal species as well as on the host tissue compartments involved.

2.2.1 Superficial Fungal Infections

Superficial fungal infections comprising mucosal, cutaneous, and corneal infections can affect all barrier tissues of the host. *Candida* spp. most frequently affect the oral and vaginal mucosa, the skin, and the nails and cause symptoms even in otherwise healthy individuals. Vulvovaginal infections are particularly frequent, even in otherwise healthy individuals, with around 70% of all women experiencing at least one episode during their lifetime and 5–10% of them developing recurrent or chronic vulvovaginal candidiasis [308]. Oral and esophageal *Candida* infections are associated with $CD4^+$ T cell defects such as those occurring in patients with progressive AIDS. More recently, specific defects in the interleukin-17 pathway were linked to chronic mucocutaneous candidiasis (CMC) with both cutaneous (skin, nails) and mucosal (oropharyngeal, genital) manifestations.

Although less studied than *Candida* spp., dermatophytes are the most frequent cause of superficial fungal infections. They give rise to well-known conditions such as athlete's foot, ringworm of the scalp, and infection of the nails [141], which are usually curable with available antimycotics. Specific immune defects however allow more severe and sometimes life-threatening forms of dermatomycoses to occur, such as deep dermatophytosis and invasive *Exophiala* infection in individuals with CARD9 deficiency [198, 200]. *Malassezia* spp. are commensal yeasts found abundantly on the human skin [344] that can be involved in various skin disorders such as atopic dermatitis, tinea versicolor, and folliculitis [11, 298]. The causative relationship between fungal overgrowth and the development of disease symptoms is not well understood [349]. *Malassezia pachydermatis* is an important opportunistic fungal pathogen in dogs with zoonotic potential [239].

Fungal infection of the cornea of the eye, called fungal keratitis, can develop as a consequence of eye trauma, e.g., caused by thorns and sticks. This disease is most often caused by *Fusarium*, *Aspergillus*, and *Candida* species [330]. If untreated, it can result in vision loss or blindness. The rural communities of the developing world are particularly affected. Contact lens wearers are also at risk.

2.2.2 Deep-Seated Fungal Infections

Deep-seated fungal infections, although much less frequent than superficial fungal infections, are much feared because of their association with high mortality rates (often >50%). They remain challenging to diagnose and to treat. Invasive fungal infections occur predominantly in hospital settings and develop when fungi penetrate unchecked the natural barriers in susceptible hosts.

Systemic candidiasis is rated the fourth common bloodstream infection among nosocomial infections. It develops in severely ill patients upon entry of *Candida* spp. from the skin (e.g., via venous catheters) or from the gastrointestinal tract (e.g., upon neutropenia, prolonged antibiotic exposure, and cytotoxic chemotherapy) via the circulation into the spleen, the liver, and/or the kidney causing organ failure and sepsis-like syndromes [213, 266]. Specific immune defects such as those observed in individuals with genetic defects in the gene CARD9 can cause rare organ-specific infections targeting the central nervous system (CNS) [85].

Cryptococcus neoformans accounts for 50% of all fungal infections in HIV patients, and it is the third most common cause of fungal infections in solid organ transplantation [134]. Systemic dissemination of *C. neoformans* from the lung and crossing of the blood-brain barrier can result in subsequent infection of the CNS [134].

Another common respiratory opportunistic pathogen is *Pneumocystis jirovecii*, which causes pneumonia in individuals with impaired immunity, especially those suffering from HIV/AIDS [43]. Other groups at risk include individuals with hematological malignancies, transplant patients, and individuals on prolonged immunosuppressive therapy, such as corticosteroids or methotrexate. Transmission occurs via aerosols from patients with pneumonia or from early-life contact with family or community members who carry the organism in their lungs [238].

Zygomycetes is the causative agent of mucormycosis (zygomycosis), a rare but severe fungal disease that develops in settings of leukemia, transplantation, diabetic ketoacidosis, neutropenia, and severe immunosuppression [314]. Herein, angioinvasion results in systemic dissemination, infarction of blood vessels, and necrosis of surrounding tissues. The associated mortality rates in transplantation patients may be as high as 80% [126]. Diabetic patients are at the risk of rhino-orbital mucormycosis, which can require eye removal [142, 306].

Thermally dimorphic fungi that are endemic to certain areas in the Americas typically infect healthy hosts and cause systemic mycoses [114, 182]. They can also reactivate from a latent state when immunity is impaired, such as in solid organ transplant recipients that are particularly at risk for respiratory failure and extrapulmonary dissemination [114, 182].

Continuous exposure to environmental molds of the *Aspergillus* spp. can translate into invasive pulmonary aspergillosis, which is associated with high mortality rates [39]. Patients at risk are those with impaired immune functions including individuals with low numbers of neutrophils, solid organ transplant recipients, patients on immunosuppressive therapies, patients with chronic obstructive pulmonary disease (COPD), and cystic fibrosis patients [187]. In addition, different forms of chronic pulmonary aspergillosis, a gradual destructive disease in the lung, are observed in non-immunocompromised patients with prior or current lung disease [77].

2.2.3 Allergic Fungal Diseases

Some fungi have allergenic potential. The most common allergic mycosis is allergic bronchopulmonary aspergillosis (ABPA) [109]. Asthma and cystic fibrosis patients are especially at risk to develop this Th2-mediated allergic disease [127, 184].

2.2.4 Compartmentalized Immune Mechanisms Act Against Different Fungal Infections

Most fungal diseases in humans are caused by environmental or commensal organisms that have coevolved with their host for millions of years without causing harm to the host under normal conditions. Disease susceptibility is attributed primarily to defects in host defense. Studying the immune defects in patients suffering from fungal infections has revealed host mechanisms that are responsible for maintaining homeostasis with different fungal species in different tissue compartments. Generally, fungal control in superficial tissues is maintained by the barrier function of the epithelium, which prevents fungal overgrowth and invasion. This function is critically complemented by the adaptive immune system, which forms memory cells (predominantly $CD4^+$ T cell memory) in response to the continuous fungal exposure and provides constant antigen-specific surveillance (Fig. 2.1). In contrast, protection from invasive and disseminated fungal disease, where fungi gain access to the circulation and to internal organs and where they usually not reside, relies primarily on the acute response of myeloid effector cells of the innate immune system, including neutrophils, monocytes, and macrophages (Fig. 2.2). The different forms/types/mechanisms of antifungal defense will be discussed in detail below.

Clinical studies on patients suffering from fungal diseases were complemented by numerous mechanistic studies with cultured cells (primary human and mouse cells and tumor cell lines) and experimental infections in animal models. Together, they have provided important insights into the cellular and molecular mechanisms of fungal recognition by the host, activation of innate and adaptive immunity, and the exertion of effector mechanisms against fungal pathogens. Animal studies are particularly valuable for revealing multicellular interactions and tissue-specific aspects of antifungal host defense in vivo. Different animal models for several types of fungal infections were established in mice [152], and zebra fish models for mucosal and disseminated infections were developed more recently [37, 125, 333]. While animal studies in mice were very informative and greatly advanced the field, animal models reflect the situation in humans only to a certain extent. Most importantly, many fungal pathogens including *C. albicans*, which are part of the microbiota in humans, are not generally commensals in SPF mice [161]. Therefore, experimental infections in mice with these species reflect in most cases primary infections that trigger acute immune responses and thus bear important differences to the responses to continuous fungal presence in humans. This discrepancy is most relevant in case of superficial infections. There is thus a need to develop refined infection models to close this gap in the future.

2.3 Fungal-Host Interactions

2.3.1 Fungal Morphological Plasticity Is an Important Determinant of the Interaction with the Host

Many pathogenic fungi exist in different morphotypes and can switch between environmental and pathogenic forms that bear a differential virulence potential. Morphotype switching is generally accompanied by major changes in the transcriptional program of the fungus that alters the behavior of the fungus in contact with the host. Most *Candida* species are thought to exist as unicellular yeasts undergoing asexual reproduction in their commensal state, while the hyphal form is associated with increased adhesion and invasion of host tissue surfaces. In case of *A. fumigatus*, conidia are inhaled, and the swelling of conidia (asexual spores) in the alveolar spaces is accompanied by increased immunogenicity that allows/promotes enhanced control by the immune system, while *A. fumigatus* hyphae are associated with host tissue invasion [69]. Thermally dimorphic fungi, a group of at least six primary human fungal pathogens, grow as a mold in soil at ambient temperature and convert to virulent yeast after infectious spores are inhaled [182]. Generally, it is believed that morphological plasticity rather than a specific fixed morphotype is the key feature of fungal pathogenicity [296].

2.3.2 Fungal Interactions with the Epithelium

Epithelial cells are usually the first cells of the host to interact with opportunistic fungal pathogens during homeostasis and for induction of disease. Depending on their route of acquisition and their tissue tropism, fungi encounter different types of epithelia, such as simple squamous epithelia (in the lung and gastrointestinal tract) or stratified squamous epithelia (in the skin and vagina). These epithelia not only serve as mere physical barriers, but they are also involved in sensing fungi and in activating host defense mechanisms in dependence of the fungal pathogenicity. The interaction of fungi with epithelial cells was studied most extensively with *C. albicans*. The progression from *C. albicans* commensalism to infection involves fungal adhesion to the epithelium, invasion, and eventually damage of epithelial cells [143], which may result in the secretion of inflammatory mediators by the epithelium.

Adhesion of *C. albicans* to epithelial cells is mediated by cell surface adhesins as well as physical properties such as cell surface hydrophobicity. A number of adhesin genes show increased expression upon *C. albicans* interaction with epithelial cells consistent with a role in adhesion to these cells. This role was clearly established for the Als3 glycosylphosphatidylinositol (GPI)-anchored cell wall protein that mediates hyphal adhesion through interaction with host cadherins [267]. Hwp1 is another GPI-anchored protein at the *C. albicans* hyphal cell surface that mediates adhesion to epithelial cells and, interestingly, is recognized by host cell transglutaminases that create covalent bonding between Hwp1 and host surface proteins [315]. Notably, the *ALS3* and *HWP1* genes and other genes encoding cell surface adhesins involved in the interaction with epithelial cells are expressed upon yeast-to-hyphae transition [356, 385], suggesting that this morphotypic switch of *C. albicans* contributes to adhesion, while at the same time, adhesion to epithelial cells promotes hyphenation. The reciprocal relationship between these two processes thus highlights that fungal morphotype and function are intricately linked.

Invasion of the oral epithelium is a critical step for the infection process. In case of *C. albicans*, it involves induced endocytosis and active penetration of epithelial cells [355]. Induced endocytosis is the consequence of the interaction of cell surface adhesins or proteins with host cell receptors, such as Als3-cadherin and Ssa1-cadherin interactions that trigger the recruitment of clathrin and other components of the endocytosis machinery at the site of interaction between the hyphal tip and the host cell [237, 267, 324]. Actin-dependent endocytosis is also observed with other fungi, such as the internalization of *A. fumigatus* conidia by lung epithelial cells [31, 121]. Active penetration of epithelial cells by *C. albicans* is less well understood but may involve the combined action of secreted aspartyl proteases (SAPs) and mechanical pressure [70]. Sap5 was reported to degrade E-cadherin, which is part of epithelial tight junctions [350]. Active penetration was also observed by *A. fumigatus* hyphae grown on a human lung biopsy, which invaded through and in between epithelial cells resulting in cell damage, loss of cilia, and cell detachment [8].

2.3.3 Fungal Interactions with Endothelial Cells

During dissemination, fungal pathogens interact with endothelial cells for invasion by distinct mechanisms. Systemic infection with *C. albicans* involves the transendothelial migration of the fungus into the bloodstream and subsequent rapid escape from the circulation for entry into target organs such as the kidney [213]. *C. albicans* (but not *C. tropicalis* and *C. glabrata*) was internalized by endothelial cells in vitro [105]. The observations that in vivo endothelial transmigration into the tissues takes only several minutes [93, 220], while morphological switching takes several hours [288], and that yeast-locked *C. albicans* is also able to enter the tissue [21], suggest that yeast-to-hyphae transition is not required for endothelial transmigration of *C. albicans*. Factors involved in adhesion and invasion of the endothelium by *C. albicans* include $\alpha_M\beta_2$ integrin-like adhesins, which likely bind to ICAM-1 [383], and members of the Als family (e.g., Als3) and Ssa1, which bind to N-cadherin on endothelial cells [267, 388].

Transendothelial migration of *Zygomycetes* was also studied in some detail. Indeed, it was shown that *Zygomycetes* adhere to and are taken up by endothelial cells in vitro [158]. This process is thought to be critical for angioinvasion of *Zygomycetes* from the lung and to enter blood vessels during pulmonary infection.

2.3.4 Fungi-Induced Damage of the Host

Tissue invasion by fungal hyphae causes epithelial (and endothelial) damage. Host cell damage appears to result from a combination of different mechanisms. Damage induction by *C. albicans*, for which this process and its significance during the infection process were studied most extensively, depends on fungal viability, although being alive is not sufficient for damage induction. Furthermore, it is not strictly coupled to invasion. Damage induction depends on many genes related to yeast-to-hyphae transition [356]. For instance, *C. albicans* SAPs were reported to contribute to alter the integrity of the epithelium through their actions on E-cadherins [107, 350]. More recently, a role for the *ECE1* gene in epithelial damage was demonstrated, whereby the hyphal-specific Ece1 protein is proteolytically processed leading to extracellular release of peptides, among which the so-called candidalysin peptide that acts as a toxin toward host cell membranes [243]. While at low concentration candidalysin peptide triggers a c-Fos- and MKP-dependent danger response pathway, at higher concentrations it forms pores in epithelial cells allowing for calcium influx and eliciting direct tissue damage. Production of Ece1 and candidalysin might in part explain why sustained hyphal growth is central to damage of epithelial cells. The capacity of a fungus to cause damage seems thus to be directly linked to its pathogenicity.

2.3.5 Activation of the Epithelium by Pathogenic Fungi

As described above, epithelia not only serve an important physical barrier to prevent fungal invasion, but they also actively respond and have the capacity to discriminate pathogenic from nonpathogenic forms [247]. Epithelial cells express pattern recognition receptors (PRRs) such as Toll-like receptors (TLRs) and dectin-1 (see below for a more detailed description of these receptors). However, PRR-independent signaling pathways are also involved in fungal recognition by epithelial cells [241]. The response of epithelial cells to fungi was studied most extensively with *C. albicans*, and we will thus focus our discussion on the interaction of the epithelium with this fungus. Although the exact nature of the receptors that link fungal recognition by epithelial cells to cytokine secretion remains unknown, downstream signaling components were identified. In fact, *C. albicans* yeast cells can induce basal NFκB and c-Jun activation, while *C. albicans* hyphae trigger a more profound MAPK response resulting in MPK1 and c-Fos phosphorylation [241] and PI3K/Akt/mTOR activation [242], which results in the secretion of cytokines, including G-CSF, GM-CSF, IL-6, and IL-1α. Quantitative and qualitative differences exist between different cytokines depending on individual signaling pathways and depending on the type of epithelial cells analyzed [240]. A key factor of *C. albicans* responsible for triggering these responses has recently been identified to be the candidalysin peptide derived from the hyphal-specific virulence factor Ece1 [243]. Importantly, low concentrations of candidalysin were shown to induce G-CSF and GM-CSF secretion, while higher concentrations were required for pore formation in the epithelial cell membrane that then led to the release of IL-1α. IL-1α is preformed in epithelial cells [80, 195], and induction of cellular damage is thought to be sufficient for its release. Similar to the situation with *C. albicans*, MAPK signaling has also been implicated in the epithelial response to *A. fumigatus* [16].

2.3.6 Antifungal Effector Mechanisms of the Epithelium

Epithelial cells are an important source of cytokines and chemokines for the recruitment of leukocytes such as neutrophils, monocytes, and T cells to the site of infection [317, 339, 340]. G-CSF has pleiotropic effects on neutrophils. Most importantly, it is a key regulator of granulopoiesis, and it mobilizes neutrophil from the bone marrow in response to infection and inflammation to meet the increased demand for neutrophils during these situations [26]. In addition, G-CSF promotes neutrophil survival by inducing Mcl-1 RNA [257]. G-CSF also enhances neutrophil function, e.g., by inducing ROS production [250, 287], and it may enhance the killing activity of human neutrophils toward *A. fumigatus* [210] and *C. albicans* [286, 376]. Neutrophil survival and function are also enhanced by GM-CSF [176, 287].

IL-1α together with the related family member IL-1β, which can also be produced by epithelial cells, at least in humans, and by leukocytes, can act in an autocrine or paracrine manner on epithelial cells to amplify cytokine and chemokine production and thereby to promote the inflammatory response. During acute pulmonary aspergillosis, IL-1α induces neutrophil recruitment via the production of CXCL1 and enhances neutrophil activity against the fungus [42]. This is also reflected by the requirement of MyD88, which is an essential signaling component downstream of the IL-1R and required in the non-hematopoietic compartment in this process [165]. Similarly, in the context of oropharyngeal candidiasis, IL-1R signaling was implicated in neutrophil recruitment and fungal control [149]. The role of IL-1 cytokines in protective immunity to fungi is not limited to barrier tissues. Indeed, *Il1a*$^{-/-}$ and *Il1b*$^{-/-}$ mice display an increased fungal burden and impaired survival in a mouse model of systemic candidiasis [353].

Epithelial cells are an important source of host defense peptides (HDPs). Active peptides are usually 10–50 amino acids in size that are generated by proteolytic processing from precursors and are mostly positively charged but can also contain a substantial portion of hydrophobic residues [137]. They kill or block the growth of pathogens by membrane permeabilization of microbial cells and by inactivation of cytoplasmic targets therein. In addition to their antimicrobial activity, many HDPs can also act as immune modulators and promote chemotaxis of immune cells [137]. The major families of HDPs include α- and β-defensins, histatins, and cathelicidins (human LL-37, murine Cramp). Expression of some HDPs by epithelial cells is constitutive, while others are inducible by microbial and inflammatory triggers. In addition, HDP production is not limited to epithelial cells; neutrophils are an important source of, e.g., cathelicidins and α-defensins.

β-Defensins, which are distinguished from α-defensins by their cysteine disulfide connectivities, are expressed almost exclusively by epithelial cells, and several of them are induced by pathogenic fungi [7, 98, 206]. The mechanism of β-defensin-mediated antifungal activity is not well studied [191], but it is believed to involve the formation of membrane pores [112] and to be energy-dependent and salt-sensitive [354]. Human β-defensin 2 (hBD2, mouse homologues mBD3 and mBD4) and hBD3 (mouse homologue mBD14) exert direct antifungal activity toward *Candida* spp. [98, 170] and *A. fumigatus* [259]. mBD1 deficiency was associated with impaired fungal control in mice in a model of mixed oropharyngeal and systemic candidiasis [334].

Expression of histatins is restricted to human salivary glands [164]. The parent protein histatin 3 undergoes multiple proteolytic cleavages during and after secretion to give rise to cascades of peptide products, including histatin 5 (Hst5). The fungicidal activity of Hst5 relies on its capacity to disrupt the cellular ionic homeostasis [272] by binding to *C. albicans* Ssa1 and Ssa2 [208, 323], intracellular translocation, disruption of the fungal Trk1 transporter function [14], and finally ATP and potassium efflux [144, 186, 375]. The loss of cytosolic ions initiates cellular shrinkage and cell cycle arrest. Hst5 also affects mitochondrial functions, causes oxidative stress [272], and may inhibit *C. albicans* adhesion to epithelial cells [234].

The cathelicidin LL-37 (called Cramp in mice) is another HDP that acts by altering the ionic homeostasis of fungal cells. In *C. albicans*, the cell wall β-1,3-exoglucanase Xog1 was identified to bind LL-37 [50], which in turn leads to processing of LL-37 by cell wall proteases, intracellular translocation, massive disruption of the *C. albicans* cell membrane [74], and induction of nucleotide and protein efflux [75]. In mice, Cramp was proposed to be responsible for *C. albicans* colonization resistance [94].

Metal-chelating agents, such as calprotectin, can also prevent fungal growth [310]. The calprotectin subunits S100A8 and S100A9 are strongly induced in response to fungal infection [63, 338]. Moreover, S100A9-deficient mice display impaired fungal clearance during barrier tissue infections with *C. albicans* [345, 380] and *A. fumigatus* [59].

The existence of a large number of different antimicrobial effectors, many of which with at least seemingly redundant effects, guarantees efficient protection of the host from a large spectrum of different microbes. The absence of a single antimicrobial effector may thus not be sufficient to disrupt efficient control of an infection by the host [101]. In summary, epithelial cells have multiple mechanisms to respond to infection including antimicrobial defense peptides that mediate direct antifungal control, alarmins such as IL-1α that report the presence of invasive pathogens, chemotactic factors that can recruit immune cells, and cytokines that signal to and activate immune cells. While many of those responses are induced directly by the fungus, they may also be stimulated and/or amplified by microbial-induced cytokines in an autocrine and/or paracrine manner. The epithelium thus integrates signals from the fungus and the host to promote efficient host defense in barrier tissues.

2.3.7 Innate Recognition of Fungal Pathogens

If fungal pathogens overcome the initial epithelial barrier and (start to) invade the host tissue, they may get in contact with immune cells in the tissue, and/or – depending on the route and degree of invasion – in the circulation. The innate immune system has evolved to sense conserved microbial structures, so-called pathogen-associated molecular patterns (PAMPs) via germline-encoded PRRs. Ligand binding by PRRs induces the activation of signaling cascades inside the cell that leads to gene expression in the nucleus. The production of cytokines, chemokines, and antimicrobial factors by innate immune cells results in the activation and recruitment of effector cells to the site of infection and in the elimination of pathogens, respectively. Here, we discuss the most common PRR pathways involved in fungal recognition, while the effect of individual cytokines, chemokines, and cellular effector mechanisms that are induced by these pathways is discussed below.

2.3.8 Fungal PAMPs

The primary fungal PAMPs that are recognized by the innate immune system of the host are components of the cell wall. The fungal cell wall is composed of skeletal and matrix components, which resemble mesh and mortar in concrete buildings [252]. The skeletal structures at the base of the cell wall consist of chitin, which is a β-(1,4)-linked polymer of N-acetylglucosamine, and β-1,3- and β-1,6-glucans that are stabilized by intermolecular hydrogen bonds. The fungal cell wall matrix is composed of mannoproteins, namely, heavily glycosylated proteins with mannose-containing polysaccharides (sometimes called mannans). These mannoproteins are attached to β-1,3-glucans or chitin by a linker structure. Important differences in cell wall composition and conformation exist between different fungal species [91]. β-1,3-glucan, which is usually hidden by other carbohydrates, is one of the most potent fungal PAMPs. The sequestration of β-1,3-glucan by less immunostimulatory cell wall components evolved as a potent immune evasion strategy in many pathogenic fungi. Examples for this are the masking of β-glucans by mannans in *Candida* spp. [365], the rodlet layer of airborne fungal spores such as in *Aspergillus* spp. [5], the presence of α-glucans in the outer cell wall of *Histoplasma* [278] and *Paracoccidioides brasiliensis* [29], and the capsule ensheathing/surrounding

Cryptococcus neoformans [189]. Consequently, exposure, or unmasking, of β-1,3-glucans enhances immunogenicity. This is achieved naturally during the infection process as the cell wall is attacked by host-derived lytic enzymes or by antifungal drugs, such as echinocandins that interfere with the natural integrity and architecture of the fungal cell wall [365]. Importantly, β-1,3-glucans are also exposed stage specifically in *C. albicans* and *A. fumigatus* as a consequence of the dynamics of the fungal cell wall in response to environmental factors [111, 117, 153, 318].

2.3.9 C-Type Lectin Receptors (CLR)

The main PRRs involved in fungal recognition belong to the family of myeloid C-type lectin receptors (CLRs) that are highly expressed by dendritic cells (DCs), neutrophils, and macrophages. CLRs are classified by the presence of one or several C-type lectin-like domains (CTLDs), many of which bind to carbohydrates such as those in the fungal cell wall. The family of CLRs encompasses soluble molecules such as the mannose-binding protein (MBP) or surfactant protein D that activate the complement cascade, endocytic receptors that internalize their ligands such as the mannose receptor (MR), and signaling receptors that act as bona fide PRRs to initiate innate and adaptive immunity, while others have immunomodulatory activities [71, 139, 261].

The prototypic signaling CLR is dectin-1. It binds to β-(1,3)-glucans in the fungal cell wall [40]. Dectin-1 contains an ITAM-like motif, also called hemITAM, in its cytoplasmic domain [285]. Receptor dimerization and phosphorylation of a tyrosine-residue of this motif by Src-family kinases lead to the recruitment of the spleen tyrosine kinase (Syk) [285], which in turn couples to the canonical NF-κB pathway via the protein kinase C δ (PKCδ) [321], and the adaptor protein CARD9 [132, 138]. Selective signaling via dectin-1 results in the induction of high levels of TNF, IL-6, and IL-23, but little IL-12, and is thus qualitatively distinct from TLR-mediated signaling [203]. Dectin-1 signaling can also engage phospholipase Cγ2 (PLCγ2)-dependent nuclear factor of activated T cell (NFAT) activation, resulting in the production of IL-2 and IL-10 [307]. Moreover, dectin-1 signaling leads to the induction of IL-1β via the activation of caspase-1, which mediates cleavage of pro-IL-1β into mature IL-1β (see below). In addition to its predominant expression by myeloid immune cells, dectin-1 was also reported to be expressed on epithelial cells and to respond to pure β-glucans and fungal cells by the release of pro-inflammatory cytokines in a Syk-dependent manner [60, 325].

Dectin-1 signaling was implicated in the response to many pathogenic fungi, and its host-protective role was demonstrated in mouse models with *C. albicans* [328], *A. fumigatus* [155, 318, 364], and *Pneumocystis* [291], among others. In humans, dectin-1 polymorphisms were associated with enhanced susceptibility to vulvovaginal candidiasis and onychomycosis [102] and with invasive pulmonary aspergillosis [67, 293]. However, the precise role of dectin-1 in protection from these human diseases deserves further investigations. The high prevalence of the Y238X polymorphism in dectin-1 in the human population [102] puts in question its causal link to disease development.

Dectin-2 and mincle are two additional Syk-coupled CLRs that recognize fungal α-mannan structures [226]. Unlike dectin-1, they lack the hemiTAM motif in their cytoplasmic tail. Instead, they assemble with FcRγ, an ITAM-containing adaptor for signaling [295]. In addition, dectin-2 and mincle have recently been shown to associate with MCL (also called dectin-3) for enhanced ligand binding [231, 389, 390]. Dectin-2 signaling promotes immunity to *C. albicans* [284, 292], *C. glabrata* [159], and *Malassezia* [163]. In contrast to the broad spectrum of fungi stimulating dectin-2 [179], mincle agonists appear more restricted among fungal pathogens, as demonstrated by the selective binding of mincle to *Malassezia* spp. among 50 fungal species tested [378]. More recently, mincle was also shown to be involved in sensing *F. pedrosoi*, the causative agent of chromoblastosis [312], and it may also recognize *C. albicans* [363]. In addition, mincle possesses a ligand in mycobacteria [162, 225] and responds to a self-ligand exposed by dying cells [377].

While defects in individual CLRs can lead to partial and/or selective defects in antifungal defense, the deficiency in Card9, a signaling component common to all myeloid signaling CLR pathways, leads to more severe defects in controlling fungal infections [132]. Likewise, CARD9 polymorphisms are associated with persistent and severe forms of fungal infections in humans that primarily localize to the skin and subcutaneous tissue, mucosal surfaces, and/or the central nervous system [83, 84, 115, 116, 120, 198–200, 209, 359]. This suggests redundancy between different fungal PRRs but also the existence of Card9-dependent functions that are independent and go beyond those of CLRs [85].

Several fungal CLRs were identified that signal via an immunoreceptor tyrosine-based inhibitory motif (ITIM) rather than an ITAM domain. Ligand binding to ITIM-containing receptors results in ITIM phosphorylation and the association of SH2 domain-containing protein tyrosine phosphatases including (SHP)-1 and SHP-2 that thereby exhibit regulatory effects on other activation pathways [279]. Examples of such receptors are DCIR, MICL, and MAH [270].

DC-specific intercellular adhesion molecule-3 grabbing non-integrin (DC-SIGN, murine homolog SIGNR1) is a mannose- and fucose-binding signaling CLR bearing di-leucine and tri-acidic motifs in its cytoplasmic tail rather than an ITAM domain. DC-SIGN can activate Raf-1, a serine/threonine MAP kinase that is involved in the acetylation of the pre-activated NF-κB subunit p65, thereby enhancing transcription of the IL-10 gene to dampen the inflammatory response [130].

The mannose receptor (MR), which was the first mannan-binding receptor that was discovered [319, 368], recognizes multiple fungi and other microbes via eight extracellular CTLDs. The extracellular domain of the MR can be cleaved to release soluble MR with preserved ligand binding capacity [172]. Although the MR was shown to promote ROS and cytokine induction, the lack of a known signaling motif in its cytoplasmic tail suggests that it may rather act as a binding coreceptor to enhance the function of (a) bona fide signal receptor(s).

2.3.10 Toll-Like Receptors (TLRs)

Besides CLRs, certain TLRs are also implicated in fungal recognition, including TLR2, TLR4, TLR7, and TLR9. The family of TLRs is the best-characterized family of PRRs. TLRs are membrane-bound receptors composed of leucine-rich repeats for ligand recognition and a conserved Toll/IL-1R-domain in the cytoplasmic domain. The latter mediates signaling via MyD88 (and/or TRIF in some cases) to couple to NF-κB activation (or IRF activation in case of TRIF-mediated signaling) and the induction of pro-inflammatory target genes. TLR2 and TLR4 are expressed at the cell surface, where they recognize fungal phospholipomannan and O-mannan structures, respectively [173, 254]. The endosomal TLRs TLR7 and TLR9 have also been implicated in fungal recognition, namely, in sensing of nucleic acids and induction of IL-12 and/or type I interferons in response to *C. neoformans*, *A. fumigatus*, and *C. albicans* [24, 233, 277]. The literature on the relative contribution of individual TLRs, in particular TLR2 and TLR4, in response to various fungi is complicated by reports on increased as well as decreased susceptibility to infection in mice. The contradictory reports may be explained by the variability in ligand expression and exposure by different fungal strains and morphotypes within each species. Moreover, the expression pattern of different TLRs varies greatly among different cell types, including both hematopoietic and non-hematopoietic cells. In humans, no increase in susceptibility to fungal infections was reported in MyD88-deficient individuals, which are broadly deficient in TLR signaling, indicating that TLRs play no central role in antifungal immunity in humans. However, TLRs may contribute to protection under immunocompromised conditions, as illustrated by the association of TLR4 polymorphisms in stem-cell transplant with aspergillosis [25]. Moreover, TLRs contribute to antifungal immunity by modulating the response induced by other PRRs.

2.3.11 Cross Talk Between TLRs and CLRs

TLR and CLR pathways interact in response to fungal stimuli with synergistic or antagonistic outcomes. Co-stimulation of dectin-1 and TLR2 leads to synergy between the two pathways resulting in enhanced production of TNF, IL-6, and IL-23. However, the synergy between dectin-1 and TLR2 also alters the quality of the overall cytokine response with a shift in the relative quantities of IL-23 versus IL-1 in comparison to TLR stimulation alone [76]. SIGNR1 and TLR2 pathways also interact, albeit with a distinct outcome, as SIGNR1 represses the activity of TLR2 and dampens the TLR2-induced response [130].

A recent study explored the possibility of harnessing PRR collaborations for therapeutic use in the context of chromoblastomycosis. Host recognition of *F. pedrosoi*, the causative agent of this severe and chronic disease, depends on mincle signaling via the Syk/Card9 pathway. However, mincle signaling is not sufficient for fungal control by the host. Exogenous administration of TLR agonists enabled the induction of pro-inflammatory cytokines and clearance of infection in mice [312]. Importantly, applying this principle in humans by treating chromoblastomycosis patients with a topical application of imiquimod (a TLR7/8 agonist) resulted in a marked improvement of the lesions [73].

The cross talk between different PRR pathways is not limited to TLRs and CLRs. Synergistic activation of different receptors across other PRR families has also been described. Such an example is provided in the sensing of chitin via TLR9, NOD2 (a member of the NOD-like receptor (NLR) family), and MR, which was shown to lead to the induction of IL-10 production [357].

Together, the induction of protective immunity against fungal pathogens thus depends on the balanced activation of different PRRs. The overall response to a particular fungal pathogen is determined by the coordinate action of qualitatively and quantitatively distinct signaling events that are further influenced by cell-type-specific peculiarities of the responding cells. The detailed molecular events that control the cross talk of PRR signaling in response to fungal recognition remain not well understood.

2.3.12 Inflammasome Activation by Fungal Pathogens

Besides other cytokines and chemokines, many fungal pathogens induce the production of IL-1β. Biosynthesis of bioactive IL-1β requires two independent signals. The first regulates transcription and translation of pro-IL-1β, and the second induces the proteolytic cleavage of pro-IL-1β into the active IL-1β [81]. Fungi trigger both steps of IL-1β synthesis. Importantly they induce proteolytic cleavage by caspase-1 via the assembly of inflammasomes with distinct subunit composition.

C. albicans stimulates the assembly of a canonical inflammasome composed of the NOD-like receptor NLRP3 and ASC to provide a scaffold for caspase-1 activation [133, 149, 169, 194]. The importance of the NLRP3 inflammasome in antifungal immunity was demonstrated in Nlrp3-deficient mice, which display an increased susceptibility to systemic and superficial candidiasis [41, 133, 149, 169]. Activation of the NLRP3 inflammasome by *C. albicans* depends on yeast-to-hyphal transition [169], which may reflect the dependence on β-glucan exposure at the fungal cell surface [56] and the secretion of secreted aspartyl proteinase (SAP) 2 and SAP6 [268]. Similar data were also reported for *A. fumigatus*-infected human monocytes [290]. In addition to the NLRP3 inflammasome, the NLRC4 inflammasome was also shown to promote protective immunity to *C. albicans* in a model of mixed oral and systemic candidiasis [335]. Interestingly, the function of NLRC4 was attributed to the stromal cell compartment in this context [335]. Finally, NLRP10 was reported to be required for fungal control and survival in disseminated candidiasis [168].

Processing of IL-1β can be achieved, at least in some cases, by enzymes other than caspase-1. In the response to *C. albicans*, it was shown that caspase-8 and ASC can be recruited into a complex with CARD9/Bcl-10/MALT1 to give rise to a noncanonical inflammasome that is able to process pro-IL-1β independently of caspase-1 [131]. It may also modulate the activity of the NLRP3 inflammasome [110]. Interestingly, assembly and activation of the noncanonical caspase-8 inflammasome by *C. albicans* were independent of fungal internalization, indicating that cytosolic NLRs are not required in this process [131].

In certain cell types, the production of IL-1β was suggested to be completely independent of inflammasome activation. This is, for instance, the case in human monocytes, which constitutively express caspase-1 and release ATP and thus are able to secrete bioactive IL-1β after stimulation through TLR2 or TLR4 alone [253] or combined stimulation of TLR2, MR, and dectin-1 [346]. In addition, IL-1β can be processed by neutrophil-derived proteinase-3 [95, 171] and by *C. albicans*-derived aspartyl proteases [19]. Release of mature IL-1β from the producing cell is achieved via nonclassical protein secretion, a process that is ER/Golgi independent [273] and remains not well understood.

IL-1β is closely related to IL-1α, which signals through the same receptor. IL-1α also depends on processing for becoming bioactive, but it is not a substrate of caspase-1 [81]. However, the NLRP3 inflammasome and caspase-1 were implicated indirectly in the secretion of IL-1α [193, 207, 326] by catalyzing the processing of IL-1β, which was proposed to bind to intracellular IL-1a and to serve as a shuttle for IL-1α release [103]. Cell surface-bound IL-1α [79, 320] can be cleaved by calpain I and II at the cell membrane [44, 185], and secreted pro-IL-1α can be processed by extracellular proteases [2, 3, 146]. IL-1α, which is constitutively expressed in some cells such as keratinocytes, is also released upon cytolytic cell death.

In addition that caspase-1 has a critical function in the processing of IL-1β, caspase-1 activation can also induce pyroptosis, an inflammatory form of programmed cell death [358]. Pyroptosis results in DNA fragmentation and chromatin condensation. However, in contrast to apoptosis, which is a non-lytic mechanism, pyroptosis involves cell swelling, pore-mediated lysis, and release of intracellular components, which usually are not exposed to the extracellular compartment, including cytoplasmic cytokines such as IL-1α and IL-1β ATP, HMGB1, and nucleic acids. Due to their inflammatory properties when released in the extracellular environment, these molecules were also called damage-associated molecular patterns (DAMPs) [52]. For some of them, cellular receptors were identified that promote inflammatory responses [197]. Activation of caspase-1 is thus an important mechanism of the host to evaluate the degree of danger arising from a particular infection insult.

2.3.13 Complement

Complement activation plays a central role during bloodstream infections [87]. Fungal pathogens rapidly activate the complement via multiple pathways including the alternative complement pathway as it was shown for *C. albicans* and also for *Zygomycetes* [122, 123, 188]. Rapid activation of the C3 convertase leads to *C. albicans* opsonization by C3b binding to β-(1,6)-glucan [289], which facilitates phagocytosis by neutrophils in a CR3-dependent manner [190, 236, 289, 331]. Importantly, complement activation also results in the induction of anaphylatoxins C3a and C5a [331] with important immunostimulatory activities, in particular on neutrophils and monocytes [157], which are abundant in the circulation, and they can act as chemoattractants for these cells in tissues [361]. Mice lacking C3 or C5 display an increased susceptibility to systemic candidiasis [12, 276, 341]. In case of C5 deficiency, the increased susceptibility is associated with an aberrant inflammatory response that is marked by an increased release of TNF and IL-6 [244, 245]. In line, C5a enhances cytokine release from human PBMCs in response to *C. albicans*

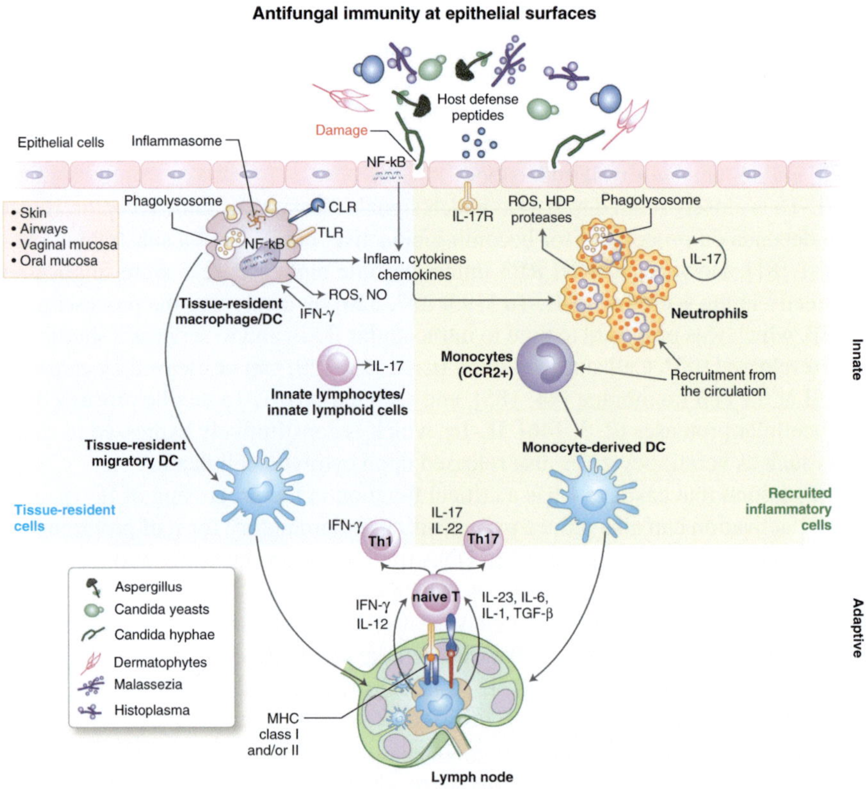

Fig. 2.1 Antifungal immunity at epithelial surfaces. The epithelium responds to the invasion of pathogenic fungi and provides important cues for the activation of innate antifungal immunity in superficial tissues, which includes the activation of tissue-resident macrophage and dendritic cells as well as the recruitment of inflammatory cells from the circulation, such as neutrophils and monocytes. Induction of adaptive immunity is coordinated in a tissue- and fungus-dependent manner by tissue-resident DCs and/or monocyte-derived DCs that migrate to the draining lymph nodes, where they activate and prime antigen-specific T cells.

[55]. Rapid activation of complement is thus critical for acute antifungal defense, especially during fungemia.

2.4 Innate Defense Mechanisms Against Fungal Pathogens

2.4.1 Tissue-Resident Immune Cells in Antifungal Defense

Within the tissue, fungal pathogens encounter different immune cells, some of which reside constitutively within peripheral tissue during homeostasis, while others only enter the tissue upon infection. Tissue-resident (TR) immune cells have gained increasing interest over recent years. Several subsets of lymphoid

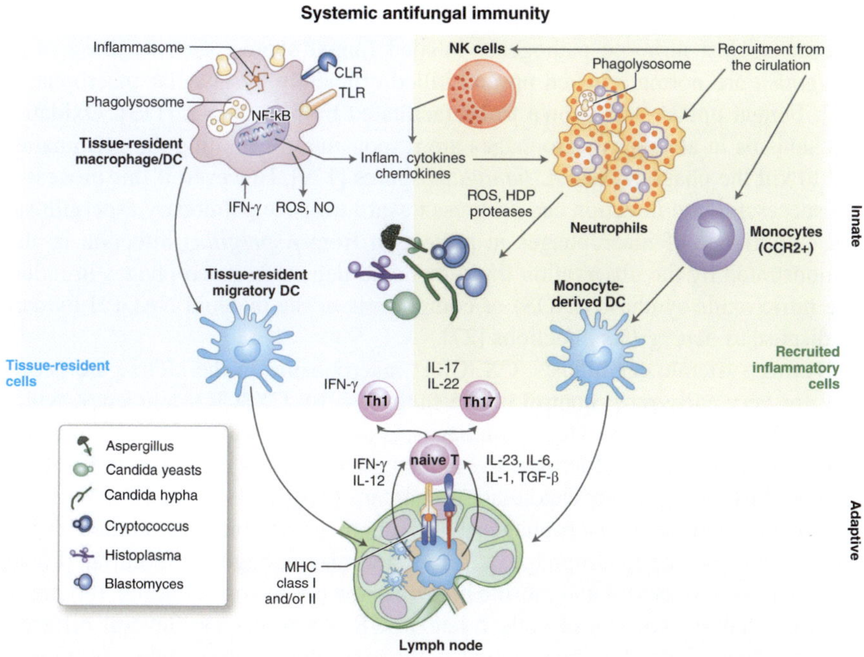

Fig. 2.2 Systemic antifungal immunity. Tissue-resident and recruited inflammatory cells both contribute to efficient innate defense against systemic fungal infections. Cells from both compartments also contribute to the activation of adaptive immunity in a tissue- and fungus-dependent manner

and myeloid TR cells were identified. Their distribution is strongly tissue-dependent with some being limited very selectively to the CNS, the epidermis of the skin, or the alveolar space of the lung. The myeloid TR cells are ontogenically distinct from myeloid cells in the bone marrow, blood, and secondary lymphoid organ. They are seeded as early as during embryonic hematopoiesis and self-renew from local precursors. For TR cells of the lymphoid lineage, this remains less clear. TR immune cells are strategically located to monitor the mucosa and the skin for the presence of invading pathogens and to provide an immediate response. In addition, they may also fulfill regulatory functions to dampen inflammation and prevent dysregulated immunity in case of harmless microbes. The difficulty to identify and to isolate these rare cells from the tissues, to maintain them in culture, or to generate them in vitro from precursors and the scarcity of genetic tools or antibody-mediated deletion strategies to study their role in vivo have greatly hampered their comprehensive investigation in the context of fungal infections. Here, we will discuss just a small selection of TR immune cells that were studied in the context of fungal infections, including TR macrophages, γδ T cells, and innate lymphoid cells. For a discussion of TR DCs, see the section on adaptive immunity.

Alveolar macrophages, which reside in the airways, play a prominent role in host defense against airborne pathogens. Inhaled fungal spores, such as those of *A. fumigatus*, are normally taken up and killed efficiently by alveolar macrophages [15]. Fungal uptake was shown to be facilitated by pentraxin-3 [113]. Oxidative mechanisms in alveolar macrophages are responsible for limiting the germination and to kill the phagocytosed *A. fumigatus* spores [129]. However, if this process is not successful, the infection can progress toward invasive pulmonary aspergillosis. The importance of macrophages in protection from *Aspergillus* infection is also demonstrated by the observation that functional defects in macrophages in inducible nitric oxide synthase (iNOS) or components of the myeloid NADPH oxidase predispose to *Aspergillus* infections [27].

During systemic candidiasis, $CX3CR1^+$ macrophages in the kidney are necessary for very early renal control of the fungus [216]. CX3CR1 deficiency, which affects the survival of the TR macrophages, is associated with defective protection from infection in mice. Moreover, the mutant allele CX3CR1-M280 is linked to an increased risk for systemic candidiasis in humans [216].

The interaction of macrophages with fungal pathogens was studied extensively in vitro using macrophage cell lines and macrophages differentiated from human blood monocytes and murine bone marrow precursors, although it remains not well defined how these cells relate to TR macrophages. Several different strategies were identified how fungal pathogens survive after uptake by phagocytes [38]. Indeed, *C. neoformans* is able to survive and replicate within macrophage phagosomes [204, 342]. *H. capsulatum*, *C. albicans*, and *C. glabrata* can inhibit phagosomal maturation by inhibiting phagolysosomal fusion and alteration of the phagolysosomal pH [88, 99, 305, 316]. Moreover, *C. albicans* and *A. fumigatus* can disrupt the phagosome by generating hyphae and thereby escape from macrophages, whereby this process often involves host cell death [192]. To what extent fungal escape from macrophages by lytic mechanisms are relevant in vivo remains unclear and contradictive. An example is provided by live imaging of *C. albicans*-macrophage interactions in a zebra fish model, which revealed that *C. albicans* filamentation inside macrophages is prevented by NADPH oxidase in vivo [36].

Macrophages have also developed strategies complementary to the ROS-mediated ones to combat fungal growth inside the phagolysosome. An example is provided by the cytokine-regulated shift in metal homeostasis during *Histoplasma capsulatum* infection [369]. GM-CSF stimulates the selective shuffling of Zn^{2+} from the phagolysosome to the Golgi and thereby leads to deprivation of the fungus from Zn^{2+} to suppress fungal replication and promote fungal clearance [322].

In addition to myeloid TR cells, the skin and mucosa also contain TR lymphocytes, including γδ T cells and RAG-independent innate lymphoid cells (ILCs, also termed helper ILCs) with tissue-specific distribution and function [66]. A common feature is that they are preprogramed to rapidly produce cytokines in response to inflammatory or infectious stimuli, which are shared with conventional T cells (in particular IFN-γ and IL-17; see below), albeit the kinetics of cytokine production are much faster. In addition to their protective role against infectious insults, innate lymphocytes are implicated in keeping the commensal microbiota in barrier tissues in check. They can also promote autoinflammatory and autoimmune disorders if dysregulated [263, 311]. In the context of fungal infections, innate lymphocytes were studied mainly for their capacity to produce IL-17 in superficial candidiasis in mice. γδ T cells provide the primary source of IL-17 for protection in an acute model of cutaneous candidiasis [148, 160, 174], while ILCs, γδ T cells, and innate αβ T cells contribute in a redundant manner to the rapid production of this key protective cytokine during an acute model of oropharyngeal candidiasis [62, 119].

2.4.2 Recruited Inflammatory Cells in Antifungal Defense

2.4.2.1 Neutrophils

Neutrophils are the most abundant circulating leukocytes and generally provide a first line of defense against invading microbes. Their key role in antifungal immunity is evidenced by the strong association between neutropenia and fungal diseases [218]. Leukemic patients undergoing neutrophil-depleting cytotoxic chemotherapy frequently develop systemic candidiasis. Likewise, defects in neutrophil functions such as leukocyte adhesion deficiency (LAG) predispose to *Pneumocystis carinii* infections [140], NADPH oxidase deficiency (chronic granulomatous disease, CGD) is associated with invasive pulmonary aspergillosis [304], and MPO-deficient individuals display an increased incidence of *C. albicans* infections [202]. While these examples clearly illustrate the key role of neutrophils in systemic fungal diseases, it remains unclear why and how different neutrophil defects are associated with different types of disease.

In the blood, neutrophils are for the fore to provide immediate protection against blood-borne microbes, while in the tissues, they reside at low numbers during steady state and are rapidly recruited upon infection and inflammation. Diverse molecules have chemotactic activity toward neutrophils, and many of them also promote neutrophil function such as CXC chemokines, anaphylatoxins, and HDPs. Neutrophils possess a broad spectrum of antimicrobial activities against intracellular and extracellular microbes that can be classified in oxidative and non-oxidative mechanisms.

Neutrophils efficiently take up small microbes, including fungal spores and yeast cells [201]. Internalization is followed by phagosome maturation and assembly of the NADPH oxidase complex at the phagosomal membrane. The NADPH oxidase complex can also form at the plasma membrane in response to non-ingestible particles. The NADPH-dependent generation of superoxide and the consecutive formation of reactive oxygen species (ROS) are referred to as the respiratory burst [303]. ROS are a key component of the antimicrobial defense against intracellular and extracellular fungi due to their high fungicidal capacity. The respiratory burst further contributes to microbial killing by inducing a potassium influx and activation of antifungal proteases within the phagosome [280]. The production of reactive nitrogen intermediates by the inducible nitric oxide synthase (iNOS) is another albeit less well-studied oxidative system of neutrophils. Its relevance for antifungal defense is not clear, and evidence from experiments with iNOS-deficient animals suggests that it may be required for the control of only a few selected pathogens, such as *C. neoformans* [4].

Neutrophils are equipped with an armory of granules filled with proteases and other antimicrobial effectors. Distinct subsets of granules, which can be distinguished by their content, are formed sequentially during neutrophil maturation in the bone marrow [30]. Azurophilic granules contain MPO, azurocidin, cathepsin G, neutrophil elastase, proteinase 3, and others, and specific granules are rich in lactoferrin and lysozyme, while tertiary granules, which are also called gelatinase granules, contain gelatinase and MMP9. Neutrophil granules also store HDPs produced by neutrophils such as cathelicidins and α-defensins (HNP1-HNP4, only in humans). Microbes are exposed to these proteases and antimicrobials upon fusion of the granules with the phagosome. Granules also fuse with the plasma membrane in a process termed degranulation to release the granule content in the extracellular space against extracellular microbes, with the downside that they can also cause tissue damage [30]. The relevance of granule proteases for fungal killing was demonstrated, in particular for cathepsin G, proteinase 3, and neutrophil elastase [255, 280, 332]. Neutrophils also secrete cytokines that support their own antifungal activities and contribute to the regulation of the immune response more generally [329]. In this context, it was proposed that neutrophils, rather than cells of the lymphoid lineage, serve as the major source of IL-17 during fungal keratitis [327].

A final mechanism of neutrophil-mediated defense discussed here is the process of NETosis. Over the past decade, an increasing number of reports have shown that neutrophils can extrude stands of DNA with microbicidal proteins attached that can act as extracellular traps for microorganisms [35]. This process, which is also seen as an alternative form of neutrophil cell death, was shown to be selectively induced in response to fungal hyphae, which are too large to be phagocytosed, but not yeast cells [33]. NETosis involves chromatin decondensation, disintegration of the nuclear envelope and granule membranes, and disruption of the cell membrane [108]. This is dependent on NADPH oxidase and MPO and on the enzyme peptidyl arginine deiminase type IV (PAD4), which modifies arginine residues of histones to promote chromatin decondensation [360]. Consistent with the dependence on NADPH, restoration of NADPH deficiency in CGD patients by gene therapy restored NET formation and relieved the patient's susceptibility to *A. nidulans* [23]. A proteomic approach revealed that NETs are decorated with granule proteases and cytoplasmic effector proteins such as calprotectin [345]. NETs may thus provide not only a physical trap for pathogens but also act as a scaffold for fungicidal and fungistatic activities. NETosis may thus represent an adaption to infection by large pathogens. However, whether NETosis is required for combating fungal infections in vivo remains a matter of debate and awaits confirmation.

2.4.2.2 Inflammatory Monocytes

Although neutrophils are undisputedly the primary inflammatory effector cells against fungal infections, it has become clear that blood-derived monocytes also contribute to host protection. This was studied primarily in a mouse model of invasive pulmonary aspergillosis. $CCR2^+$ inflammatory monocytes contribute to innate protection from *A. fumigatus* in three ways. First, monocytes ingest conidia [92]; second, they are required for the production of IL-1α that promotes chemokine production and neutrophil recruitment [42]; and third, they shape the inflammatory milieu of the lung to enhance neutrophil candidacidal activity [42, 92]. Inflammatory monocytes also play a protective role during systemic candidiasis. *Ccr2*$^{-/-}$ mice display increased fungal burden at early time points and impaired survival, and adoptive transfer of monocytes prior to infection restores protection [256]. Inflammatory monocytes further contribute to host defense against fungal infection through their capacity to differentiate into macrophages and/or DCs under inflammatory conditions. Monocyte-derived macrophages are thought to be functionally similar to TR macrophages [38] (see above). Monocyte-derived DCs on the other hand contribute to adaptive immunity against *A. fumigatus*, *C. albicans*, and *B. dermatitidis* by priming $CD4^+$ T cells [90, 154, 337] (see below). Finally, monocytes themselves are able to confer protection from secondary infection through a process termed "trained immunity" [274]. Monocyte training is associated with epigenetic reprogramming in response to *C. albicans* and fungal cell wall β-glucans resulting in a shift in metabolism that is dependent on the activation of mammalian target of rapamycin (mTOR) and hypoxia-inducible factor-1α (HIF-1α) [54].

2.4.2.3 Natural Killer (NK) Cells and Natural Killer T (NKT) Cells

NK cells belong to the family of ILCs. To distinguish them from the family "helper ILCs" (see above), NK cells are also termed "killing ILCs" to account for their capacity to kill target cells by perforin- and death ligand-mediated mechanisms [78]. During steady state, NK cells are only sparsely found in tissues (with the exception of the liver where they reside constitutively at comparably large numbers [384]), but they can become recruited into tissues under inflammatory and infectious conditions [215]. The activity of NK cells against diverse fungal pathogens was first tested in vitro. Thereby, NK cells were found to kill *Paracoccidioides brasiliensis* [166], *Coccidioides immitis* [265], *Cryptococcus neoformans* [219, 246], Mucormycetes [301], and the hyphal form of *A. fumigatus* [32, 300]. Moreover, NK cells isolated from mice were shown to exert antifungal activity against *C. albicans* yeast [224], while their human counterparts display no or very limited antifungal activity against the same fungus [9, 10, 22]. The molecular basis and specificity of the interaction between NK cells and the different fungi have not been established. In addition to directly killing pathogens, NK cells can also act by secreting cytokines, in particular TNF, IFN-γ, and GM-CSF [351], which can enhance the survival and antimicrobial activity of neutrophils and macrophages [65, 82, 100, 223]. Indeed, it was shown that cytokines from *C. albicans*-stimulated NK cells could enhance the antifungal activity of neutrophils [18, 352].

During infection in vivo, NK cells can act as a rapid source of IFN-γ, which is required for protection from *A. fumigatus* in neutropenic mice [264]. Similarly, NK cells are required for fungal control in a mouse model of *C. neoformans* infection [147]. NK cells also play a critical role during systemic candidiasis through the secretion of GM-CSF, which is induced by IL-23p19 derived from $CD11c^+$ cells [18, 367]. NK cell-derived GM-CSF production in turn promotes neutrophil survival and function [18]. The role of NK cells in systemic candidiasis was challenged by a contradictive report suggesting that the depletion of NK cells protects mice via attenuation of systemic inflammation [275]. Consistent/reminiscent with the primary role of NK cells in systemic immunity, NK cells appear to have no impact on fungal defense in barrier tissues such as during OPC [62].

NKT cells, which share common features with both NK cells and T cells, are involved in host defense against *A. fumigatus* [61]. NKT cells are activated via the recognition of β-glucans and production of IL-12 by DCs, while fungal lipids appear not to be involved for direct NKT cell stimulation [61]. This mechanism may thus broadly apply to antifungal NKT cell responses. However, contradictory reports on the role of NKT cells in antifungal defense also exist suggesting that cytokine production by NKT cells is reduced in the presence of *A. fumigatus* [20].

2.4.2.4 Uncontrolled Inflammatory Responses

Although evolved for host protection, the armory of antimicrobial effector molecules including ROS and proteases has the potential to harm the host. Therefore, to benefit the host, inflammatory responses depend on tight regulation. We still lack a comprehensive understanding of how inflammation is resolved after pathogen clearance [309]. That inflammation induced by fungal pathogens can be deleterious to the host, rather than beneficial, is exemplified by the case of vulvovaginal candidiasis (VVC). Disease symptoms do not correlate with fungal load and are a consequence of overt inflammation, rather than of the presence of the fungus. Indeed, the inflammatory infiltrate during symptomatic infection consists of neutrophils [104]. Using a mouse model of VVC, it was demonstrated that neutrophil recruitment is regulated independently of IL-23, IL-17, and IL-22 [379], but rather depends on the NLRP3 inflammasome, which is triggered by *C. albicans*-derived secreted aspartyl proteases (SAPs) [41, 268]. The role of IL-1R signaling versus pyroptosis has however not been tested in this context.

Similarly, immunopathological functions of neutrophils were described during systemic candidiasis. Whereas early neutrophil recruitment to the infected organs is associated with fungal clearance, the prolonged presence of neutrophils in the kidney is associated with immunopathology [215]. Recruitment of neutrophils to the kidney at late time points and immunopathology depend on CCR1, the absence of which leads to improved renal function and host survival [214]. IFN type I signaling can also be deleterious for the host as it was shown in the context of systemic candidiasis in mice, where it promoted an overt neutrophil response [221]. Similarly, neutrophils may contribute to susceptibility rather than protection from infection during pulmonary cryptococcosis, despite the fact that these cells show fungicidal activity toward this pathogen in vitro [227].

2.5 Adaptive Antifungal Mechanisms

Adaptive immunity and $CD4^+$ T cells in particular are key for protection from many fungal infections, as illustrated by the strong link between defects in T cell immunity and severe fungal infections such as superficial candidiasis, pneumocystosis, histoplasmosis, and cryptococcal infections. One of the most prominent examples are HIV/AIDS patients, in which low $CD4^+$ T cell counts correlate with the occurrence of OPC and pneumocystis pneumonia [43, 183]. Other T cell defects predisposing for fungal infections include primary immunodeficiencies that result in impaired T cell development or function such as severe combined immunodeficiency (SCID) [181], ZAP70 deficiency [180], and, albeit less specifically, corticosteroid therapy [181].

T cell immunity to fungal infections was studied for many years. Here, we summarize the most important aspects of how antifungal T cell responses are initiated and regulated and how T cells contribute to protection.

2.5.1 Antigenic Specificity of Antifungal $CD4^+$ T Cells

T cells carry antigen receptors that recognize antigenic peptides presented in the context of MHC class II molecules on antigen-presenting cells. Each T cell carries antigen receptors of a different specificity, and thereby the overall T cell population displays thereby a nearly unlimited diversity of different antigenic specificities. The T cell repertoire is generated through somatic recombination of germline-encoded gene segments. This process underlies a strict quality control and selection process to avoid the generation of self-reactive T cells. Antigen recognition by $CD4^+$ T cells is limited to peptide antigens that are presented in the context of MHC class II molecules. To become fully functional, naïve T cells require stimulation by cognate antigen-MHC-II complexes that are presented by antigen-presenting cells to induce their activation and clonal expansion, which precedes their differentiation into effector T cells.

Although theoretically, the spectrum of antigenic peptides that can be generated from a complex microbe such as a fungus is nearly unlimited, the specificities of T cells that respond to a given pathogen during infection are limited to a restricted number of epitopes. Often, a significant proportion of all pathogen-specific T cells are directed toward only a few distinct peptides that are termed immunodominant T cell epitopes [6].

Only a few fungal T cell epitopes were identified to date. These include the *C. albicans*-derived $pALS3_{236-253}$ and $pADH_{126-140}$ epitopes, which are functionally conserved in diverse non-albicans species of *Candida* [17, 337]. $pALS3_{236-253}$ is recognized by a major population of all *C. albicans*-specific $CD4^+$ T cells in mice and humans, and it provides protection against experimental infection with *C. albicans* if used as a vaccine [17]. Several other fungal antigens, such as the 65-kDa mannoprotein MP65 from *C. albicans* and heat shock protein from *H. capsulatum* and *Paracoccidioides* [250] were shown to act as a T cell antigens, although the precise range of amino acids binding to MHC-II molecules have not been determined in most cases. Recently, fungal calnexin, which is usually found in the ER but can also be displayed at the fungal cell surface, was identified as a novel T cell antigen shared across *Ascomycota* including the thermally dimorphic fungi, opportunistic molds, as well as *Pseudogymnoascus destructans*, the fungus causing the white nose syndrome in bats [370]. Vaccination experiments in mice have demonstrated the immunogenicity of the calnexin-derived peptide epitope and its potential as a vaccine candidate against multiple fungal pathogens. Importantly, human T cells from individuals with a prior history of infection with thermally dimorphic fungi displayed an enhanced response to calnexin compared to control subjects [370].

Of the several vaccine candidates that were reported in recent years [249], only two were taken forward and studied in human clinical trials so far [251]. One of them directed against *C. albicans* contains an N-terminal portion of Als3p (NDV-3) and may also act against methicillin-resistant *Staphylococcus aureus* [211, 382]. While NDV-3 mediates protection via Th1 and Th17 cells in preclinical studies [211], the vaccine also induces specific antibodies in humans [299].

The identification of fungal T cell epitopes not only opens new perspectives toward the development of novel vaccination approaches but also allows studying the generation and regulation of antifungal T cell immunity in more details. To this aim, MHC-II tetramers bound to the *C. albicans*-derived pALS3 or the *H. capsulatum*-derived calnexin peptide epitope were generated for the detection of antigen-specific T cells within the endogenous T cell repertoire [86, 370]. An alternative approach for studying antigen-specific T cell responses in vivo in experimental mouse models relies on adoptively transferred fungus-specific TCR-transgenic T cells. TRC-transgenic models were developed for *A. fumigatus* [283], *C. albicans* [337], and multiple thermally dimorphic fungi [372, 373]. Moreover, in case of unknown epitopes, fungal strains expressing model antigens, such as ovalbumin or I-Eα, were used in combination with established TCR-transgenic T cells specific for these model antigens to explore the antifungal T cell response in vivo [160]. However, caution should be taken as the processing of model antigens might be different and might result in ineffective or altered generation of effector and memory T cells if compared to the response to endogenous antigens [371].

2.5.2 Effector T Cell Differentiation

Activation and differentiation of naïve T cells into effector and memory T cells is induced by DCs, which act as professional antigen-presenting cells (APCs). The APC function of DCs is regulated by PRR signaling in response to microbial stimuli promoting antigen uptake, processing, and presentation as well as enhanced expression of costimulatory molecules and secretion of inflammatory cytokines [167, 281]. This coordinated process, also called DC maturation, is coupled to the migration of the DCs from the peripheral site of infection to the draining lymph node and is a prerequisite for efficient T cell priming.

The quality of the signals provided by the APCs, which is determined by the combination of PRRs triggered, instructs the polarization of the newly activated T cell into different subsets of effector cells, including Th1, Th2, Th17, and regulatory T cells (T_{reg}). For an example, IL-12 promotes differentiation of $CD4^+$ T cells into Th1 cells, whereas TGF-β and IL-6 promote their differentiation into Th17 cells. Moreover, maintenance of the Th17 fate requires IL-23 [222, 362]. Each effector T cell subset produces a set of effector cytokines with Th1 cells secreting IFN-γ and

Th17 cells secreting IL-17. These cytokines in turn mediate distinct effector responses that contribute to the elimination of pathogens but can also promote immunopathology if dysregulated. Thereby, the activation of a particular effector response to a specific pathogen is coupled to the induction of a particular (sets of) innate signaling pathway(s) in the APCs [167]. This is exemplified by Syk and Card9-coupled signaling in response to fungal PAMPs, which promotes preferential production of IL-6 and IL-23 and was linked to Th17 differentiation [203]. While activation of dectin-1 is sufficient for instructing this response, dectin-1 appears redundant in the context of infection with complex fungal pathogens that express a plethora of different PAMPs, by which multiple PRRs can be engaged simultaneously [203, 284, 372]. In addition to the Syk/Card9 pathway, MyD88-dependent signaling can also contribute to the promotion of Th17 differentiation [348, 372]. Moreover, environmental and tissue-specific factors can influence the polarization of T cell responses. This is highlighted by the example of *C. albicans*, which activates distinct effector T cell responses upon infection via different routes. A selective Th17 response is induced in the oral mucosa [17, 145], a mixed but balanced Th17/Th1 response in the skin [148, 160], and a predominant Th1 response with only a minor proportion of Th17 cells in response to systemic infection [337]. The reasons underlying these tissue-specific differences are not well understood, but they are thought to be due to differences in the DC composition between tissues and to the differential contribution of (secreted) factors from third-party cells that can modulate the overall response. The presence of regulatory T cells (Tregs) also appears to impact on the development of Th17 responses. They were shown to promote the differentiation of Th17 cells in response to *C. albicans* by consuming IL-2, which can have Th17-inhibitory effects [262]. Moreover, Tregs can themselves convert into IL-17-producing cells in response to fungal stimuli [260]. Besides their role in maintaining tolerance and immune homeostasis, Tregs can thus also participate in protective immunity against fungal infections.

2.5.3 Dendritic Cell Subsets Regulating Effector T Cell Differentiation During Fungal Infections

DCs encompass heterogeneous subsets of mononuclear phagocytes (MNPs). They generally express high levels of CD11c and MHC-II and constitutively reside in secondary lymphoid organs or in peripheral tissue such as the skin and mucosa. DC subsets arise from precursors via distinct developmental programs [58]. Conventional DCs develop in a Flt3-dependent manner from a common macrophage and DC progenitor (MDP) via a common DC progenitor (CDP) [229]. They exist as Batf3-independent or Batf3-dependent subsets that can also be distinguished by functional differences [229]. Langerhans cells, the prototypic DCs in the skin, originate from fetal liver precursors that are seeded prenatally and retain self-renewal capacity [151, 228]. Under inflammatory conditions, Ly6C^{hi}CCR2^{+} monocytes differentiate into inflammatory DCs in an M-CSF-dependent manner and infiltrate into the tissue where they can take over bona fide APC functions [128]. The relative contribution of distinct DC subsets for activation of adaptive immunity varies between different types of infections and differs between tissues.

Studies in mice have suggested that TR Langerhans cells are necessary and sufficient for the development of Th17 responses against cutaneous candidiasis [160]. This was linked to the capacity of Langerhans cells to induce IL-6 in response to *C. albicans* yeast via dectin-1 [177]. The Th17-polarizing activity of Langerhans cells comes as a surprise as it was suggested that this DC subset has immunoregulatory rather than immunoactivatory functions in other models [175]. Indeed, during OPC in mice, Langerhans cells were not required for the activation of Th17 cells in the oral mucosa [337]. Instead, Flt3-dependent conventional DCs and CCR2-dependent monocyte-derived inflammatory DCs were shown to cooperate in transporting and presenting fungal antigens in the draining lymph nodes for T cell activation and differentiation [337].

Monocyte-derived DCs are also critically involved in priming T cell responses during pulmonary fungal infections because depletion of $CCR2^+$ inflammatory monocytes during experimental *A. fumigatus* infection resulted in reduced antigen transport to the lymph nodes and impaired priming of CD4 T cells [154]. The situation appears to be somewhat more complicated in case of infection with the thermally dimorphic fungi. During subcutaneous infection with a vaccine strain of *B. dermatitidis*, monocyte-derived DCs were shown to be required for antigen transport to the draining lymph nodes but insufficient for T cell priming, suggesting the involvement of antigen transfer to lymph node-resident conventional DCs [90].

2.5.4 T Cell Effector Functions Against Fungal Infections

In line with the differential activation of T cell subsets during fungal infections, distinct T cell subsets appear to have a selective capacity to protect against different forms of disease. Generally, Th1 cells are thought to protect against intracellular pathogens by promoting phagocyte function, while Th17 cells are effective against extracellular bacteria and fungi in barrier tissues. However, in most cases, the division in labor is likely not restricted to a single cellular subset, and protection is rather achieved by the combined action of Th1 and Th17 cells with variable contribution of the two subsets. In this context, it should also be noted that Th17 cells can display a significant degree of plasticity [294], although it remains unclear to what degree this applies to antifungal Th17 cells.

Over the last years, Th17 cells gained much attention for their nonredundant role in protection from superficial candidiasis. Since the first report linking defective Th17 immunity to CMC [120], an increasing number of primary immunodeficiencies were identified in CMC patients, most of which lead to a reduced Th17 response. Mutations include loss-of-function mutations in the genes for *STAT3*, *DOCK8,* and *RORC*, as well as gain-of-function mutations in *STAT1*, all of which affect the differentiation of Th17 cells [13, 72, 89, 217, 230, 282, 347, 387]. The link between CMC and the IL-17 pathway was confirmed with the discovery of mutations affecting the IL-17 pathway more directly, namely, those in the genes encoding *IL-17F*, *IL-17RA*, *IL-17RC,* and *ACT1* [28, 212, 258, 271].

The key role of the IL-17 pathway and more specifically the IL-17 family cytokines IL-17A and IL-17F in protection from superficial candidiasis was also confirmed in mouse models of OPC and cutaneous candidiasis [63, 64, 118, 150, 178, 366]. In contrast, the role of IL-17 during VVC still remains controversial [269, 379]. Adoptive transfer of Th17 cells into a T cell-deficient host can enhance fungal control during murine OPC [145]. Vaccine-induced Th17 cells have also been implicated in protection from lethal pulmonary infection with *B. dermatitidis* [372] or in protection against systemic candidiasis [17, 211]. These studies provide direct evidence for the protective capacity of Th17 cells against different fungal infections.

In addition to $CD4^+$ T cells, a number of other cell types can also produce IL-17. This may be particularly relevant in settings of CD4 deficiency such as in HIV/AIDS patients. Experiments in mice have provided evidence that $CD8^+$ T cells can confer protection and prevent fungal overgrowth in the absence of $CD4^+$ T cells [145, 248]. In addition, innate lymphocytes have emerged as important alternative sources of IL-17. Their protective role was revealed in the context of OPC and cutaneous candidiasis in mice, both of which represent acute infections. The rapid production of IL-17 by innate lymphocytes thus fills a gap at the onset of infection prior to the activation of the adaptive immune system ([313]). While $\gamma\delta$ T cells act as an essential source of IL-17 in the skin [148, 160], ILCs, $\gamma\delta$ T cells, and innate $\alpha\beta$ T cells (also referred to as natural Th17 cell) can provide IL-17 in the oral mucosa of infected mice [62, 119]. The contribution of innate lymphocytes to IL-17-mediated antifungal defense in humans remains unclear. Given the continuous exposure to *C. albicans*, which is a commensal in humans, and the existence of *C. albicans*-responsive memory Th17 cells in most healthy individuals [1], the relative roles of innate and adaptive IL-17 cellular sources are difficult to distinguish. Moreover, many immunodeficiencies associated with CMC or other forms of superficial candidiasis may affect IL-17 production beyond conventional Th17 cells. Indeed, recent studies revealed that ILCs are also depleted during HIV infection [135, 374], and cytokine production by ILCs in the oral mucosa was found to be decreased during simian immunodeficiency virus (SIV) infection [205]. Moreover, the functional defects of many polymorphisms affecting IL-17 signaling such as those of the *IL-17RA*, *IL-17RC*, and *ACT1* genes cannot be attributed to any particular source of IL-17 and thus leave open the possibility that different cell types beyond Th17 cells may contribute to IL-17 production in humans.

Irrespective of its cellular source, the mechanism(s), by which IL-17 mediates protection, remains not well understood. Early studies on the biology of IL-17 found a direct link of IL-17 to neutrophil trafficking via the induction of granulopoietic factors and neutrophil chemokines [106, 196]. Administration of recombinant IL-17 or exogenous expression of the cytokine promotes neutrophil recruitment [196, 232, 302], while IL-17 deficiency led to impaired neutrophil responses under various infectious conditions [53, 57, 343, 381]. In contrast, the IL-17 pathway was found to be redundant for the neutrophil response to *C. albicans* during OPC in mice [338]. Although neutrophils are critical for preventing fungal dissemination during the acute phase of infection, disruption of the IL-17 pathway did not affect neutrophil trafficking to the site of infection in the oral mucosa. Instead, IL-17 might exert its protective effects by regulating the production of HDP from the epithelium [63, 338].

The observation that CMC is often an isolated disease in patients with defects in the IL-17 pathway suggests that IL-17 plays a unique role for defense against *Candida* in barrier tissues, while it seems to be less important for the control of other fungal (and generally microbial) infections. It may even play a pathological role in some cases [386]. In mice, IL-17 deficiency leads to an increased susceptibility for systemic candidiasis [156]. However, this is thought to be due to a developmental defect in these mice rather than to a direct effect of IL-17 or Th17 cells during the course of infection [18]. It was recently proposed that the failure of T helper cell to contribute to protection from systemic candidiasis might be due to their inefficient recruitment to the kidney [86]. However, the kinetics of the disease suggest that fungal control depends primarily on innate immunity, primarily mediated by myeloid cells.

In pulmonary fungal infections, type 1 may be more important for protection than type 17 immunity. Adoptive transfer of IFN-γ-producing Th1 cells can promote protection from *H. capsulatum* and *A. fumigatus* in experimental settings [49, 297]. IFN-γ deficiency on the other hand impairs fungal control during experimental invasive pulmonary aspergillosis and *C. neoformans* infection [34, 51]. Whether the requirement for IFN-γ relied on Th1 cells or innate sources of IFN-γ, e.g., by NK cells, was not assessed in these early studies. Importantly, although Th1 cells may provide protection from *A. fumigatus* in some cases, natural defense against invasive pulmonary aspergillosis relies primarily on innate mechanisms, in particular those conveyed by neutrophils and macrophages [38].

Together, a picture of compartmentalized and tissue-specific antifungal immunity emerges where T helper cells protect from opportunistic fungal pathogens, to which we are continuously exposed at epithelial barriers, whereby distinct Th cell subsets act at different body sites. In contrast, innate mechanisms of myeloid cells prevail for natural immunity against invasive and acute infections. Understanding the mechanisms of antifungal T cell activation, maintenance, and function remains an area of intense research and a prerequisite for future advances in the development of antifungal vaccines.

2.5.5 Antibody-Mediated Protection from Fungal Infections

Antibody-mediated immunity is generally thought to play a minor role for natural protection from fungal infections. Although antibodies are generated in response to commensal or environmental fungi and can be detected in the serum, their specificities are not usually protective to the host [68]. More recently, it has become clear that depending on the specificity and isotype, certain antibodies can modulate the course of fungal infections and thereby benefit or harm the host [47]. Antibody-mediated immunity is now viewed as a promising therapeutic approach against fungal infections, and several protective antibodies to fungi have now been developed [47]. They may act via different mechanisms. Antibodies directed against β-glucan

can inhibit fungal growth and biofilm formation by *C. albicans* and *A. fumigatus* [48, 124, 336]. Anti-cell wall mannoprotein antibodies can block adhesion of *C. albicans* [136, 235]. In contrast, antibodies directed against *C. neoformans* glucuronoxylomannan (GXM) [45, 46] protect via enhancing cellular immunity including phagocytosis and antibody-mediated cellular cytotoxicity, [47] but also the modulation of the inflammatory response [96, 97].

The protective effect of several antifungal antibodies was demonstrated in animal models. Promising candidates include antibodies targeting β-glucans, which act against different fungal pathogens because these carbohydrate structures are phylogenetically conserved [336]. How antifungal vaccines are explored for vaccination approaches in humans is discussed in more details in the chapter "Vaccination Against Fungal Diseases."

References

1. Acosta-Rodriguez EV, Rivino L, Geginat J, Jarrossay D, Gattorno M, Lanzavecchia A, Sallusto F, Napolitani G. Surface phenotype and antigenic specificity of human interleukin 17-producing T helper memory cells. Nat Immunol. 2007;8:639–46.
2. Afonina IS, Muller C, Martin SJ, Beyaert R. Proteolytic processing of interleukin-1 family cytokines: variations on a common theme. Immunity. 2015;42:991–1004.
3. Afonina IS, Tynan GA, Logue SE, Cullen SP, Bots M, Luthi AU, Reeves EP, McElvaney NG, Medema JP, Lavelle EC, Martin SJ. Granzyme B-dependent proteolysis acts as a switch to enhance the proinflammatory activity of IL-1alpha. Mol Cell. 2011;44:265–78.
4. Aguirre KM, Gibson GW. Differing requirement for inducible nitric oxide synthase activity in clearance of primary and secondary *Cryptococcus neoformans* infection. Med Mycol. 2000;38:343–53.
5. Aimanianda V, Bayry J, Bozza S, Kniemeyer O, Perruccio K, Elluru SR, Clavaud C, Paris S, Brakhage AA, Kaveri SV, et al. Surface hydrophobin prevents immune recognition of airborne fungal spores. Nature. 2009;460:1117–21.
6. Akram A, Inman RD. Immunodominance: a pivotal principle in host response to viral infections. Clin Immunol. 2012;143:99–115.
7. Alekseeva L, Huet D, Femenia F, Mouyna I, Abdelouahab M, Cagna A, Guerrier D, Tichanne-Seltzer V, Baeza-Squiban A, Chermette R, et al. Inducible expression of beta defensins by human respiratory epithelial cells exposed to Aspergillus fumigatus organisms. BMC Microbiol. 2009;9:33.
8. Amitani R, Kawanami R. Interaction of Aspergillus with human respiratory mucosa: a study with organ culture model. Med Mycol. 2009;47(Suppl 1):S127–31.
9. Arancia G, Molinari A, Crateri P, Stringaro A, Ramoni C, Dupuis ML, Gomez MJ, Torosantucci A, Cassone A. Noninhibitory binding of human interleukin-2-activated natural killer cells to the germ tube forms of *Candida albicans*. Infect Immun. 1995;63:280–8.
10. Arancia G, Stringaro A, Crateri P, Torosantucci A, Ramoni C, Urbani F, Ausiello CM, Cassone A. Interaction between human interleukin-2-activated natural killer cells and heat-killed germ tube forms of *Candida albicans*. Cell Immunol. 1998;186:28–38.
11. Ashbee HR. Recent developments in the immunology and biology of Malassezia species. Fems Immunol Med Mic. 2006;47:14–23.
12. Ashman RB, Bolitho EM, Papadimitriou JM. Patterns of resistance to *Candida albicans* in inbred mouse strains. Immunol Cell Biol. 1993;71(Pt 3):221–5.
13. Aydin SE, Kilic SS, Aytekin C, Kumar A, Porras O, Kainulainen L, Kostyuchenko L, Genel F, Kutukculer N, Karaca N, et al. DOCK8 deficiency: clinical and immunological phenotype and treatment options – a review of 136 patients. J Clin Immunol. 2015;35:189–98.

14. Baev D, Rivetta A, Vylkova S, Sun JN, Zeng GF, Slayman CL, Edgerton M. The TRK1 potassium transporter is the critical effector for killing of *Candida albicans* by the cationic protein, Histatin 5. J Biol Chem. 2004;279:55060–72.
15. Balloy V, Chignard M. The innate immune response to Aspergillus fumigatus. Microbes Infect. 2009;11:919–27.
16. Balloy V, Sallenave JM, Wu Y, Touqui L, Latge JP, Si-Tahar M, Chignard M. Aspergillus fumigatus-induced interleukin-8 synthesis by respiratory epithelial cells is controlled by the phosphatidylinositol 3-kinase, p38 MAPK, and ERK1/2 pathways and not by the toll-like receptor-MyD88 pathway. J Biol Chem. 2008;283:30513–21.
17. Bar E, Gladiator A, Bastidas S, Roschitzki B, Acha-Orbea H, Oxenius A, LeibundGut-Landmann S. A novel Th cell epitope of *Candida albicans* mediates protection from fungal infection. J Immunol. 2012;188:5636–43.
18. Bar E, Whitney PG, Moor K, Reis e Sousa C, LeibundGut-Landmann S. IL-17 regulates systemic fungal immunity by controlling the functional competence of NK cells. Immunity. 2014;40:117–27.
19. Beausejour A, Grenier D, Goulet JP, Deslauriers N. Proteolytic activation of the interleukin-1beta precursor by *Candida albicans*. Infect Immun. 1998;66:676–81.
20. Beitzen-Heineke A, Bouzani M, Schmitt AL, Kurzai O, Hunniger K, Einsele H, Loeffler J. Human invariant natural killer T cells possess immune-modulating functions during Aspergillus infection. Med Mycol. 2016;54:169–76.
21. Bendel CM, Hess DJ, Garni RM, Henry-Stanley M, Wells CL. Comparative virulence of *Candida albicans* yeast and filamentous forms in orally and intravenously inoculated mice. Crit Care Med. 2003;31:501–7.
22. Beno DW, Stover AG, Mathews HL. Growth inhibition of *Candida albicans* hyphae by CD8+ lymphocytes. J Immunol. 1995;154:5273–81.
23. Bianchi M, Hakkim A, Brinkmann V, Siler U, Seger RA, Zychlinsky A, Reichenbach J. Restoration of NET formation by gene therapy in CGD controls aspergillosis. Blood. 2009;114:2619–22.
24. Biondo C, Malara A, Costa A, Signorino G, Cardile F, Midiri A, Galbo R, Papasergi S, Domina M, Pugliese M, et al. Recognition of fungal RNA by TLR7 has a nonredundant role in host defense against experimental candidiasis. Eur J Immunol. 2012;42:2632–43.
25. Bochud PY, Chien JW, Marr KA, Leisenring WM, Upton A, Janer M, Rodrigues SD, Li S, Hansen JA, Zhao LP, et al. Toll-like receptor 4 polymorphisms and aspergillosis in stem-cell transplantation. N Engl J Med. 2008;359:1766–77.
26. Boettcher S, Gerosa RC, Radpour R, Bauer J, Ampenberger F, Heikenwalder M, Kopf M, Manz MG. Endothelial cells translate pathogen signals into G-CSF-driven emergency granulopoiesis. Blood. 2014;124:1393–403.
27. Bogdan C, Rollinghoff M, Diefenbach A. Reactive oxygen and reactive nitrogen intermediates in innate and specific immunity. Curr Opin Immunol. 2000;12:64–76.
28. Boisson B, Wang C, Pedergnana V, Wu L, Cypowyj S, Rybojad M, Belkadi A, Picard C, Abel L, Fieschi C, et al. An ACT1 mutation selectively abolishes interleukin-17 responses in humans with chronic mucocutaneous candidiasis. Immunity. 2013;39:676–86.
29. Borges-Walmsley MI, Chen D, Shu X, Walmsley AR. The pathobiology of Paracoccidioides brasiliensis. Trends Microbiol. 2002;10:80–7.
30. Borregaard N. Neutrophils, from marrow to microbes. Immunity. 2010;33:657–70.
31. Botterel F, Gross K, Ibrahim-Granet O, Khoufache K, Escabasse V, Coste A, Cordonnier C, Escudier E, Bretagne S. Phagocytosis of Aspergillus fumigatus conidia by primary nasal epithelial cells in vitro. BMC Microbiol. 2008;8:97.
32. Bouzani M, Ok M, McCormick A, Ebel F, Kurzai O, Morton CO, Einsele H, Loeffler J. Human NK cells display important antifungal activity against Aspergillus fumigatus, which is directly mediated by IFN-gamma release. J Immunol. 2011;187:1369–76.
33. Branzk N, Lubojemska A, Hardison SE, Wang Q, Gutierrez MG, Brown GD, Papayannopoulos V. Neutrophils sense microbe size and selectively release neutrophil extracellular traps in response to large pathogens. Nat Immunol. 2014;15:1017–25.

34. Brieland JK, Jackson C, Menzel F, Loebenberg D, Cacciapuoti A, Halpern J, Hurst S, Muchamuel T, Debets R, Kastelein R, et al. Cytokine networking in lungs of immunocompetent mice in response to inhaled Aspergillus fumigatus. Infect Immun. 2001;69:1554–60.
35. Brinkmann V, Reichard U, Goosmann C, Fauler B, Uhlemann Y, Weiss DS, Weinrauch Y, Zychlinsky A. Neutrophil extracellular traps kill bacteria. Science. 2004;303:1532–5.
36. Brothers KM, Newman ZR, Wheeler RT. Live imaging of disseminated candidiasis in zebrafish reveals role of phagocyte oxidase in limiting filamentous growth. Eukaryot Cell. 2011;10:932–44.
37. Brothers KM, Wheeler RT. Non-invasive imaging of disseminated candidiasis in zebrafish larvae. J Vis Exp. 2012.
38. Brown GD. Innate antifungal immunity: the key role of phagocytes. Annu Rev Immunol. 2011;29:1–21.
39. Brown GD, Denning DW, Gow NA, Levitz SM, Netea MG, White TC. Hidden killers: human fungal infections. Sci Transl Med. 2012;4:165rv113.
40. Brown GD, Gordon S. Immune recognition. A new receptor for beta-glucans. Nature. 2001;413:36–7.
41. Bruno VM, Shetty AC, Yano J, Fidel PL Jr, Noverr MC, Peters BM. Transcriptomic analysis of vulvovaginal candidiasis identifies a role for the NLRP3 inflammasome. MBio. 2015;6.
42. Caffrey AK, Lehmann MM, Zickovich JM, Espinosa V, Shepardson KM, Watschke CP, Hilmer KM, Thammahong A, Barker BM, Rivera A, et al. IL-1alpha signaling is critical for leukocyte recruitment after pulmonary Aspergillus fumigatus challenge. PLoS Pathog. 2015;11:e1004625.
43. Carmona EM, Limper AH. Update on the diagnosis and treatment of Pneumocystis pneumonia. Ther Adv Respir Dis. 2011;5:41–59.
44. Carruth LM, Demczuk S, Mizel SB. Involvement of a calpain-like protease in the processing of the murine interleukin 1 alpha precursor. J Biol Chem. 1991;266:12162–7.
45. Casadevall A, Cleare W, Feldmesser M, Glatman-Freedman A, Goldman DL, Kozel TR, Lendvai N, Mukherjee J, Pirofski LA, Rivera J, et al. Characterization of a murine monoclonal antibody to *Cryptococcus neoformans* polysaccharide that is a candidate for human therapeutic studies. Antimicrob Agents Chemother. 1998;42:1437–46.
46. Casadevall A, Mukherjee J, Devi SJ, Schneerson R, Robbins JB, Scharff MD. Antibodies elicited by a *Cryptococcus neoformans*-tetanus toxoid conjugate vaccine have the same specificity as those elicited in infection. J Infect Dis. 1992;165:1086–93.
47. Casadevall A, Pirofski LA. Immunoglobulins in defense, pathogenesis, and therapy of fungal diseases. Cell Host Microbe. 2012;11:447–56.
48. Casanova M, Martinez JP, Chaffin WL. Fab fragments from a monoclonal antibody against a germ tube mannoprotein block the yeast-to-mycelium transition in *Candida albicans*. Infect Immun. 1990;58:3810–2.
49. Cenci E, Mencacci A, Bacci A, Bistoni F, Kurup VP, Romani L. T cell vaccination in mice with invasive pulmonary aspergillosis. J Immunol. 2000;165:381–8.
50. Chang HT, Tsai PW, Huang HH, Liu YS, Chien TS, Lan CY. LL37 and hBD-3 elevate the beta-1,3-exoglucanase activity of *Candida albicans* Xog1p, resulting in reduced fungal adhesion to plastic. Biochem J. 2012;441:963–70.
51. Chen GH, McDonald RA, Wells JC, Huffnagle GB, Lukacs NW, Toews GB. The gamma interferon receptor is required for the protective pulmonary inflammatory response to *Cryptococcus neoformans*. Infect Immun. 2005;73:1788–96.
52. Chen GY, Nunez G. Sterile inflammation: sensing and reacting to damage. Nat Rev Immunol. 2010;10:826–37.
53. Cheng P, Liu T, Zhou WY, Zhuang Y, Peng LS, Zhang JY, Yin ZN, Mao XH, Guo G, Shi Y, Zou QM. Role of gamma-delta T cells in host response against *Staphylococcus aureus*-induced pneumonia. BMC Immunol. 2012;13:38.
54. Cheng SC, Quintin J, Cramer RA, Shepardson KM, Saeed S, Kumar V, Giamarellos-Bourboulis EJ, Martens JH, Rao NA, Aghajanirefah A, et al. MTOR- and HIF-1alpha-

mediated aerobic glycolysis as metabolic basis for trained immunity. Science. 2014;345:1250684.
55. Cheng SC, Sprong T, Joosten LA, van der Meer JW, Kullberg BJ, Hube B, Schejbel L, Garred P, van Deuren M, Netea MG. Complement plays a central role in *Candida albicans*-induced cytokine production by human PBMCs. Eur J Immunol. 2012;42:993–1004.
56. Cheng SC, van de Veerdonk FL, Lenardon M, Stoffels M, Plantinga T, Smeekens S, Rizzetto L, Mukaremera L, Preechasuth K, Cavalieri D, et al. The dectin-1/inflammasome pathway is responsible for the induction of protective T-helper 17 responses that discriminate between yeasts and hyphae of *Candida albicans*. J Leukoc Biol. 2011;90:357–66.
57. Cho JS, Pietras EM, Garcia NC, Ramos RI, Farzam DM, Monroe HR, Magorien JE, Blauvelt A, Kolls JK, Cheung AL, et al. IL-17 is essential for host defense against cutaneous *Staphylococcus aureus* infection in mice. J Clin Invest. 2010;120:1762–73.
58. Chow A, Brown BD, Merad M. Studying the mononuclear phagocyte system in the molecular age. Nat Rev Immunol. 2011;11:788–98.
59. Clark HL, Jhingran A, Sun Y, Vareechon C, de Jesus Carrion S, Skaar EP, Chazin WJ, Calera JA, Hohl TM, Pearlman E. Zinc and manganese chelation by neutrophil S100A8/A9 (calprotectin) limits extracellular aspergillus fumigatus hyphal growth and corneal infection. J Immunol. 2016;196:336–44.
60. Cohen-Kedar S, Baram L, Elad H, Brazowski E, Guzner-Gur H, Dotan I. Human intestinal epithelial cells respond to beta-glucans via Dectin-1 and Syk. Eur J Immunol. 2014;44:3729–40.
61. Cohen NR, Tatituri RV, Rivera A, Watts GF, Kim EY, Chiba A, Fuchs BB, Mylonakis E, Besra GS, Levitz SM, et al. Innate recognition of cell wall beta-glucans drives invariant natural killer T cell responses against fungi. Cell Host Microbe. 2011;10:437–50.
62. Conti HR, Peterson AC, Brane L, Huppler AR, Hernandez-Santos N, Whibley N, Garg AV, Simpson-Abelson MR, Gibson GA, Mamo AJ, et al. Oral-resident natural Th17 cells and gammadelta T cells control opportunistic *Candida albicans* infections. J Exp Med. 2014;211:2075–84.
63. Conti HR, Shen F, Nayyar N, Stocum E, Sun JN, Lindemann MJ, Ho AW, Hai JH, Yu JJ, Jung JW, et al. Th17 cells and IL-17 receptor signaling are essential for mucosal host defense against oral candidiasis. J Exp Med. 2009;206:299–311.
64. Conti HR, Whibley N, Coleman BM, Garg AV, Jaycox JR, Gaffen SL. Signaling through IL-17C/IL-17RE is dispensable for immunity to systemic, oral and cutaneous candidiasis. PLoS One. 2015;10:e0122807.
65. Costantini C, Micheletti A, Calzetti F, Perbellini O, Pizzolo G, Cassatella MA. Neutrophil activation and survival are modulated by interaction with NK cells. Int Immunol. 2010;22:827–38.
66. Cua DJ, Tato CM. Innate IL-17-producing cells: the sentinels of the immune system. Nat Rev Immunol. 2010;10:479–89.
67. Cunha C, Di Ianni M, Bozza S, Giovannini G, Zagarella S, Zelante T, D'Angelo C, Pierini A, Pitzurra L, Falzetti F, et al. Dectin-1 Y238X polymorphism associates with susceptibility to invasive aspergillosis in hematopoietic transplantation through impairment of both recipient- and donor-dependent mechanisms of antifungal immunity. Blood. 2010;116:5394–402.
68. Cutler JE, Deepe Jr GS, Klein BS. Advances in combating fungal diseases: vaccines on the threshold. Nat Rev Microbiol. 2007;5:13–28.
69. Dagenais TRT, Keller NP. Pathogenesis of Aspergillus fumigatus in Invasive Aspergillosis. Clin Microbiol Rev. 2009;22:447–65.
70. Dalle F, Wachtler B, L'Ollivier C, Holland G, Bannert N, Wilson D, Labruere C, Bonnin A, Hube B. Cellular interactions of *Candida albicans* with human oral epithelial cells and enterocytes. Cell Microbiol. 2010;12:248–71.
71. Dambuza IM, Brown GD. C-type lectins in immunity: recent developments. Curr Opin Immunol. 2015;32:21–7.
72. de Beaucoudrey L, Puel A, Filipe-Santos O, Cobat A, Ghandil P, Chrabieh M, Feinberg J, von Bernuth H, Samarina A, Janniere L, et al. Mutations in STAT3 and IL12RB1 impair the development of human IL-17-producing T cells. J Exp Med. 2008;205:1543–50.

73. de Sousa Mda G, Belda Jr W, Spina R, Lota PR, Valente NS, Brown GD, Criado PR, Benard G. Topical application of imiquimod as a treatment for chromoblastomycosis. Clin Infect Dis. 2014;58:1734–7.
74. den Hertog AL, van Marle J, van Veen HA, Van't Hof W, Bolscher JG, Veerman EC, Nieuw Amerongen AV. Candidacidal effects of two antimicrobial peptides: histatin 5 causes small membrane defects, but LL-37 causes massive disruption of the cell membrane. Biochem J. 2005;388:689–95.
75. den Hertog AL, van Marle J, Veerman EC, Valentijn-Benz M, Nazmi K, Kalay H, Grun CH, Van't Hof W, Bolscher JG, Nieuw Amerongen AV. The human cathelicidin peptide LL-37 and truncated variants induce segregation of lipids and proteins in the plasma membrane of *Candida albicans*. Biol Chem. 2006;387:1495–502.
76. Dennehy KM, Willment JA, Williams DL, Brown GD. Reciprocal regulation of IL-23 and IL-12 following co-activation of Dectin-1 and TLR signaling pathways. Eur J Immunol. 2009;39:1379–86.
77. Denning DW, Cadranel J, Beigelman-Aubry C, Ader F, Chakrabarti A, Blot S, Ullmann AJ, Dimopoulos G, Lange C, European Society for Clinical, M, et al. Chronic pulmonary aspergillosis: rationale and clinical guidelines for diagnosis and management. Eur Respir J. 2016;47:45–68.
78. Diefenbach A, Colonna M, Koyasu S. Development, differentiation, and diversity of innate lymphoid cells. Immunity. 2014;41:354–65.
79. Dinarello CA. The interleukin-1 family: 10 years of discovery. FASEB J. 1994;8:1314–25.
80. Dinarello CA. Interleukin-1. Cytokine Growth Factor Rev. 1997;8:253–65.
81. Dinarello CA. Interleukin-1 beta, interleukin-18, and the interleukin-1 beta converting enzyme. Ann N Y Acad Sci. 1998;856:1–11.
82. Djeu JY, Blanchard DK, Halkias D, Friedman H. Growth inhibition of *Candida albicans* by human polymorphonuclear neutrophils: activation by interferon-gamma and tumor necrosis factor. J Immunol. 1986;137:2980–4.
83. Drewniak A, Gazendam RP, Tool AT, van Houdt M, Jansen MH, van Hamme JL, van Leeuwen EM, Roos D, Scalais E, de Beaufort C, et al. Invasive fungal infection and impaired neutrophil killing in human CARD9 deficiency. Blood. 2013;121:2385–92.
84. Drummond RA, Collar AL, Swamydas M, Rodriguez CA, Lim JK, Mendez LM, Fink DL, Hsu AP, Zhai B, Karauzum H, et al. CARD9-Dependent Neutrophil Recruitment Protects against Fungal Invasion of the Central Nervous System. PLoS Pathog. 2015;11:e1005293.
85. Drummond RA, Lionakis MS. Mechanistic insights into the role of C-type lectin receptor/CARD9 signaling in human antifungal immunity. Front Cell Infect Microbiol. 2016;6:39.
86. Drummond RA, Wallace C, Reid DM, Way SS, Kaplan DH, Brown GD. Cutting edge: failure of antigen-specific CD4+ T cell recruitment to the kidney during systemic candidiasis. J Immunol. 2014;193:5381–5.
87. Duggan S, Leonhardt I, Hunniger K, Kurzai O. Host response to *Candida albicans* bloodstream infection and sepsis. Virulence. 2015;6:316–26.
88. Eissenberg LG, Goldman WE, Schlesinger PH. Histoplasma capsulatum modulates the acidification of phagolysosomes. J Exp Med. 1993;177:1605–11.
89. Engelhardt KR, McGhee S, Winkler S, Sassi A, Woellner C, Lopez-Herrera G, Chen A, Kim HS, Lloret MG, Schulze I, et al. Large deletions and point mutations involving the dedicator of cytokinesis 8 DOCK8 in the autosomal-recessive form of hyper-IgE syndrome. J Allergy Clin Immunol. 2009;124(1289–1302):e1284.
90. Ersland K, Wuthrich M, Klein BS. Dynamic interplay among monocyte-derived, dermal, and resident lymph node dendritic cells during the generation of vaccine immunity to fungi. Cell Host Microbe. 2010;7:474–87.
91. Erwig LP, Gow NAR. Interactions of fungal pathogens with phagocytes. Nat Rev Microbiol. 2016;14:163–76.
92. Espinosa V, Jhingran A, Dutta O, Kasahara S, Donnelly R, Du P, Rosenfeld J, Leiner I, Chen CC, Ron Y, et al. Inflammatory monocytes orchestrate innate antifungal immunity in the lung. PLoS Pathog. 2014;10:e1003940.

93. Evans ZA, Mardon DN. Organ localization in mice challenged with a typical *Candida albicans* strain and a pseudohyphal variant. Proc Soc Exp Biol Med. 1977;155:234–8.
94. Fan D, Coughlin LA, Neubauer MM, Kim J, Kim MS, Zhan X, Simms-Waldrip TR, Xie Y, Hooper LV, Koh AY. Activation of HIF-1alpha and LL-37 by commensal bacteria inhibits *Candida albicans* colonization. Nat Med. 2015;21:808–14.
95. Fantuzzi G, Ku G, Harding MW, Livingston DJ, Sipe JD, Kuida K, Flavell RA, Dinarello CA. Response to local inflammation of IL-1 beta-converting enzyme- deficient mice. J Immunol. 1997;158:1818–24.
96. Feldmesser M, Casadevall A. Effect of serum IgG1 to *Cryptococcus neoformans* glucuronoxylomannan on murine pulmonary infection. J Immunol. 1997;158:790–9.
97. Feldmesser M, Mednick A, Casadevall A. Antibody-mediated protection in murine *Cryptococcus neoformans* infection is associated with pleotrophic effects on cytokine and leukocyte responses. Infect Immun. 2002;70:1571–80.
98. Feng Z, Jiang B, Chandra J, Ghannoum M, Nelson S, Weinberg A. Human beta-defensins: differential activity against candidal species and regulation by *Candida albicans*. J Dent Res. 2005;84:445–50.
99. Fernandez-Arenas E, Bleck CK, Nombela C, Gil C, Griffiths G, Diez-Orejas R. *Candida albicans* actively modulates intracellular membrane trafficking in mouse macrophage phagosomes. Cell Microbiol. 2009;11:560–89.
100. Ferrante A. Tumor necrosis factor alpha potentiates neutrophil antimicrobial activity: increased fungicidal activity against *Torulopsis glabrata* and *Candida albicans* and associated increases in oxygen radical production and lysosomal enzyme release. Infect Immun. 1989;57:2115–22.
101. Ferreira MC, Whibley N, Mamo AJ, Siebenlist U, Chan YR, Gaffen SL. Interleukin-17-induced protein lipocalin 2 is dispensable for immunity to oral candidiasis. Infect Immun. 2014;82:1030–5.
102. Ferwerda B, Ferwerda G, Plantinga TS, Willment JA, van Spriel AB, Venselaar H, Elbers CC, Johnson MD, Cambi A, Huysamen C, et al. Human dectin-1 deficiency and mucocutaneous fungal infections. N Engl J Med. 2009;361:1760–7.
103. Fettelschoss A, Kistowska M, LeibundGut-Landmann S, Beer HD, Johansen P, Senti G, Contassot E, Bachmann MF, French LE, Oxenius A, Kundig TM. Inflammasome activation and IL-1beta target IL-1alpha for secretion as opposed to surface expression. Proc Natl Acad Sci U S A. 2011;108:18055–60.
104. Fidel Jr PL, Barousse M, Espinosa T, Ficarra M, Sturtevant J, Martin DH, Quayle AJ, Dunlap K. An intravaginal live Candida challenge in humans leads to new hypotheses for the immunopathogenesis of vulvovaginal candidiasis. Infect Immun. 2004;72:2939–46.
105. Filler SG, Swerdloff JN, Hobbs C, Luckett PM. Penetration and damage of endothelial cells by *Candida albicans*. Infect Immun. 1995;63:976–83.
106. Fossiez F, Djossou O, Chomarat P, Flores-Romo L, Ait-Yahia S, Maat C, Pin JJ, Garrone P, Garcia E, Saeland S, et al. T cell interleukin-17 induces stromal cells to produce proinflammatory and hematopoietic cytokines. J Exp Med. 1996;183:2593–603.
107. Frank CF, Hostetter MK. Cleavage of E-cadherin: a mechanism for disruption of the intestinal epithelial barrier by *Candida albicans*. Transl Res. 2007;149:211–22.
108. Fuchs TA, Abed U, Goosmann C, Hurwitz R, Schulze I, Wahn V, Weinrauch Y, Brinkmann V, Zychlinsky A. Novel cell death program leads to neutrophil extracellular traps. J Cell Biol. 2007;176:231–41.
109. Fukutomi Y, Taniguchi M. Sensitization to fungal allergens: Resolved and unresolved issues. Allergol Int. 2015;64:321–31.
110. Ganesan S, Rathinam VA, Bossaller L, Army K, Kaiser WJ, Mocarski ES, Dillon CP, Green DR, Mayadas TN, Levitz SM, et al. Caspase-8 modulates dectin-1 and complement receptor 3-driven IL-1beta production in response to beta-glucans and the fungal pathogen, *Candida albicans*. J Immunol. 2014;193:2519–30.
111. Gantner BN, Simmons RM, Underhill DM. Dectin-1 mediates macrophage recognition of *Candida albicans* yeast but not filaments. EMBO J. 2005;24:1277–86.

112. Ganz T. Defensins: antimicrobial peptides of innate immunity. Nat Rev Immunol. 2003;3:710–20.
113. Garlanda C, Hirsch E, Bozza S, Salustri A, De Acetis M, Nota R, Maccagno A, Riva F, Bottazzi B, Peri G, et al. Non-redundant role of the long pentraxin PTX3 in anti-fungal innate immune response. Nature. 2002;420:182–6.
114. Gauthier GM. Dimorphism in fungal pathogens of mammals, plants, and insects. PLoS Pathog. 2015;11:e1004608.
115. Gavino C, Cotter A, Lichtenstein D, Lejtenyi D, Fortin C, Legault C, Alirezaie N, Majewski J, Sheppard DC, Behr MA, et al. CARD9 deficiency and spontaneous central nervous system candidiasis: complete clinical remission with GM-CSF therapy. Clin Infect Dis. 2014; 59:81–4.
116. Gazendam RP, van Hamme JL, Tool AT, van Houdt M, Verkuijlen PJ, Herbst M, Liese JG, van de Veerdonk FL, Roos D, van den Berg TK, Kuijpers TW. Two independent killing mechanisms of *Candida albicans* by human neutrophils: evidence from innate immunity defects. Blood. 2014;124:590–7.
117. Gersuk GM, Underhill DM, Zhu L, Marr KA. Dectin-1 and TLRs permit macrophages to distinguish between different Aspergillus fumigatus cellular states. J Immunol. 2006;176:3717–24.
118. Gladiator A, LeibundGut-Landmann S. Innate lymphoid cells: new players in IL-17-mediated antifungal immunity. PLoS Pathog. 2013;9:e1003763.
119. Gladiator A, Wangler N, Trautwein-Weidner K, LeibundGut-Landmann S. Cutting edge: IL-17-secreting innate lymphoid cells are essential for host defense against fungal infection. J Immunol. 2013;190:521–5.
120. Glocker EO, Hennigs A, Nabavi M, Schaffer AA, Woellner C, Salzer U, Pfeifer D, Veelken H, Warnatz K, Tahami F, et al. A homozygous CARD9 mutation in a family with susceptibility to fungal infections. N Engl J Med. 2009;361:1727–35.
121. Gomez P, Hackett TL, Moore MM, Knight DA, Tebbutt SJ. Functional genomics of human bronchial epithelial cells directly interacting with conidia of Aspergillus fumigatus. BMC Genomics. 2010;11:358.
122. Granja LF, Pinto L, Almeida CA, Alviano DS, Da Silva MH, Ejzemberg R, Alviano CS. Spores of mucor ramosissimus, mucor plumbeus and mucor circinelloides and their ability to activate human complement system in vitro. Med Mycol. 2010;48:278–84.
123. Granja LF, Pinto L, Silvestre JS, Almeida CA, Alviano DS, Takaki GMC, Da Silva MH, Ejzemberg R, Alviano CS. Spores and yeasts of mucor polymorphosporus and their ability to activate human complement system in vitro. Arch Clin Microbiol. 2016;7
124. Grappel SF, Calderone RA. Effect of antibodies on the respiration and morphology of *Candida albicans*. Sabouraudia. 1976;14:51–60.
125. Gratacap RL, Bergeron AC, Wheeler RT. Modeling mucosal candidiasis in larval zebrafish by swimbladder injection. J Vis Exp. 2014;93:e52182.
126. Greenberg RN, Scott LJ, Vaughn HH, Ribes JA. Zygomycosis mucormycosis: emerging clinical importance and new treatments. Curr Opin Infect Dis. 2004;17:517–25.
127. Greenberger PA, Bush RK, Demain JG, Luong A, Slavin RG, Knutsen AP. Allergic bronchopulmonary aspergillosis. J Allergy Clin Immunol Pract. 2014;2:703–8.
128. Greter M, Helft J, Chow A, Hashimoto D, Mortha A, Agudo-Cantero J, Bogunovic M, Gautier EL, Miller J, Leboeuf M, et al. GM-CSF controls nonlymphoid tissue dendritic cell homeostasis but is dispensable for the differentiation of inflammatory dendritic cells. Immunity. 2012;36:1031–46.
129. Grimm MJ, Vethanayagam RR, Almyroudis NG, Dennis CG, Khan AN, D'Auria AC, Singel KL, Davidson BA, Knight PR, Blackwell TS, et al. Monocyte- and macrophage-targeted NADPH oxidase mediates antifungal host defense and regulation of acute inflammation in mice. J Immunol. 2013;190:4175–84.
130. Gringhuis SI, den Dunnen J, Litjens M, van Het Hof B, van Kooyk Y, Geijtenbeek TB. C-type lectin DC-SIGN modulates Toll-like receptor signaling via Raf-1 kinase-dependent acetylation of transcription factor NF-kappaB. Immunity. 2007;26:605–16.

131. Gringhuis SI, Kaptein TM, Wevers BA, Theelen B, van der Vlist M, Boekhout T, Geijtenbeek TB. Dectin-1 is an extracellular pathogen sensor for the induction and processing of IL-1beta via a noncanonical caspase-8 inflammasome. Nat Immunol. 2012;13:246–54.
132. Gross O, Gewies A, Finger K, Schafer M, Sparwasser T, Peschel C, Forster I, Ruland J. Card9 controls a non-TLR signalling pathway for innate anti-fungal immunity. Nature. 2006;442:651–6.
133. Gross O, Poeck H, Bscheider M, Dostert C, Hannesschlager N, Endres S, Hartmann G, Tardivel A, Schweighoffer E, Tybulewicz V, et al. Syk kinase signalling couples to the Nlrp3 inflammasome for anti-fungal host defence. Nature. 2009;459:433–6.
134. Guegan S, Lanternier F, Rouzaud C, Dupin N, Lortholary O. Fungal skin and soft tissue infections. Curr Opin Infect Dis. 2016;29:124–30.
135. Guo X, Fu YX. The tragic fate of group 3 innate lymphoid cells during HIV-1 infection. J Clin Invest. 2015;125:3992.
136. Han Y, Kozel TR, Zhang MX, MacGill RS, Carroll MC, Cutler JE. Complement is essential for protection by an IgM and an IgG3 monoclonal antibody against experimental, hematogenously disseminated candidiasis. J Immunol. 2001;167:1550–7.
137. Hancock RE, Haney EF, Gill EE. The immunology of host defence peptides: beyond antimicrobial activity. Nat Rev Immunol. 2016;16:321–34.
138. Hara H, Ishihara C, Takeuchi A, Imanishi T, Xue L, Morris SW, Inui M, Takai T, Shibuya A, Saijo S, et al. The adaptor protein CARD9 is essential for the activation of myeloid cells through ITAM-associated and Toll-like receptors. Nat Immunol. 2007;8:619–29.
139. Hardison SE, Brown GD. C-type lectin receptors orchestrate antifungal immunity. Nat Immunol. 2012;13:817–22.
140. Harris ES, Shigeoka AO, Li W, Adams RH, Prescott SM, McIntyre TM, Zimmerman GA, Lorant DE. A novel syndrome of variant leukocyte adhesion deficiency involving defects in adhesion mediated by beta1 and beta2 integrins. Blood. 2001;97:767–76.
141. Havlickova B, Czaika VA, Friedrich M. Epidemiological trends in skin mycoses worldwide. Mycoses. 2008;51(Suppl 4):2–15.
142. Hayat M, Mushtaq S, Saba S, Saif R. Rhino-orbital-mucormycosis as a presenting manifestation of gestational diabetes mellitus. Indian J Endocrinol Metab. 2011;15:S65–6.
143. Hebecker B, Naglik JR, Hube B, Jacobsen ID. Pathogenicity mechanisms and host response during oral *Candida albicans* infections. Expert Rev Anti-Infect Ther. 2014;12:867–79.
144. Helmerhorst EJ, Breeuwer P, van't Hof W, Walgreen-Weterings E, Oomen LC, Veerman EC, Amerongen AV, Abee T. The cellular target of histatin 5 on *Candida albicans* is the energized mitochondrion. J Biol Chem. 1999;274:7286–91.
145. Hernandez-Santos N, Huppler AR, Peterson AC, Khader SA, McKenna KC, Gaffen SL. Th17 cells confer long-term adaptive immunity to oral mucosal *Candida albicans* infections. Mucosal Immunol. 2013;6:900–10.
146. Heutinck KM, ten Berge IJ, Hack CE, Hamann J, Rowshani AT. Serine proteases of the human immune system in health and disease. Mol Immunol. 2010;47:1943–55.
147. Hidore MR, Murphy JW. Natural cellular resistance of beige mice against *Cryptococcus neoformans*. J Immunol. 1986;137:3624–31.
148. Hirota K, Duarte JH, Veldhoen M, Hornsby E, Li Y, Cua DJ, Ahlfors H, Wilhelm C, Tolaini M, Menzel U, et al. Fate mapping of IL-17-producing T cells in inflammatory responses. Nat Immunol. 2011;12:255–63.
149. Hise AG, Tomalka J, Ganesan S, Patel K, Hall BA, Brown GD, Fitzgerald KA. An essential role for the NLRP3 inflammasome in host defense against the human fungal pathogen *Candida albicans*. Cell Host Microbe. 2009;5:487–97.
150. Ho AW, Shen F, Conti HR, Patel N, Childs EE, Peterson AC, Hernandez-Santos N, Kolls JK, Kane LP, Ouyang W, Gaffen SL. IL-17RC is required for immune signaling via an extended SEF/IL-17R signaling domain in the cytoplasmic tail. J Immunol. 2010;185:1063–70.
151. Hoeffel G, Wang Y, Greter M, See P, Teo P, Malleret B, Leboeuf M, Low D, Oller G, Almeida F, et al. Adult Langerhans cells derive predominantly from embryonic fetal liver monocytes with a minor contribution of yolk sac-derived macrophages. J Exp Med. 2012;209:1167–81.

152. Hohl TM. Overview of vertebrate animal models of fungal infection. J Immunol Methods. 2014;410:100–12.
153. Hohl TM, Feldmesser M, Perlin DS, Pamer EG. Caspofungin modulates inflammatory responses to Aspergillus fumigatus through stage-specific effects on fungal beta-glucan exposure. J Infect Dis. 2008;198:176–85.
154. Hohl TM, Rivera A, Lipuma L, Gallegos A, Shi C, Mack M, Pamer EG. Inflammatory monocytes facilitate adaptive CD4 T cell responses during respiratory fungal infection. Cell Host Microbe. 2009;6:470–81.
155. Hohl TM, Van Epps HL, Rivera A, Morgan LA, Chen PL, Feldmesser M, Pamer EG. Aspergillus fumigatus triggers inflammatory responses by stage-specific beta-glucan display. PLoS Pathog. 2005;1:e30.
156. Huang W, Na L, Fidel PL, Schwarzenberger P. Requirement of interleukin-17A for systemic anti-*Candida albicans* host defense in mice. J Infect Dis. 2004;190:624–31.
157. Hunniger K, Bieber K, Martin R, Lehnert T, Figge MT, Loffler J, Guo RF, Riedemann NC, Kurzai O. A second stimulus required for enhanced antifungal activity of human neutrophils in blood is provided by anaphylatoxin C5a. J Immunol. 2015;194:1199–210.
158. Ibrahim AS, Spellberg B, Avanessian V, Fu Y, Edwards Jr JE. Rhizopus oryzae adheres to, is phagocytosed by, and damages endothelial cells in vitro. Infect Immun. 2005;73:778–83.
159. Ifrim DC, Bain JM, Reid DM, Oosting M, Verschueren I, Gow NA, van Krieken JH, Brown GD, Kullberg BJ, Joosten LA, et al. Role of Dectin-2 for host defense against systemic infection with Candida glabrata. Infect Immun. 2014;82:1064–73.
160. Igyarto BZ, Haley K, Ortner D, Bobr A, Gerami-Nejad M, Edelson BT, Zurawski SM, Malissen B, Zurawski G, Berman J, Kaplan DH. Skin-resident murine dendritic cell subsets promote distinct and opposing antigen-specific T helper cell responses. Immunity. 2011;35:260–72.
161. Iliev ID, Funari VA, Taylor KD, Nguyen Q, Reyes CN, Strom SP, Brown J, Becker CA, Fleshner PR, Dubinsky M, et al. Interactions between commensal fungi and the C-type lectin receptor Dectin-1 influence colitis. Science. 2012;336:1314–7.
162. Ishikawa E, Ishikawa T, Morita YS, Toyonaga K, Yamada H, Takeuchi O, Kinoshita T, Akira S, Yoshikai Y, Yamasaki S. Direct recognition of the mycobacterial glycolipid, trehalose dimycolate, by C-type lectin Mincle. J Exp Med. 2009;206:2879–88.
163. Ishikawa T, Itoh F, Yoshida S, Saijo S, Matsuzawa T, Gonoi T, Saito T, Okawa Y, Shibata N, Miyamoto T, Yamasaki S. Identification of distinct ligands for the C-type lectin receptors Mincle and Dectin-2 in the pathogenic fungus Malassezia. Cell Host Microbe. 2013;13:477–88.
164. Jang W, Edgerton M. Salivary histatins: structure, function, and mechanisms of antifungal activity. In: Calderone R, Clancy C, editors. Candida and candidiasis. 2 ed. Washington, DC: ASM Press; 2012. p. 185–94.
165. Jhingran A, Kasahara S, Shepardson KM, Junecko BA, Heung LJ, Kumasaka DK, Knoblaugh SE, Lin X, Kazmierczak BI, Reinhart TA, et al. Compartment-specific and sequential role of MyD88 and CARD9 in chemokine induction and innate defense during respiratory fungal infection. PLoS Pathog. 2015;11:e1004589.
166. Jimenez BE, Murphy JW. In vitro effects of natural killer cells against Paracoccidioides brasiliensis yeast phase. Infect Immun. 1984;46:552–8.
167. Joffre O, Nolte MA, Sporri R, Reis e Sousa C. Inflammatory signals in dendritic cell activation and the induction of adaptive immunity. Immunol Rev. 2009;227:234–247.
168. Joly S, Eisenbarth SC, Olivier AK, Williams A, Kaplan DH, Cassel SL, Flavell RA, Sutterwala FS. Cutting edge: Nlrp10 is essential for protective antifungal adaptive immunity against *Candida albicans*. J Immunol. 2012;189:4713–7.
169. Joly S, Ma N, Sadler JJ, Soll DR, Cassel SL, Sutterwala FS. Cutting edge: *Candida albicans* hyphae formation triggers activation of the Nlrp3 inflammasome. J Immunol. 2009;183:3578–81.
170. Joly S, Maze C, McCray Jr PB, Guthmiller JM. Human beta-defensins 2 and 3 demonstrate strain-selective activity against oral microorganisms. J Clin Microbiol. 2004;42:1024–9.

171. Joosten LA, Netea MG, Fantuzzi G, Koenders MI, Helsen MM, Sparrer H, Pham CT, van der Meer JW, Dinarello CA, van den Berg WB. Inflammatory arthritis in caspase 1 gene-deficient mice: contribution of proteinase 3 to caspase 1-independent production of bioactive interleukin-1beta. Arthritis Rheum. 2009;60:3651–62.
172. Jordens R, Thompson A, Amons R, Koning F. Human dendritic cells shed a functional, soluble form of the mannose receptor. Int Immunol. 1999;11:1775–80.
173. Jouault T, Ibata-Ombetta S, Takeuchi O, Trinel PA, Sacchetti P, Lefebvre P, Akira S, Poulain D. *Candida albicans* phospholipomannan is sensed through toll-like receptors. J Infect Dis. 2003;188:165–72.
174. Kagami S, Rizzo HL, Kurtz SE, Miller LS, Blauvelt A. IL-23 and IL-17A, but not IL-12 and IL-22, are required for optimal skin host defense against *Candida albicans*. J Immunol. 2010;185:5453–62.
175. Kaplan DH, Kissenpfennig A, Clausen BE. Insights into Langerhans cell function from Langerhans cell ablation models. Eur J Immunol. 2008;38:2369–76.
176. Kapp A, Zeck-Kapp G, Danner M, Luger TA. Human granulocyte-macrophage colony stimulating factor: an effective direct activator of human polymorphonuclear neutrophilic granulocytes. J Invest Dermatol. 1988;91:49–55.
177. Kashem SW, Igyarto BZ, Gerami-Nejad M, Kumamoto Y, Mohammed J, Jarrett E, Drummond RA, Zurawski SM, Zurawski G, Berman J, et al. *Candida albicans* morphology and dendritic cell subsets determine T helper cell differentiation. Immunity. 2015;42:356–66.
178. Kashem SW, Riedl MS, Yao C, Honda CN, Vulchanova L, Kaplan DH. Nociceptive sensory fibers drive interleukin-23 production from CD301b+ dermal dendritic cells and drive protective cutaneous immunity. Immunity. 2015;43:515–26.
179. Kerscher B, Willment JA, Brown GD. The Dectin-2 family of C-type lectin-like receptors: an update. Int Immunol. 2013;25:271–7.
180. Kim VH, Murguia L, Schechter T, Grunebaum E, Roifman CM. Emergency treatment for zeta chain-associated protein of 70 kDa ZAP70 deficiency. J Allergy Clin Immunol. 2013;131:1233–5.
181. Kirkpatrick CH. Chronic mucocutaneous candidiasis. Pediatr Infect Dis J. 2001; 20:197–206.
182. Klein BS, Tebbets B. Dimorphism and virulence in fungi. Curr Opin Microbiol. 2007;10:314–9.
183. Klein RS, Harris CA, Small CB, Moll B, Lesser M, Friedland GH. Oral candidiasis in high-risk patients as the initial manifestation of the acquired immunodeficiency syndrome. N Engl J Med. 1984;311:354–8.
184. Knutsen AP, Chauhan B, Slavin RG. Cell-mediated immunity in allergic bronchopulmonary aspergillosis. Immunol Allergy Clin. 1998;18:575.
185. Kobayashi Y, Yamamoto K, Saido T, Kawasaki H, Oppenheim JJ, Matsushima K. Identification of calcium-activated neutral protease as a processing enzyme of human interleukin 1 alpha. Proc Natl Acad Sci U S A. 1990;87:5548–52.
186. Koshlukova SE, Lloyd TL, Araujo MW, Edgerton M. Salivary histatin 5 induces non-lytic release of ATP from *Candida albicans* leading to cell death. J Biol Chem. 1999;274:18872–9.
187. Kosmidis C, Denning DW. The clinical spectrum of pulmonary aspergillosis. Thorax. 2015;70:270–7.
188. Kozel TR. Activation of the complement system by pathogenic fungi. Clin Microbiol Rev. 1996;9:34–46.
189. Kozel TR, Mastroianni RP. Inhibition of phagocytosis by cryptococcal polysaccharide: dissociation of the attachment and ingestion phases of phagocytosis. Infect Immun. 1976;14:62–7.
190. Kozel TR, Weinhold LC, Lupan DM. Distinct characteristics of initiation of the classical and alternative complement pathways by *Candida albicans*. Infect Immun. 1996;64:3360–8.
191. Krishnakumari V, Rangaraj N, Nagaraj R. Antifungal activities of human beta-defensins HBD-1 to HBD-3 and their C-terminal analogs Phd1 to Phd3. Antimicrob Agents Chemother. 2009;53:256–60.

192. Krysan DJ, Sutterwala FS, Wellington M. Catching fire: *Candida albicans*, macrophages, and pyroptosis. PLoS Pathog. 2014;10:e1004139.
193. Kuida K, Lippke JA, Ku G, Harding MW, Livingston DJ, Su MS, Flavell RA. Altered cytokine export and apoptosis in mice deficient in interleukin-1 beta converting enzyme. Science. 1995;267:2000–3.
194. Kumar H, Kumagai Y, Tsuchida T, Koenig PA, Satoh T, Guo Z, Jang MH, Saitoh T, Akira S, Kawai T. Involvement of the NLRP3 inflammasome in innate and humoral adaptive immune responses to fungal beta-glucan. J Immunol. 2009;183:8061–7.
195. Kupper TS. The activated keratinocyte: a model for inducible cytokine production by non-bone marrow-derived cells in cutaneous inflammatory and immune responses. J Invest Dermatol. 1990;94:146S–50S.
196. Laan M, Cui ZH, Hoshino H, Lotvall J, Sjostrand M, Gruenert DC, Skoogh BE, Linden A. Neutrophil recruitment by human IL-17 via C-X-C chemokine release in the airways. J Immunol. 1999;162:2347–52.
197. Lamkanfi M, Sarkar A, Vande Walle L, Vitari AC, Amer AO, Wewers MD, Tracey KJ, Kanneganti TD, Dixit VM. Inflammasome-dependent release of the alarmin HMGB1 in endotoxemia. J Immunol. 2010;185:4385–92.
198. Lanternier F, Barbati E, Meinzer U, Liu L, Pedergnana V, Migaud M, Heritier S, Chomton M, Fremond ML, Gonzales E, et al. Inherited CARD9 deficiency in 2 unrelated patients with invasive Exophiala infection. J Infect Dis. 2015;211:1241–50.
199. Lanternier F, Mahdaviani SA, Barbati E, Chaussade H, Koumar Y, Levy R, Denis B, Brunel AS, Martin S, Loop M, et al. Inherited CARD9 deficiency in otherwise healthy children and adults with Candida species-induced meningoencephalitis, colitis, or both. J Allergy Clin Immunol. 2015;135:1558–68.e2.
200. Lanternier F, Pathan S, Vincent QB, Liu L, Cypowyj S, Prando C, Migaud M, Taibi L, Ammar-Khodja A, Boudghene Stambouli O, et al. Deep dermatophytosis and inherited CARD9 deficiency. N Engl J Med. 2013;369:1704–14.
201. Lehrer RI, Cline MJ. Interaction of *Candida albicans* with human leukocytes and serum. J Bacteriol. 1969;98:996–1004.
202. Lehrer RI, Cline MJ. Leukocyte myeloperoxidase deficiency and disseminated candidiasis: the role of myeloperoxidase in resistance to Candida infection. J Clin Invest. 1969;48:1478–88.
203. LeibundGut-Landmann S, Gross O, Robinson MJ, Osorio F, Slack EC, Tsoni SV, Schweighoffer E, Tybulewicz V, Brown GD, Ruland J, Reis e Sousa C. Syk- and CARD9-dependent coupling of innate immunity to the induction of T helper cells that produce interleukin 17. Nat Immunol. 2007;8, 630–638.
204. Levitz SM, Harrison TS, Tabuni A, Liu X. Chloroquine induces human mononuclear phagocytes to inhibit and kill *Cryptococcus neoformans* by a mechanism independent of iron deprivation. J Clin Invest. 1997;100:1640–6.
205. Li H, Reeves RK. Functional perturbation of classical natural killer and innate lymphoid cells in the oral mucosa during SIV infection. Front Immunol. 2012;3:417.
206. Li M, Chen Q, Tang R, Shen Y, Liu WD. The expression of beta-defensin-2, 3 and LL-37 induced by *Candida albicans* phospholipomannan in human keratinocytes. J Dermatol Sci. 2011;61:72–5.
207. Li P, Allen H, Banerjee S, Franklin S, Herzog L, Johnston C, McDowell J, Paskind M, Rodman L, Salfeld J, et al. Mice deficient in IL-1 beta-converting enzyme are defective in production of mature IL-1 beta and resistant to endotoxic shock. Cell. 1995;80:401–11.
208. Li XS, Reddy MS, Baev D, Edgerton M. *Candida albicans* Ssa1/2p is the cell envelope binding protein for human salivary histatin 5. J Biol Chem. 2003;278:28553–61.
209. Liang P, Wang X, Wang R, Wan Z, Han W, Li R. CARD9 deficiencies linked to impaired neutrophil functions against Phialophora verrucosa. Mycopathologia. 2015;179: 347–57.
210. Liles WC, Huang JE, van Burik JA, Bowden RA, Dale DC. Granulocyte colony-stimulating factor administered in vivo augments neutrophil-mediated activity against opportunistic fungal pathogens. J Infect Dis. 1997;175:1012–5.

211. Lin L, Ibrahim AS, Xu X, Farber JM, Avanesian V, Baquir B, Fu Y, French SW, Edwards Jr JE, Spellberg B. Th1-Th17 cells mediate protective adaptive immunity against *Staphylococcus aureus* and *Candida albicans* infection in mice. PLoS Pathog. 2009;5:e1000703.
212. Ling Y, Cypowyj S, Aytekin C, Galicchio M, Camcioglu Y, Nepesov S, Ikinciogullari A, Dogu F, Belkadi A, Levy R, et al. Inherited IL-17RC deficiency in patients with chronic mucocutaneous candidiasis. J Exp Med. 2015;212:619–31.
213. Lionakis MS. New insights into innate immune control of systemic candidiasis. Med Mycol. 2014;52:555–64.
214. Lionakis MS, Fischer BG, Lim JK, Swamydas M, Wan W, Richard Lee CC, Cohen JI, Scheinberg P, Gao JL, Murphy PM. Chemokine receptor Ccr1 drives neutrophil-mediated kidney immunopathology and mortality in invasive candidiasis. PLoS Pathog. 2012;8:e1002865.
215. Lionakis MS, Lim JK, Lee CC, Murphy PM. Organ-specific innate immune responses in a mouse model of invasive candidiasis. J Innate Immun. 2011;3:180–99.
216. Lionakis MS, Swamydas M, Fischer BG, Plantinga TS, Johnson MD, Jaeger M, Green NM, Masedunskas A, Weigert R, Mikelis C, et al. CX3CR1-dependent renal macrophage survival promotes Candida control and host survival. J Clin Invest. 2013;123:5035–51.
217. Liu L, Okada S, Kong XF, Kreins AY, Cypowyj S, Abhyankar A, Toubiana J, Itan Y, Audry M, Nitschke P, et al. Gain-of-function human STAT1 mutations impair IL-17 immunity and underlie chronic mucocutaneous candidiasis. J Exp Med. 2011;208:1635–48.
218. Lortholary O, Dupont B. Antifungal prophylaxis during neutropenia and immunodeficiency. Clin Microbiol Rev. 1997;10:477–504.
219. Ma LL, Wang CL, Neely GG, Epelman S, Krensky AM, Mody CH. NK cells use perforin rather than granulysin for anticryptococcal activity. J Immunol. 2004;173:3357–65.
220. MacCallum DM, Odds FC. Temporal events in the intravenous challenge model for experimental *Candida albicans* infections in female mice. Mycoses. 2005;48:151–61.
221. Majer O, Bourgeois C, Zwolanek F, Lassnig C, Kerjaschki D, Mack M, Muller M, Kuchler K. Type I interferons promote fatal immunopathology by regulating inflammatory monocytes and neutrophils during Candida infections. PLoS Pathog. 2012;8:e1002811.
222. Mangan PR, Harrington LE, O'Quinn DB, Helms WS, Bullard DC, Elson CO, Hatton RD, Wahl SM, Schoeb TR, Weaver CT. Transforming growth factor-beta induces development of the T17 lineage. Nature. 2006;441:231–4.
223. Marodi L, Schreiber S, Anderson DC, MacDermott RP, Korchak HM, Johnston Jr RB. Enhancement of macrophage candidacidal activity by interferon-gamma. Increased phagocytosis, killing, and calcium signal mediated by a decreased number of mannose receptors. J Clin Invest. 1993;91:2596–601.
224. Mathews HL, Witek-Janusek L. Antifungal activity of interleukin-2-activated natural killer (NK1.1)+ lymphocytes against *Candida albicans*. J Med Microbiol. 1998;47:1007–14.
225. Matsunaga I, Moody DB. Mincle is a long sought receptor for mycobacterial cord factor. J Exp Med. 2009;206:2865–8.
226. McGreal EP, Rosas M, Brown GD, Zamze S, Wong SY, Gordon S, Martinez-Pomares L, Taylor PR. The carbohydrate-recognition domain of Dectin-2 is a C-type lectin with specificity for high mannose. Glycobiology. 2006;16:422–30.
227. Mednick AJ, Feldmesser M, Rivera J, Casadevall A. Neutropenia alters lung cytokine production in mice and reduces their susceptibility to pulmonary cryptococcosis. Eur J Immunol. 2003;33:1744–53.
228. Merad M, Manz MG, Karsunky H, Wagers A, Peters W, Charo I, Weissman IL, Cyster JG, Engleman EG. Langerhans cells renew in the skin throughout life under steady-state conditions. Nat Immunol. 2002;3:1135–41.
229. Merad M, Sathe P, Helft J, Miller J, Mortha A. The dendritic cell lineage: ontogeny and function of dendritic cells and their subsets in the steady state and the inflamed setting. Annu Rev Immunol. 2013;31:563–604.
230. Milner JD, Brenchley JM, Laurence A, Freeman AF, Hill BJ, Elias KM, Kanno Y, Spalding C, Elloumi HZ, Paulson ML, et al. Impaired T(H)17 cell differentiation in subjects with autosomal dominant hyper-IgE syndrome. Nature. 2008;452:773–6.

231. Miyake Y, Masatsugu OH, Yamasaki S. C-type lectin receptor MCL facilitates mincle expression and signaling through complex formation. J Immunol. 2015;194:5366–74.
232. Miyamoto M, Prause O, Sjostrand M, Laan M, Lotvall J, Linden A. Endogenous IL-17 as a mediator of neutrophil recruitment caused by endotoxin exposure in mouse airways. J Immunol. 2003;170:4665–72.
233. Miyazato A, Nakamura K, Yamamoto N, Mora-Montes HM, Tanaka M, Abe Y, Tanno D, Inden K, Gang X, Ishii K, et al. Toll-like receptor 9-dependent activation of myeloid dendritic cells by Deoxynucleic acids from *Candida albicans*. Infect Immun. 2009;77:3056–64.
234. Moffa EB, Mussi MC, Xiao Y, Garrido SS, Machado MA, Giampaolo ET, Siqueira WL. Histatin 5 inhibits adhesion of *C. albicans* to reconstructed human oral epithelium. Front Microbiol. 2015;6:885.
235. Moragues MD, Omaetxebarria MJ, Elguezabal N, Sevilla MJ, Conti S, Polonelli L, Ponton J. A monoclonal antibody directed against a *Candida albicans* cell wall mannoprotein exerts three anti-*C. albicans* activities. Infect Immun. 2003;71:5273–9.
236. Morelli R, Rosenberg LT. The role of complement in the phagocytosis of *Candida albicans* by mouse peripheral blood leukocytes. J Immunol. 1971;107:476–80.
237. Moreno-Ruiz E, Galan-Diez M, Zhu WD, Fernandez-Ruiz E, d'Enfert C, Filler SG, Cossart P, Veiga E. *Candida albicans* internalization by host cells is mediated by a clathrin-dependent mechanism. Cell Microbiol. 2009;11:1179–89.
238. Morris A, Wei K, Afshar K, Huang L. Epidemiology and clinical significance of pneumocystis colonization. J Infect Dis. 2008;197:10–7.
239. Morris DO, O'Shea K, Shofer FS, Rankin S. Malassezia pachydermatis carriage in dog owners. Emerg Infect Dis. 2005;11:83–8.
240. Moyes DL, Murciano C, Runglall M, Islam A, Thavaraj S, Naglik JR. *Candida albicans* yeast and hyphae are discriminated by MAPK signaling in vaginal epithelial cells. PLoS One. 2011;6:e26580.
241. Moyes DL, Runglall M, Murciano C, Shen CG, Nayar D, Thavaraj S, Kohli A, Islam A, Mora-Montes H, Challacombe SJ, Naglik JR. A biphasic innate immune MAPK response discriminates between the yeast and hyphal forms of *Candida albicans* in epithelial cells. Cell Host Microbe. 2010;8:225–35.
242. Moyes DL, Shen C, Murciano C, Runglall M, Richardson JP, Arno M, Aldecoa-Otalora E, Naglik JR. Protection against epithelial damage during *Candida albicans* infection is mediated by PI3K/Akt and mammalian target of rapamycin signaling. J Infect Dis. 2014;209:1816–26.
243. Moyes DL, Wilson D, Richardson JP, Mogavero S, Tang SX, Wernecke J, Hofs S, Gratacap RL, Robbins J, Runglall M, et al. Candidalysin is a fungal peptide toxin critical for mucosal infection. Nature. 2016;532(7597):64–8.
244. Mullick A, Elias M, Picard S, Bourget L, Jovcevski O, Gauthier S, Tuite A, Harakidas P, Bihun C, Massie B, Gros P. Dysregulated inflammatory response to *Candida albicans* in a C5-deficient mouse strain. Infect Immun. 2004;72:5868–76.
245. Mullick A, Leon Z, Min-Oo G, Berghout J, Lo R, Daniels E, Gros P. Cardiac failure in C5-deficient A/J mice after *Candida albicans* infection. Infect Immun. 2006;74:4439–51.
246. Murphy JW, McDaniel DO. In vitro reactivity of natural killer (NK) cells against *Cryptococcus neoformans*. J Immunol. 1982;128:1577–83.
247. Naglik JR, Moyes DL, Wachtler B, Hube B. *Candida albicans* interactions with epithelial cells and mucosal immunity. Microbes Infection/Institut Pasteur. 2011;13:963–76.
248. Nanjappa SG, Heninger E, Wuthrich M, Gasper DJ, Klein BS. Tc17 cells mediate vaccine immunity against lethal fungal pneumonia in immune deficient hosts lacking CD4+ T cells. PLoS Pathog. 2012;8:e1002771.
249. Nanjappa SG, Klein BS. Vaccine immunity against fungal infections. Curr Opin Immunol. 2014;28:27–33.
250. Nathan CF. Respiratory burst in adherent human neutrophils: triggering by colony-stimulating factors CSF-GM and CSF-G. Blood. 1989;73:301–6.
251. NCT01926028, and NCT01067131. https://clinicaltrials.gov/ct2/show/NCT01926028 and https://clinicaltrials.gov/ct2/show/NCT01067131.

252. Netea MG, Brown GD, Kullberg BJ, Gow NA. An integrated model of the recognition of *Candida albicans* by the innate immune system. Nat Rev Microbiol. 2008;6:67–78.
253. Netea MG, Nold-Petry CA, Nold MF, Joosten LA, Opitz B, van der Meer JH, van de Veerdonk FL, Ferwerda G, Heinhuis B, Devesa I, et al. Differential requirement for the activation of the inflammasome for processing and release of IL-1beta in monocytes and macrophages. Blood. 2009;113:2324–35.
254. Netea MG, Van Der Graaf CA, Vonk AG, Verschueren I, Van der Meer JW, Kullberg BJ. The role of toll-like receptor (TLR) 2 and TLR4 in the host defense against disseminated candidiasis. J Infect Dis. 2002;185:1483–9.
255. Newman SL, Gootee L, Gabay JE, Selsted ME. Identification of constituents of human neutrophil azurophil granules that mediate fungistasis against Histoplasma capsulatum. Infect Immun. 2000;68:5668–72.
256. Ngo LY, Kasahara S, Kumasaka DK, Knoblaugh SE, Jhingran A, Hohl TM. Inflammatory monocytes mediate early and organ-specific innate defense during systemic candidiasis. J Infect Dis. 2014;209:109–19.
257. Oguma K, Sano J, Kano R, Watari T, Moritomo T, Hasegawa A. In vitro effect of recombinant human granulocyte colony-stimulating factor on canine neutrophil apoptosis. Vet Immunol Immunopathol. 2005;108:307–14.
258. Okada S, Markle JG, Deenick EK, Mele F, Averbuch D, Lagos M, Alzahrani M, Al-Muhsen S, Halwani R, Ma CS, et al. IMMUNODEFICIENCIES Impairment of immunity to candida and Mycobacterium in humans with bi-allelic RORC mutations. Science. 2015;349:606–13.
259. Okamoto T, Tanida T, Wei B, Ueta E, Yamamoto T, Osaki T. Regulation of fungal infection by a combination of amphotericin B and peptide 2, a lactoferrin peptide that activates neutrophils. Clin Diagn Lab Immunol. 2004;11:1111–9.
260. Osorio F, LeibundGut-Landmann S, Lochner M, Lahl K, Sparwasser T, Eberl G, Reis e Sousa C. DC activated via dectin-1 convert Treg into IL-17 producers. Eur J Immunol. 2008;38:3274–81.
261. Osorio F, Reis e Sousa C. Myeloid C-type lectin receptors in pathogen recognition and host defense. Immunity. 2011;34:651–64.
262. Pandiyan P, Conti HR, Zheng L, Peterson AC, Mathern DR, Hernandez-Santos N, Edgerton M, Gaffen SL, Lenardo MJ. CD4(+)CD25(+)Foxp3(+) regulatory T cells promote Th17 cells in vitro and enhance host resistance in mouse *Candida albicans* Th17 cell infection model. Immunity. 2011;34:422–34.
263. Pantelyushin S, Haak S, Ingold B, Kulig P, Heppner FL, Navarini AA, Becher B. Rorgammat+ innate lymphocytes and gammadelta T cells initiate psoriasiform plaque formation in mice. J Clin Invest. 2012;122:2252–6.
264. Park SJ, Hughes MA, Burdick M, Strieter RM, Mehrad B. Early NK cell-derived IFN-gamma is essential to host defense in neutropenic invasive aspergillosis. J Immunol. 2009;182:4306–12.
265. Petkus AF, Baum LL. Natural killer cell inhibition of young spherules and endospores of Coccidioides immitis. J Immunol. 1987;139:3107–11.
266. Pfaller MA, Diekema DJ. Epidemiology of invasive candidiasis: a persistent public health problem. Clin Microbiol Rev. 2007;20:133–63.
267. Phan QT, Myers CL, Fu Y, Sheppard DC, Yeaman MR, Welch WH, Ibrahim AS, Edwards Jr JE, Filler SG. Als3 is a *Candida albicans* invasin that binds to cadherins and induces endocytosis by host cells. PLoS Biol. 2007;5:e64.
268. Pietrella D, Pandey N, Gabrielli E, Pericolini E, Perito S, Kasper L, Bistoni F, Cassone A, Hube B, Vecchiarelli A. Secreted aspartic proteases of *Candida albicans* activate the NLRP3 inflammasome. Eur J Immunol. 2013;43:679–92.
269. Pietrella D, Rachini A, Pines M, Pandey N, Mosci P, Bistoni F, d'Enfert C, Vecchiarelli A. Th17 cells and IL-17 in protective immunity to vaginal candidiasis. PLoS One. 2011;6:e22770.
270. Plato A, Willment JA, Brown GD. C-type lectin-like receptors of the dectin-1 cluster: ligands and signaling pathways. Int Rev Immunol. 2013;32:134–56.

271. Puel A, Cypowyj S, Bustamante J, Wright JF, Liu LY, Lim HK, Migaud M, Israel L, Chrabieh M, Audry M, et al. Chronic mucocutaneous candidiasis in humans with inborn errors of interleukin-17 immunity. Science. 2011;332:65–8.
272. Puri S, Edgerton M. How does it kill?: understanding the candidacidal mechanism of salivary histatin 5. Eukaryot Cell. 2014;13:958–64.
273. Qu Y, Franchi L, Nunez G, Dubyak GR. Nonclassical IL-1 beta secretion stimulated by P2X7 receptors is dependent on inflammasome activation and correlated with exosome release in murine macrophages. J Immunol. 2007;179:1913–25.
274. Quintin J, Saeed S, Martens JH, Giamarellos-Bourboulis EJ, Ifrim DC, Logie C, Jacobs L, Jansen T, Kullberg BJ, Wijmenga C, et al. *Candida albicans* infection affords protection against reinfection via functional reprogramming of monocytes. Cell Host Microbe. 2012;12:223–32.
275. Quintin J, Voigt J, van der Voort R, Jacobsen ID, Verschueren I, Hube B, Giamarellos-Bourboulis EJ, van der Meer JW, Joosten LA, Kurzai O, Netea MG. Differential role of NK cells against *Candida albicans* infection in immunocompetent or immunocompromised mice. Eur J Immunol. 2014;44:2405–14.
276. Radovanovic I, Mullick A, Gros P. Genetic control of susceptibility to infection with *Candida albicans* in mice. PLoS One. 2011;6:e18957.
277. Ramirez-Ortiz ZG, Specht CA, Wang JP, Lee CK, Bartholomeu DC, Gazzinelli RT, Levitz SM. Toll-like receptor 9-dependent immune activation by unmethylated CpG motifs in Aspergillus fumigatus DNA. Infect Immun. 2008;76:2123–9.
278. Rappleye CA, Eissenberg LG, Goldman WE. Histoplasma capsulatum alpha-(1, 3)-glucan blocks innate immune recognition by the beta-glucan receptor. P Natl Acad Sci USA. 2007;104:1366–70.
279. Redelinghuys P, Brown GD. Inhibitory C-type lectin receptors in myeloid cells. Immunol Lett. 2011;136:1–12.
280. Reeves EP, Lu H, Jacobs HL, Messina CG, Bolsover S, Gabella G, Potma EO, Warley A, Roes J, Segal AW. Killing activity of neutrophils is mediated through activation of proteases by K+ flux. Nature. 2002;416:291–7.
281. Reis e Sousa C. Activation of dendritic cells: translating innate into adaptive immunity. Curr Opin Immunol. 2004;16:21–5.
282. Renner ED, Rylaarsdam S, Anover-Sombke S, Rack AL, Reichenbach J, Carey JC, Zhu Q, Jansson AF, Barboza J, Schimke LF, et al. Novel signal transducer and activator of transcription 3 (STAT3) mutations, reduced T(H)17 cell numbers, and variably defective STAT3 phosphorylation in hyper-IgE syndrome. J Allergy Clin Immunol. 2008;122:181–7.
283. Rivera A, Ro G, Van Epps HL, Simpson T, Leiner I, Sant'Angelo DB, Pamer EG. Innate immune activation and CD4+ T cell priming during respiratory fungal infection. Immunity. 2006;25:665–75.
284. Robinson MJ, Osorio F, Rosas M, Freitas RP, Schweighoffer E, Gross O, Verbeek JS, Ruland J, Tybulewicz V, Brown GD, et al. Dectin-2 is a Syk-coupled pattern recognition receptor crucial for Th17 responses to fungal infection. J Exp Med. 2009;206:2037–51.
285. Rogers NC, Slack EC, Edwards AD, Nolte MA, Schulz O, Schweighoffer E, Williams DL, Gordon S, Tybulewicz VL, Brown GD, Reis e Sousa C. Syk-dependent cytokine induction by Dectin-1 reveals a novel pattern recognition pathway for C type lectins. Immunity. 2005;22:507–17.
286. Roilides E, Holmes A, Blake C, Pizzo PA, Walsh TJ. Effects of granulocyte colony-stimulating factor and interferon-gamma on antifungal activity of human polymorphonuclear neutrophils against pseudohyphae of different medically important Candida species. J Leukoc Biol. 1995;57:651–6.
287. Root RK, Dale DC. Granulocyte colony-stimulating factor and granulocyte-macrophage colony-stimulating factor: comparisons and potential for use in the treatment of infections in nonneutropenic patients. J Infect Dis. 1999;179(Suppl 2):S342–52.
288. Rotrosen D, Edwards Jr JE, Gibson TR, Moore JC, Cohen AH, Green I. Adherence of Candida to cultured vascular endothelial cells: mechanisms of attachment and endothelial cell penetration. J Infect Dis. 1985;152:1264–74.

289. Rubin-Bejerano I, Abeijon C, Magnelli P, Grisafi P, Fink GR. Phagocytosis by human neutrophils is stimulated by a unique fungal cell wall component. Cell Host Microbe. 2007;2:55–67.
290. Said-Sadier N, Padilla E, Langsley G, Ojcius DM. Aspergillus fumigatus stimulates the NLRP3 inflammasome through a pathway requiring ROS production and the Syk tyrosine kinase. PLoS One. 2010;5:e10008.
291. Saijo S, Fujikado N, Furuta T, Chung SH, Kotaki H, Seki K, Sudo K, Akira S, Adachi Y, Ohno N, et al. Dectin-1 is required for host defense against Pneumocystis carinii but not against *Candida albicans*. Nat Immunol. 2007;8:39–46.
292. Saijo S, Ikeda S, Yamabe K, Kakuta S, Ishigame H, Akitsu A, Fujikado N, Kusaka T, Kubo S, Chung SH, et al. Dectin-2 recognition of alpha-mannans and induction of Th17 cell differentiation is essential for host defense against *Candida albicans*. Immunity. 2010;32:681–91.
293. Sainz J, Lupianez CB, Segura-Catena J, Vazquez L, Rios R, Oyonarte S, Hemminki K, Forsti A, Jurado M. Dectin-1 and DC-SIGN Polymorphisms Associated with Invasive Pulmonary Aspergillosis Infection. Plos One. 2012;7(2):e32273.
294. Saito S, Rosol TJ, Saito M, Ngan PW, Shanfeld J, Davidovitch Z. Bone-resorbing activity and prostaglandin E produced by human periodontal ligament cells in vitro. J Bone Miner Res. 1990;5:1013–8.
295. Sato K, Yang XL, Yudate T, Chung JS, Wu J, Luby-Phelps K, Kimberly RP, Underhill D, Cruz Jr PD, Ariizumi K. Dectin-2 is a pattern recognition receptor for fungi that couples with the Fc receptor gamma chain to induce innate immune responses. J Biol Chem. 2006;281:38854–66.
296. Saville SP, Lazzell AL, Monteagudo C, Lopez-Ribot JL. Engineered control of cell morphology in vivo reveals distinct roles for yeast and filamentous forms of *Candida albicans* during infection. Eukaryot Cell. 2003;2:1053–60.
297. Scheckelhoff M, Deepe Jr GS. A deficiency in gamma interferon or interleukin-10 modulates T-Cell-dependent responses to heat shock protein 60 from Histoplasma capsulatum. Infect Immun. 2005;73:2129–34.
298. Scheynius A, Johansson C, Buentke E, Zargari A, Linder MT. Atopic eczema/dermatitis syndrome and Malassezia. Int Arch Allergy Immunol. 2002;127:161–9.
299. Schmidt CS, White CJ, Ibrahim AS, Filler SG, Fu Y, Yeaman MR, Edwards Jr JE, Hennessey Jr JP. NDV-3, a recombinant alum-adjuvanted vaccine for Candida and *Staphylococcus aureus*, is safe and immunogenic in healthy adults. Vaccine. 2012;30:7594–600.
300. Schmidt S, Tramsen L, Hanisch M, Latge JP, Huenecke S, Koehl U, Lehrnbecher T. Human natural killer cells exhibit direct activity against Aspergillus fumigatus hyphae, but not against resting conidia. J Infect Dis. 2011;203:430–5.
301. Schmidt S, Tramsen L, Perkhofer S, Lass-Florl C, Hanisch M, Roger F, Klingebiel T, Koehl U, Lehrnbecher T. Rhizopus oryzae hyphae are damaged by human natural killer NK cells, but suppress (NK) cell mediated immunity. Immunobiology. 2013;218:939–44.
302. Schwarzenberger P, La Russa V, Miller A, Ye P, Huang W, Zieske A, Nelson S, Bagby GJ, Stoltz D, Mynatt RL, et al. IL-17 stimulates granulopoiesis in mice: use of an alternate, novel gene therapy-derived method for in vivo evaluation of cytokines. J Immunol. 1998;161:6383–9.
303. Segal BH, Leto TL, Gallin JI, Malech HL, Holland SM. Genetic, biochemical, and clinical features of chronic granulomatous disease. Medicine (Baltimore). 2000;79:170–200.
304. Segal BH, Romani LR. Invasive aspergillosis in chronic granulomatous disease. Med Mycol. 2009;47(Suppl 1):S282–90.
305. Seider K, Brunke S, Schild L, Jablonowski N, Wilson D, Majer O, Barz D, Haas A, Kuchler K, Schaller M, Hube B. The facultative intracellular pathogen Candida glabrata subverts macrophage cytokine production and phagolysosome maturation. J Immunol. 2011;187:3072–86.
306. Shinde RV, Karande GS, Mohite ST, Patil SR. Rhino-orbital mucormycosis in diabetes mellitus. J Clin Diagn Res: JCDR. 2013;7:1145–7.

307. Slack EC, Robinson MJ, Hernanz-Falcon P, Brown GD, Williams DL, Schweighoffer E, Tybulewicz VL, Reis e Sousa C. Syk-dependent ERK activation regulates IL-2 and IL-10 production by DC stimulated with zymosan. Eur J Immunol. 2007;37:1600–12.
308. Sobel JD. Vulvovaginal candidosis. Lancet. 2007;369:1961–71.
309. Soehnlein O, Lindbom L. Phagocyte partnership during the onset and resolution of inflammation. Nat Rev Immunol. 2010;10:427–39.
310. Sohnle PG, Hunter MJ, Hahn B, Chazin WJ. Zinc-reversible antimicrobial activity of recombinant calprotectin (migration inhibitory factor-related proteins 8 and 14). J Infect Dis. 2000;182:1272–5.
311. Sonnenberg GF, Artis D. Innate lymphoid cells in the initiation, regulation and resolution of inflammation. Nat Med. 2015;21:698–708.
312. Sousa Mda G, Reid DM, Schweighoffer E, Tybulewicz V, Ruland J, Langhorne J, Yamasaki S, Taylor PR, Almeida SR, Brown GD. Restoration of pattern recognition receptor costimulation to treat chromoblastomycosis, a chronic fungal infection of the skin. Cell Host Microbe. 2011;9:436–43.
313. Sparber F, LeibundGut-Landmann S. Interleukin 17-mediated host defense against *Candida albicans*. Pathogens. 2015;4:606–19.
314. Spellberg B, Edwards Jr J, Ibrahim A. Novel perspectives on mucormycosis: pathophysiology, presentation, and management. Clin Microbiol Rev. 2005;18:556–69.
315. Staab JF, Bradway SD, Fidel PL, Sundstrom P. Adhesive and mammalian transglutaminase substrate properties of *Candida albicans* Hwp1. Science. 1999;283:1535–8.
316. Stalla GK, Stalla J, von Werder K, Muller OA, Gerzer R, Hollt V, Jakobs KH. Nitroimidazole derivatives inhibit anterior pituitary cell function apparently by a direct effect on the catalytic subunit of the adenylate cyclase holoenzyme. Endocrinology. 1989;125:699–706.
317. Steele C, Fidel Jr PL. Cytokine and chemokine production by human oral and vaginal epithelial cells in response to *Candida albicans*. Infect Immun. 2002;70:577–83.
318. Steele C, Rapaka RR, Metz A, Pop SM, Williams DL, Gordon S, Kolls JK, Brown GD. The beta-glucan receptor dectin-1 recognizes specific morphologies of Aspergillus fumigatus. PLoS Pathog. 2005;1:e42.
319. Stephenson JD, Shepherd VL. Purification of the human alveolar macrophage mannose receptor. Biochem Biophys Res Commun. 1987;148:883–9.
320. Stevenson FT, Bursten SL, Fanton C, Locksley RM, Lovett DH. The 31-kDa precursor of interleukin 1 alpha is myristoylated on specific lysines within the 16-kDa N-terminal propiece. Proc Natl Acad Sci U S A. 1993;90:7245–9.
321. Strasser D, Neumann K, Bergmann H, Marakalala MJ, Guler R, Rojowska A, Hopfner KP, Brombacher F, Urlaub H, Baier G, et al. Syk kinase-coupled C-type lectin receptors engage protein kinase C-sigma to elicit Card9 adaptor-mediated innate immunity. Immunity. 2012;36:32–42.
322. Subramanian Vignesh K, Landero Figueroa JA, Porollo A, Caruso JA, Deepe Jr GS. Granulocyte macrophage-colony stimulating factor induced Zn sequestration enhances macrophage superoxide and limits intracellular pathogen survival. Immunity. 2013;39:697–710.
323. Sun JN, Li W, Jang WS, Nayyar N, Sutton MD, Edgerton M. Uptake of the antifungal cationic peptide Histatin 5 by *Candida albicans* Ssa2p requires binding to non-conventional sites within the ATPase domain. Mol Microbiol. 2008;70:1246–60.
324. Sun JN, Solis NV, Phan QT, Bajwa JS, Kashleva H, Thompson A, Liu Y, Dongari-Bagtzoglou A, Edgerton M, Filler SG. Host cell invasion and virulence mediated by *Candida albicans* Ssa1. PLoS Pathog. 2010;6:e1001181.
325. Sun WK, Lu X, Li X, Sun QY, Su X, Song Y, Sun HM, Shi Y. Dectin-1 is inducible and plays a crucial role in Aspergillus-induced innate immune responses in human bronchial epithelial cells. Eur J Clin Microbiol Infect Dis. 2012;31:2755–64.
326. Sutterwala FS, Ogura Y, Szczepanik M, Lara-Tejero M, Lichtenberger GS, Grant EP, Bertin J, Coyle AJ, Galan JE, Askenase PW, Flavell RA. Critical role for NALP3/CIAS1/Cryopyrin in innate and adaptive immunity through its regulation of caspase-1. Immunity. 2006;24:317–27.

327. Taylor PR, Roy S, Leal Jr SM, Sun Y, Howell SJ, Cobb BA, Li X, Pearlman E. Activation of neutrophils by autocrine IL-17A-IL-17RC interactions during fungal infection is regulated by IL-6, IL-23, RORgammat and dectin-2. Nat Immunol. 2014;15:143–51.
328. Taylor PR, Tsoni SV, Willment JA, Dennehy KM, Rosas M, Findon H, Haynes K, Steele C, Botto M, Gordon S, Brown GD. Dectin-1 is required for beta-glucan recognition and control of fungal infection. Nat Immunol. 2007;8:31–8.
329. Tecchio C, Micheletti A, Cassatella MA. Neutrophil-derived cytokines: facts beyond expression. Front Immunol. 2014;5:508.
330. Thomas PA, Kaliamurthy J. Mycotic keratitis: epidemiology, diagnosis and management. Clin Microbiol Infect. 2013;19:210–20.
331. Thong YH, Ferrante A. Alternative pathway of complement activation by *Candida albicans*. Aust NZ J Med. 1978;8:620–2.
332. Tkalcevic J, Novelli M, Phylactides M, Iredale JP, Segal AW, Roes J. Impaired immunity and enhanced resistance to endotoxin in the absence of neutrophil elastase and cathepsin G. Immunity. 2000;12:201–10.
333. Tobin DM, May RC, Wheeler RT. Zebrafish: a see-through host and a fluorescent toolbox to probe host-pathogen interaction. PLoS Pathog. 2012;8:e1002349.
334. Tomalka J, Azodi E, Narra HP, Patel K, O'Neill S, Cardwell C, Hall BA, Wilson JM, Hise AG. Beta-Defensin 1 plays a role in acute mucosal defense against *Candida albicans*. J Immunol. 2015;194:1788–95.
335. Tomalka J, Ganesan S, Azodi E, Patel K, Majmudar P, Hall BA, Fitzgerald KA, Hise AG. A novel role for the NLRC4 inflammasome in mucosal defenses against the fungal pathogen *Candida albicans*. PLoS Pathog. 2011;7:e1002379.
336. Torosantucci A, Bromuro C, Chiani P, De Bernardis F, Berti F, Galli C, Norelli F, Bellucci C, Polonelli L, Costantino P, et al. A novel glyco-conjugate vaccine against fungal pathogens. J Exp Med. 2005;202:597–606.
337. Trautwein-Weidner K, Gladiator A, Kirchner FR, Becattini S, Rulicke T, Sallusto F, LeibundGut-Landmann S. Antigen-specific Th17 cells are primed by distinct and complementary dendritic cell subsets in oropharyngeal candidiasis. PLoS Pathog. 2015;11:e1005164.
338. Trautwein-Weidner K, Gladiator A, Nur S, Diethelm P, LeibundGut-Landmann S. IL-17-mediated antifungal defense in the oral mucosa is independent of neutrophils. Mucosal Immunol. 2015;8:221–31.
339. Traynor TR, Herring AC, Dorf ME, Kuziel WA, Toews GB, Huffnagle GB. Differential roles of CC chemokine ligand 2/monocyte chemotactic protein-1 and CCR2 in the development of T1 immunity. J Immunol. 2002;168:4659–66.
340. Traynor TR, Kuziel WA, Toews GB, Huffnagle GB. CCR2 expression determines T1 versus T2 polarization during pulmonary *Cryptococcus neoformans* infection. J Immunol. 2000;164:2021–7.
341. Tsoni SV, Kerrigan AM, Marakalala MJ, Srinivasan N, Duffield M, Taylor PR, Botto M, Steele C, Brown GD. Complement C3 plays an essential role in the control of opportunistic fungal infections. Infect Immun. 2009;77:3679–85.
342. Tucker SC, Casadevall A. Replication of *Cryptococcus neoformans* in macrophages is accompanied by phagosomal permeabilization and accumulation of vesicles containing polysaccharide in the cytoplasm. Proc Natl Acad Sci U S A. 2002;99:3165–70.
343. Umemura M, Yahagi A, Hamada S, Begum MD, Watanabe H, Kawakami K, Suda T, Sudo K, Nakae S, Iwakura Y, Matsuzaki G. IL-17-mediated regulation of innate and acquired immune response against pulmonary Mycobacterium bovis bacille Calmette-Guerin infection. J Immunol. 2007;178:3786–96.
344. Underhill DM, Iliev ID. The mycobiota: interactions between commensal fungi and the host immune system. Nat Rev Immunol. 2014;14:405–16.
345. Urban CF, Ermert D, Schmid M, Abu-Abed U, Goosmann C, Nacken W, Brinkmann V, Jungblut PR, Zychlinsky A. Neutrophil extracellular traps contain calprotectin, a cytosolic

protein complex involved in host defense against *Candida albicans*. PLoS Pathog. 2009;5:e1000639.

346. van de Veerdonk FL, Joosten LAB, Devesa I, Mora-Montes HM, Kanneganti T-D, Dinarello CA, van der Meer JWM, Gow NAR, Kullberg BJ, Netea MG. Bypassing pathogen-induced inflammasome activation for the regulation of interleukin-1beta production by the fungal pathogen *Candida albicans*. J Infect Dis. 2009;199:1087–96.
347. van de Veerdonk FL, Plantinga TS, Hoischen A, Smeekens SP, Joosten LA, Gilissen C, Arts P, Rosentul DC, Carmichael AJ, Smits-van der Graaf CA, et al. STAT1 mutations in autosomal dominant chronic mucocutaneous candidiasis. N Engl J Med. 2011;365:54–61.
348. Veldhoen M, Hocking RJ, Atkins CJ, Locksley RM, Stockinger B. TGFbeta in the context of an inflammatory cytokine milieu supports de novo differentiation of IL-17-producing T cells. Immunity. 2006;24:179–89.
349. Velegraki A, Cafarchia C, Gaitanis G, Iatta R, Boekhout T. Malassezia infections in humans and animals: pathophysiology, detection, and treatment. PLoS Pathog. 2015;11:e1004523.
350. Villar CC, Kashleva H, Nobile CJ, Mitchell AP, Dongari-Bagtzoglou A. Mucosal tissue invasion by *Candida albicans* is associated with E-cadherin degradation, mediated by transcription factor Rim101p and protease Sap5p. Infect Immun. 2007;75:2126–35.
351. Vivier E, Tomasello E, Baratin M, Walzer T, Ugolini S. Functions of natural killer cells. Nat Immunol. 2008;9:503–10.
352. Voigt J, Hunniger K, Bouzani M, Jacobsen ID, Barz D, Hube B, Loffler J, Kurzai O. Human natural killer cells acting as phagocytes against *Candida albicans* and mounting an inflammatory response that modulates neutrophil antifungal activity. J Infect Dis. 2014;209:616–26.
353. Vonk AG, Netea MG, van Krieken JH, Iwakura Y, van der Meer JW, Kullberg BJ. Endogenous interleukin IL-1 alpha and IL-1 beta are crucial for host defense against disseminated candidiasis. J Infect Dis. 2006;193:1419–26.
354. Vylkova S, Nayyar N, Li W, Edgerton M. Human beta-defensins kill *Candida albicans* in an energy-dependent and salt-sensitive manner without causing membrane disruption. Antimicrob Agents Chemother. 2007;51:154–61.
355. Wachtler B, Citiulo F, Jablonowski N, Forster S, Dalle F, Schaller M, Wilson D, Hube B. *Candida albicans*-epithelial interactions: dissecting the roles of active penetration, induced endocytosis and host factors on the infection process. PLoS One. 2012;7:e36952.
356. Wachtler B, Wilson D, Haedicke K, Dalle F, Hube B. From attachment to damage: defined genes of *Candida albicans* mediate adhesion, invasion and damage during interaction with oral epithelial cells. PLoS One. 2011;6:e17046.
357. Wagener J, Malireddi RK, Lenardon MD, Koberle M, Vautier S, MacCallum DM, Biedermann T, Schaller M, Netea MG, Kanneganti TD, et al. Fungal chitin dampens inflammation through IL-10 induction mediated by NOD2 and TLR9 activation. PLoS Pathog. 2014;10:e1004050.
358. Wallach D, Kang TB, Dillon CP, Green DR. Programmed necrosis in inflammation: Toward identification of the effector molecules. Science. 2016;352:aaf2154.
359. Wang X, Wang W, Lin Z, Wang X, Li T, Yu J, Liu W, Tong Z, Xu Y, Zhang J, et al. CARD9 mutations linked to subcutaneous phaeohyphomycosis and TH17 cell deficiencies. J Allergy Clin Immunol. 2014;133:905–8. e903
360. Wang Y, Li M, Stadler S, Correll S, Li P, Wang D, Hayama R, Leonelli L, Han H, Grigoryev SA, et al. Histone hypercitrullination mediates chromatin decondensation and neutrophil extracellular trap formation. J Cell Biol. 2009;184:205–13.
361. Ward PA, Gao H. Sepsis, complement and the dysregulated inflammatory response. J Cell Mol Med. 2009;13:4154–60.
362. Weaver CT, Harrington LE, Mangan PR, Gavrieli M, Murphy KM. Th17: an effector CD4 T cell lineage with regulatory T cell ties. Immunity. 2006;24:677–88.
363. Wells CA, Salvage-Jones JA, Li X, Hitchens K, Butcher S, Murray RZ, Beckhouse AG, Lo YL, Manzanero S, Cobbold C, et al. The macrophage-inducible C-type lectin, mincle, is an

essential component of the innate immune response to *Candida albicans*. J Immunol. 2008;180:7404–13.
364. Werner JL, Metz AE, Horn D, Schoeb TR, Hewitt MM, Schwiebert LM, Faro-Trindade I, Brown GD, Steele C. Requisite role for the dectin-1 beta-glucan receptor in pulmonary defense against Aspergillus fumigatus. J Immunol. 2009;182:4938–46.
365. Wheeler RT, Fink GR. A drug-sensitive genetic network masks fungi from the immune system. PLoS Pathog. 2006;2:e35.
366. Whibley N, Tritto E, Traggiai E, Kolbinger F, Moulin P, Brees D, Coleman BM, Mamo AJ, Garg AV, Jaycox JR, et al. Antibody blockade of IL-17 family cytokines in immunity to acute murine oral mucosal candidiasis. J Leukoc Biol. 2016;99(6):1153–64.
367. Whitney PG, Bar E, Osorio F, Rogers NC, Schraml BU, Deddouche S, LeibundGut-Landmann S, Reise Sousa C. Syk signaling in dendritic cells orchestrates innate resistance to systemic fungal infection. PLoS Pathog. 2014;10:e1004276.
368. Wileman TE, Lennartz MR, Stahl PD. Identification of the macrophage mannose receptor as a 175-kDa membrane protein. Proc Natl Acad Sci U S A. 1986;83:2501–5.
369. Winters MS, Chan Q, Caruso JA, Deepe Jr GS. Metallomic analysis of macrophages infected with Histoplasma capsulatum reveals a fundamental role for zinc in host defenses. J Infect Dis. 2010;202:1136–45.
370. Wuthrich M, Brandhorst TT, Sullivan TD, Filutowicz H, Sterkel A, Stewart D, Li M, Lerksuthirat T, LeBert V, Shen ZT, et al. Calnexin induces expansion of antigen-specific CD4+ T cells that confer immunity to fungal ascomycetes via conserved epitopes. Cell Host Microbe. 2015;17:452–65.
371. Wuthrich M, Ersland K, Pick-Jacobs JC, Gern BH, Frye CA, Sullivan TD, Brennan MB, Filutowicz HI, O'Brien K, Korthauer KD, et al. Limited model antigen expression by transgenic fungi induces disparate fates during differentiation of adoptively transferred T cell receptor transgenic CD4+ T cells: robust activation and proliferation with weak effector function during recall. Infect Immun. 2012;80:787–97.
372. Wuthrich M, Gern B, Hung CY, Ersland K, Rocco N, Pick-Jacobs J, Galles K, Filutowicz H, Warner T, Evans M, et al. Vaccine-induced protection against 3 systemic mycoses endemic to North America requires Th17 cells in mice. J Clin Invest. 2011;121:554–68.
373. Wuthrich M, Hung CY, Gern BH, Pick-Jacobs JC, Galles KJ, Filutowicz HI, Cole GT, Klein BS. A TCR transgenic mouse reactive with multiple systemic dimorphic fungi. J Immunol. 2011;187:1421–31.
374. Xu H, Wang X, Liu DX, Moroney-Rasmussen T, Lackner AA, Veazey RS. IL-17-producing innate lymphoid cells are restricted to mucosal tissues and are depleted in SIV-infected macaques. Mucosal Immunol. 2012;5:658–69.
375. Xu Y, Ambudkar I, Yamagishi H, Swaim W, Walsh TJ, O'Connell BC. Histatin 3-mediated killing of *Candida albicans*: effect of extracellular salt concentration on binding and internalization. Antimicrob Agents Chemother. 1999;43:2256–62.
376. Yamamoto Y, Klein TW, Friedman H, Kimura S, Yamaguchi H. Granulocyte colony-stimulating factor potentiates anti-*Candida albicans* growth inhibitory activity of polymorphonuclear cells. FEMS Immunol Med Microbiol. 1993;7:15–22.
377. Yamasaki S, Ishikawa E, Sakuma M, Hara H, Ogata K, Saito T. Mincle is an ITAM-coupled activating receptor that senses damaged cells. Nat Immunol. 2008;9:1179–88.
378. Yamasaki S, Matsumoto M, Takeuchi O, Matsuzawa T, Ishikawa E, Sakuma M, Tateno H, Uno J, Hirabayashi J, Mikami Y, et al. C-type lectin Mincle is an activating receptor for pathogenic fungus, Malassezia. Proc Natl Acad Sci U S A. 2009;106:1897–902.
379. Yano J, Kolls JK, Happel KI, Wormley F, Wozniak KL, Fidel Jr PL. The acute neutrophil response mediated by S100 alarmins during vaginal Candida infections is independent of the Th17-pathway. PLoS One. 2012;7:e46311.
380. Yano J, Palmer GE, Eberle KE, Peters BM, Vogl T, McKenzie AN, Fidel Jr PL. Vaginal epithelial cell-derived S100 alarmins induced by *Candida albicans* via pattern recognition receptor interactions are sufficient but not necessary for the acute neutrophil response during experimental vaginal candidiasis. Infect Immun. 2014;82:783–92.

381. Ye P, Rodriguez FH, Kanaly S, Stocking KL, Schurr J, Schwarzenberger P, Oliver P, Huang W, Zhang P, Zhang J, et al. Requirement of interleukin 17 receptor signaling for lung CXC chemokine and granulocyte colony-stimulating factor expression, neutrophil recruitment, and host defense. J Exp Med. 2001;194:519–27.
382. Yeaman MR, Filler SG, Chaili S, Barr K, Wang H, Kupferwasser D, Hennessey Jr JP, Fu Y, Schmidt CS, Edwards Jr JE, et al. Mechanisms of NDV-3 vaccine efficacy in MRSA skin versus invasive infection. Proc Natl Acad Sci U S A. 2014;111:E5555–63.
383. Yokomura I, Iwasaki Y, Nagata K, Nakanishi M, Natsuhara A, Harada H, Kubota Y, Ueda M, Inaba T, Nakagawa M. Role of intercellular adhesion molecule 1 in acute lung injury induced by candidemia. Exp Lung Res. 2001;27:417–31.
384. Yokoyama WM, Sojka DK, Peng H, Tian Z. Tissue-resident natural killer cells. Cold Spring Harb Symp Quant Biol. 2013;78:149–56.
385. Zakikhany K, Naglik JR, Schmidt-Westhausen A, Holland G, Schaller M, Hube B. In vivo transcript profiling of *Candida albicans* identifies a gene essential for interepithelial dissemination. Cell Microbiol. 2007;9:2938–54.
386. Zelante T, De Luca A, Bonifazi P, Montagnoli C, Bozza S, Moretti S, Belladonna ML, Vacca C, Conte C, Mosci P, et al. IL-23 and the Th17 pathway promote inflammation and impair antifungal immune resistance. Eur J Immunol. 2007;37:2695–706.
387. Zhang Q, Davis JC, Lamborn IT, Freeman AF, Jing H, Favreau AJ, Matthews HF, Davis J, Turner ML, Uzel G, et al. Combined immunodeficiency associated with DOCK8 mutations. N Engl J Med. 2009;361:2046–55.
388. Zhao X, Oh SH, Cheng G, Green CB, Nuessen JA, Yeater K, Leng RP, Brown AJ, Hoyer LL. ALS3 and ALS8 represent a single locus that encodes a *Candida albicans* adhesin; functional comparisons between Als3p and Als1p. Microbiology. 2004;150:2415–28.
389. Zhao XQ, Zhu LL, Chang Q, Jiang C, You Y, Luo T, Jia XM, Lin X. C-type lectin receptor dectin-3 mediates trehalose 6, 6′-dimycolate (TDM)-induced Mincle expression through CARD9/Bcl10/MALT1-dependent nuclear factor (NF)-kappaB activation. J Biol Chem. 2014;289:30052–62.
390. Zhu LL, Zhao XQ, Jiang C, You Y, Chen XP, Jiang YY, Jia XM, Lin X. C-type lectin receptors Dectin-3 and Dectin-2 form a heterodimeric pattern-recognition receptor for host defense against fungal infection. Immunity. 2013;39:324–34.

Genetics of Chronic Mucocutaneous Candidiasis

3

Xiaowen Wang, Mihai G. Netea,
and Frank L. van de Veerdonk

Abstract
Chronic mucocutaneous candidiasis (CMC) is a group of disorders characterized by recurrent and persistent infections of the skin, nails, and mucosal membranes with *Candida* species. Genetic factors play a critical role in the pathogenesis of CMC. Various disorders that impair the sensing of *Candida* or downstream IL-17 signaling may cause CMC. This review will highlight novel findings regarding the genetics and pathogenesis of CMC in past few years.

3.1 Introduction

Chronic mucocutaneous candidiasis (CMC) is a group of disorders characterized by recurrent and persistent infections of the skin, nails, and mucosal membranes with *Candida* species, mainly *Candida albicans* (*C. albicans*) [1]. It was first described by Thorpe and Handley in 1929 [2]. CMC may present itself as a distinct clinical

Conflicts of Interest None declared.

X. Wang, MD
Department of Internal Medicine, Radboud University Nijmegen Medical Center, PO Box 9101, Nijmegen 6500 HB, The Netherlands

Department of Dermatology, Peking University First Hospital, Beijing, China

M.G. Netea, MD, PhD • F.L. van de Veerdonk, MD, PhD (✉)
Radboud Center for Infectious Diseases (RCI), Nijmegen, The Netherlands

Department of Internal Medicine, Radboud University Nijmegen Medical Center, PO Box 9101, Nijmegen 6500 HB, The Netherlands
e-mail: frank.vandeveerdonk@radboudumc.nl

A. Carvalho (ed.), *Immunogenetics of Fungal Diseases*,
DOI 10.1007/978-3-319-50842-9_3

entity called isolated CMC or CMC disease, in which CMC is the only or principal manifestation. It may also present as part of other immunodeficiencies, which is known as syndromic CMC. Moreover, CMC can be observed in addition to other infections in patients with acquired or inherited immunodeficiencies [3].

CMC was initially considered a genetic disease with defective cellular immunity in 1969 [4]. With the development of novel human genetics screening tools, genetic factors of CMC have been extensively studied in the past decide. Various defects that impair the sensing of *Candida* or downstream IL-17 signaling may lead to CMC [3]. These breakthroughs have led to novel insights in the genetic and molecular pathogenesis of CMC as well as other infections. In the present overview, we will summarize findings of the genetics of CMC, which may facilitate the diagnosis and genetic counseling in both familial and sporadic CMC patients, and this can pave the way for developing precise immunotherapeutic strategies for these patients in the future. An overview of the genetics and mechanisms of CMC are depicted in Table 3.1.

3.2 Inheritance of Isolated CMC

3.2.1 STAT1 Mutation

In 2011, heterozygous gain-of-function (GOF) mutations in signal transducer and activator of transcription 1 (*STAT1*) were first described to cause autosomal dominant (AD) CMC [37, 38], which was confirmed by many other studies as the main hereditary cause of isolated CMC. Due to the high frequency of mutations, it is suggested that all patients suspected of AD-CMC should be sequenced for STAT1 mutations [5]. Up till now, more than 123 patients with 32 different STAT1 variants have been reported in the literature [3, 5, 6, 39–49]. The majority of GOF-STAT1 mutations are confirmed to be in the coiled-coil domain (CCD), with 22 different variants and 98 patients infected, whereas 10 variants involving 25 patients in the DNA-binding domain (DBD) were also described (Table 3.2).

STAT1 is the major signaling molecule downstream of interferon (IFN) receptors. Triggered by IFNs, STAT1 translocates to the nucleus and triggers the transcription of IFNs-inducible genes, which play a pivotal role in the defense against pathogens [50]. GOF *STAT1* mutations, located in either in CCD or DBD, lead to hyperphosphorylation of STAT1 upon IFN-α, IFN-γ, and IL-27 stimulations and accumulation of phosphorylated STAT1 in the nucleus, which may shift the immune response away from a STAT3-mediated induction of Th17 cell generation [5, 37, 38]. Recent reports explained that GOF-STAT1 mutations do not impair STAT3 phosphorylation, homodimer formation, nuclear translocation, or DNA binding, but impair STAT3-dependent gene transcription, needed to induce optimal Th17 responses, which could be further reversed by preventing STAT1 phosphorylation directly or by inhibiting histone deacetylases (HDACs) [37, 51].

It was described in a recent study that the main clinical feature of these CMC patients with GOF of STAT1 mutations is oral candidiasis, in 73% of patients, with

Table 3.1 Summary of genetics of chronic mucocutaneous candidiasis

Gene	Mode of inheritance	Disease	Immunological phenotype	Refs.
Isolated CMC				
STAT1	AD	CMC	Impaired IL-17A and IL-22 production and Th17 differentiation	[5, 6]
CARD9	AR	CMC, *Candida* meningoencephalitis	Reduced TNF-α production and circulating IL-17-producing T cells	[4]
IL-17F	AD	CMC	Defective IL-17F bioactivity	[7]
IL-17RA/C	AR	CMC	Lack of cellular responses to IL-17A and IL-17F	[7, 8]
ACT1	AR	CMC	Impaired IL-17 signaling	[9]
Syndromic CMC				
STAT3	AD	HIES	Impaired Th17 differentiation and IL-17A and IL-22 production	[10, 11]
DOCK8	AR	HIES, combined immunodeficiencies	Impaired Th17 differentiation	[12]
PGM3	AR	HIES	Abnormal Th1/Th2 differentiation	2014JACI
AIRE	AR	APECED	Autoantibodies against IL-17 and IL-22	[13]
CMC associated PIDs				
TYK2	AR	Increased risk for mycobacterial and viral infections	Reduced Th1 and type I IFN responses	[14, 15]
IL-12RB1	AR	Increased risk for CMC and mycobacterial and *Salmonella* infections	Loss of function of IL-12 and IL-23 receptor, diminished IFN- γ and IL-17	[16, 17]
IL-12p40	AR	Increased risk for CMC and mycobacterial and *Salmonella* infections	Impaired IL-17 immunity	2013 medicine

(continued)

Table 3.1 (continued)

Gene	Mode of inheritance	Disease	Immunological phenotype	Refs.
RORC	AR	Increased risk for candidiasis and mycobacteriosis	Absence of IL-17A/F--producing T cells	[18]
MALT1, BCL10, CARD11	AR	Combined immunodeficiencies	Defects of the 3 components of the CBM complex	[19]
IL2RA	AR	Candida esophagitis	Reduced number of CD4+ cells	[20]
NEMO, IKBA, MST1/STK4, CRACM1, etc.	AT/AD/X--linked	Combined immunodeficiencies	T-cell deficiency	[21–27]
JAK3, RAG1, RAG2, ARTEMIS, etc.	AR/XR	Severe combined immunodeficiencies	T-cell deficiency, lymphopenia	[28]
UNC119, MAGT1, RAG1	AT/AD/X--linked	Idiopathic CD4 lymphopenia	Lymphopenia	[29–31]
GJB2	AD	KID syndrome	Unknown	2013JAAD
CMC susceptibility				
Dectin-1	AR	Candida colonization, RVVC, onychomycosis	Cytokine responses deficiency of β-glucan recognition	[32, 33]
TLR3	AR	CMC and Bacterial and CMV infections	Decreased IFN-γ levels	[34, 35]
PTPN22	AD	CMC and microbial infections	Unknown	[36]

PID primary immunodeficiency, *CMC* chronic mucocutaneous candidiasis, *HIES* Hyper-IgE syndrome, *APECED* autoimmune polyendocrinopathy-candidiasis-ectodermal dystrophy, *CGD* Chronic granulomatous disease, *STAT* signal transducer and activator of transcription, *CARD* caspase recruitment domain-containing protein, *IL* interleukin, *DOCK8* dedicator of cytokinesis 8, *AIRE* autoimmune regulator, *TYK2* tyrosine kinase 2, *MALT* mucosa-associated lymphoid tissue, *BCL10* B-cell lymphoma10, *CBM* CARD-BCL10-MALT1 complex, *JAK* Janus kinase, *CD* cluster of differentiation, *IFN* interferon, *NADPH* nicotinamide adenine dinucleotide phosphate, *TNF* tumor necrosis factor, *AD* autosomal dominant, *AR* autosomal recessive, *Th* T helper

Table 3.2 Summary of STAT1 GOF mutation reports

	Mutation	Domain	Patient number	Autoimmune disease	Other infection	Death	References
1	R274W	CC	28	Hypothyroidism/AI hepatitis/ irritable bowel syndrome/none/ inflammatory aortic aneurysms	Dermatophytosis /chest infections/herpetic whitlow/ orf	Squamous cell carcinoma	2011 NEJM, 2011 JEM, 2011 plos one, 2013JMG, 2015JACI, 2015IJC, 2016JCI, 2015CEI
2	A267V	CC	20	Hypothyroidism/none		Squamous cell carcinoma	2011 NEJM, 2011 JEM, 2013JMG, 2016JCI, 2015CI
3	M202V	CC	4	Hypothyroidism/none		Squamous cell carcinoma	2011 JEM, 2016JCI
4	R274Q	CC	14	Hypothyroidism/AI hepatitis/none	Pneumonia/aphthous stomatitis/furunculosis	Cerebral aneurysm	2011 JEM, 2012JCI, 2013JMG, 2016JCI
5	K286I	CC	2			Cerebral aneurysm	2011 JEM
6	C174R	CC	6	Hypothyroidism /none		Squamous cell carcinoma	2011 JEM
7	D165G	CC	2		Pneumonia/aphthous stomatitis/HSV infection		2011 JEM
8	T288A	CC	3				2011 JEM
9	Y170N	CC	1	Hypothyroidism			2011 JEM
10	D165H	CC	1	Hypothyroidism			2011 JEM
11	M202I	CC	3	SLE			2011 JEM
12	Q271P	CC	1			Squamous cell carcinoma	2011 JEM
13	T385M	DBD	10	Hypothyroidism/hemophagocytic lymphohistiocytosis/dental anomalies, diaphragmatic hernia, and esophageal dysmotility	Recurrent pneumonia, bronchitis, and otitis media	DIC/pulmonary insufficiency	2012JI, 2013JMG, 2014JACI, 2016JCI, 2015CI

(continued)

Table 3.2 (continued)

	Mutation	Domain	Patient number	Autoimmune disease	Other infection	Death	References
14	K388E	DBD	2	Dental anomalies, diaphragmatic hernia, and esophageal dysmotility			2014JACI, 2016JCI
15	N179K	CC	1		Pneumonia/renal abscess/ blepharitis		2013JMG
16	Q285R	CC	1		Pneumonia/aphthous stomatitis		2013JMG
17	N397D	DBD	2		Pneumonia/diarrhea		2013JIC, 2016JCI
18	K278E	CC	1		Recurrent herpes zoster		2014JI
19	G384D	DBD	2	Iron deficiency anemia/esophageal stenosis	Herpes zoster / bronchiectasis		2014JI
20	L163R	CC	1				2014JID
21	Y289C	CC	1		*Pneumocystis jiroveci* pneumonia		2014JACI
22	T387A	DBD	3	AA	Suppurative infections		2015JACI, 2015PAI, 2015CI
23	K298 N	CC	3				2015 Molecular Immunology
24	P293S	CC	1				2016JCI
25	F404Y	DBD	1				2016JCI
26	Y287D	CC	1				2016JCI
27	T385K	DBD	1				2016JCI
28	S466R	DBD	1				2016JCI
29	L283M	CCD	2				2015CI
30	L351F	DBD	2				2015CI
31	L400V	DBD	1				2015CI
32	R210K	CC	1				2015CEI
			123	10DBD-25patients			

	Mutation	Domain	Patient number	Autoimmune disease	Other infection	Death	References
1	M202 V	CC	1		Fusariosis		2013JACI
2	E353K	DBD	1		Disseminated coccidioidomycosis and histoplasmosis		2013JACI
3	A267V	CC	1				
4	T385 M	DBD	1				
5	R274G	CC	1				
6	F172L	CC	2				2016JCI
7	R210I	CC	1		Immune dysregulation-polyendocrinopathy-enteropathy-X-linked-like syndrome		2013JACI
8	L358W	DBD	1				
9	V266I	CC	1				
10	T385M	DBD	1				
11	E235A	CC	4		PD-L1 overexpression and a defect in B-cell survival		2013JACI
12	A267V	CC	1		Penicillium marneffei		2013JACI
13	L358F	DBD	1				
14	T288I	CC	1				
15	E370D	DBD	1		Disseminated mucormycosis		2014JACI
16	T385A	DBD	3		Fatal combined immunodeficiency		2014JACI
17	I294T	CC	1				
18	C284R	CC	1				
19	L400Q	DBD	3		Progressive multifocal leukencephalopathy		2016CID

a tendency to become chronic if untreated [5]. Antifungal treatment with azoles led to a partial remission in 62% of patients, with complete response in 38% of patients [5]. Autoimmune conditions, such as hypothyroidism, were also common, with 44% of patients affected [5]. One important issue that is still not clear is whether there is a genotype-phenotype association. Until now the patient cohorts have been too small to answer this question. GOF mutation of *STAT1* is also associated with a spectrum of other fungal infections such as cutaneous fusariosis, disseminated coccidioidomycosis and histoplasmosis, *Penicillium marneffei* infections, and disseminated mucormycosis [7, 52–54], highlighting the important role of STAT1 in fungal infections.

All these genetic and functional studies have important clinical implications, which contribute to the development of new approaches to treat CMC. Hematopoietic stem cell transplantation (HSCT) has been tried in patients with CMC with non-successful outcome [8]. Pilot studies of continuous G-CSF therapy [9] and oral Janus kinase [55] family protein tyrosine kinase inhibitor ruxolitinib [10, 11] have been described to successively treat CMC patients harboring *STAT1* mutations, which are considered as promising immunotherapies in the future, although treatment with G-CSF has also been reported to fail in two patients with *STAT1* GOF mutation [56].

3.2.2 CARD9 Mutation

In 2009, autosomal recessive (AR) caspase recruitment domain-containing protein 9 (*CARD9*) deficiencies were discovered to cause isolated CMC, which for the first time reported isolated CMC as a monogenic disease [57]. CARD9 is a key adaptor molecule expressed in myeloid cells downstream of the pattern recognition receptors (PRRs) that recognize fungal cell wall components and subsequently activate spleen tyrosine kinase (SYK) [58]. After phosphorylation, CARD9 binds B-cell lymphoma 10 (BCL10) and mucosa-associated lymphoid tissue lymphoma-translocation gene 1 (MALT1) to form CBM complex, resulting in nuclear factor κB (NF-κB) activation and innate antifungal immunity, thereby triggering the differentiation of naïve T cells into T helper (Th) 17 cells [12]. *CARD9*-deficient patients show reduced TNF-α production and circulating interleukin (IL)-17-producing T cells [57], underscoring the importance of CARD9-dependent pattern recognition signaling in mucocutaneous antifungal host defense.

Besides, *CARD9* deficiencies also predispose to invasive fungal infections, such as *Candida dubliniensis* meningoencephalitis [59] and relapsing *C. albicans* meningoencephalitis [60, 61]. Patients showed normal IL-17 but reduced GM-CSF production, which had a complete clinical remission with GM-CSF therapy [60]. Moreover, idiopathic deep dermatophytosis, subcutaneous pheohyphomycosis, and invasive *Exophiala* infections have also been reported in AR *CARD9* deficient patients [62–65], underscoring the importance of CARD9-dependent pattern recognition signaling in both mucocutaneous and invasive antifungal host defense.

3.2.3 IL-17 and IL-17R Mutations

Th17 cells are characterized by their production of IL-17A and IL-17F that signal through the IL-17RA/RC heterodimer complex, triggering downstream formation of the IL-17R-Act1-TRAF6 complex leading to NF-κB activation [66]. IL-17A and IL-17F, together with IL-22, promote mucocutaneous antifungal immunity through activating epithelial cells, increasing neutrophil recruitment, and inducing the production of chemokines and antimicrobial peptides [3]. The crucial role of the IL-17 cytokines and IL-17R signaling in antifungal defense is further underscored by the discovery of mutations in these cytokines and its signaling pathway. Partial AD IL-17F deficiency was reported to be the cause of CMC in one family, with mutant IL-17F displaying impaired activity [67].

Moreover, complete AR deficiency in IL-17RA and recently AR deficiency in IL-17RC were reported in several kindreds of isolated CMC from two studies [67, 68]. A recent study reported a family of two siblings with recurrent CMC, *Staphylococcus aureus* infections, chronic inflammatory disease, and vasculitis since early childhood. They both harbored homozygous deletion of IL-17RA and CECR1 (ADA2) mutations, showing a severe malfunction in the IL-17 signaling pathway and in vitro and in vivo upregulation of proinflammatory cytokines [13]. All these patients are homozygous for different alleles that abolish the expression of IL-17RA or IL-17RC that prevents cellular responses of IL-17A and IL-17F signaling [67, 68].

3.2.4 ACT1 Mutation

In addition to IL-17 and its receptors, a deficiency in *ACT1*, a key adaptor molecule downstream of IL-17R signaling, has also been reported, and the clinical phenotype was characterized by CMC. This missense mutation, located in the SEFIR domain, impaired the interaction of ACT1 with the IL-17 receptor units, subsequently leading to deficient IL-17 signaling [69], which demonstrates once more the importance of IL-17 signaling in CMC.

3.3 Inheritance of Syndromic CMC

3.3.1 AD-HIES

Hyper-IgE syndrome (HIES) is characterized by CMC, elevated serum IgE, eosinophilia, eczema, skeletal abnormalities, and recurrent staphylococcal infections, first described as Job's syndrome in 1966 [70]. In 2007, loss-of-function mutation in *STAT3* was first discovered to cause AD-HIES [16, 71]. Since then *STAT3* mutations have been identified in more AD-HIES patients, and these mutations now account for the cause of disease in 60–70% of patients with HIES [17]. STAT3, another STAT family member, regulates multiple cytokine signaling pathways, including IL-6,

IL-21, and IL-23, which are all involved in the development of Th17 cell cells [16]. In AD-HIES patients with dominant-negative *STAT3* mutations, peripheral blood cells showed defective IL-6, IL-10, and IL-21 signaling, with impaired induction of RORγt mRNA, which resulted in greatly diminished Th17 cells differentiation [14, 16, 71, 72]. Impaired Th17 responses are associated with impaired neutrophil chemoattractive factors and epithelial antimicrobial peptides, which in this way increases the susceptibility to *Candida* and staphylococcal infections [16, 71].

3.3.2 AR-HIES

Besides AD trait, HIES was also reported to be AR, with homozygous or compound heterozygous mutations in *Dedicator of cytokinesis 8 (DOCK8)* as the most common cause [15]. AR-HIES is a severe entity with a mortality of 48%, characterized by elevated serum IgE, eosinophilia, eczema, recurrent bacterial infections, and CMC, as classic AD-HIES, but lack connective tissue and skeletal affection, while in addition these patients have a clear increased susceptibility to recurrent viral infections (herpes simplex, varicella zoster, human papilloma, and molluscum contagiosum viruses), asthma, severe allergies, and malignancies at young age [18–20]. DOCK8 is a member of the DOCK180-related family of atypical guanine nucleotide exchange factors, which interacts with Rho GTPases. It has regulatory functions in cell migration, morphology, adhesion, and growth [73]. It is expressed by monocytes, B lymphocytes, and T lymphocytes and is associated with the cytoskeleton formation [21]. DOCK8-deficient patients usually have CD4 and CD8 T-cell lymphopenias and to a lesser extent decreased NK cells and B cells. These patients have mildly to moderately decreased percentages of IL-17-producing cells after activation with anti-CD3 and anti-CD28, although the induction of RORγt expression in naive T cells was intact, suggesting a defect in late differentiation or long-term survival of Th17 cells. These findings could, to some extent, explain an increased susceptibility to CMC [21]. In patients with DOCK8-deficient AR-HIES, several studies suggest HSCT as a curative option that decreases the high mortality associated with this severe immunodeficiency [22–26].

Besides DOCK8 accounting for 80% of affected AR-HIES patients, phosphoglucomutase 3 (PGM3) mutations were also reported to cause AR-HIES in a recent study [55]. PGM3 is a key enzyme in the glycosylation pathway, which catalyzes a crucial step in the synthesis of uridine diphosphate N-acetylglucosamine, which is required for the biosynthesis of N-glycans. Patients were demonstrated to have an abnormal Th1/Th2 differentiation and decreased B-cell numbers, but the exact mechanism remains elusive [55].

3.3.3 APECED

The syndrome of autoimmune polyendocrinopathy-candidiasis-ectodermal dystrophy (APECED), or autoimmune polyendocrine syndrome 1 (APS-1), is a rare AR syndrome characterized by CMC (which is often the earliest manifestation of the syndrome), multiple autoimmune endocrinopathies, hypoparathyroidism, and adrenal insufficiency. The identification of the genetic cause of APECED was found to be due to mutations in the *autoimmune regulator (AIRE)* gene discovered in 1997 [27]. AIRE is a transcription factor expressed by medullary thymic epithelial cells and is responsible for the expression of a wide variety of tissue-specific antigens in the thymus. Nonfunctional AIRE in patients leads to impaired central T-cell tolerance, with the generation of autoantibodies. High levels of neutralizing autoantibodies against IL-17A, IL-17F, and/or IL-22 have been detected in APECED patients, which might account for CMC observed in these patients [28, 29].

3.4 Inheritance of CMC Associated with PIDs

3.4.1 MSMD and CMC

Mendelian susceptibility to mycobacterial disease (MSMD) is associated with monogenic inheritance, which is characterized by selective susceptibility to atypical mycobacteria. Several genetic etiologies of MSMD have been reported so far, mainly with inborn errors of IFNγ immunity. Interestingly, a subset of patients with MSMD displays susceptibility to both candidiasis and mycobacteria.

Tyrosine kinase 2 (Tyk2) is a member of the Janus kinase [55] family that signals downstream of IL-12 and IL-23 and hence might link to reduced Th1 and type I IFN responses [30]. One case of AR-HIES has been reported to carry a homozygous nonsense mutation in *Tyk2* with mild CMC [30]. However, eight case of Tyk2 deficiencies without HIES but with mycobacterial and viral infections have been reported recently [31, 74]. It is suggested that the core clinical phenotype of Tyk2 deficiency is increased susceptibility to mycobacterial and/or viral infections, caused by impaired responses to IL-12 and IFN-α/β [74].

IL-12Rβ1 deficiency is the most common genetic cause underlying MSMD [75]. *IL-12RB1* gene encodes the first chain of the IL-12 and IL-23 receptors. IL-12 is important for the development of IFNγ-producing T cells and IFNγ production, whereas IL-23 is important for the development and maintenance of the Th17 cell population [76]. Therefore, IL-12Rβ1 deficiencies predispose not only to mycobacteria and *Salmonella* infections but also mild forms of CMC, which indeed have been reported with a frequency of 25% in patients with IL-12Rβ1 deficiency [77].

Autosomal recessive IL-12p40 deficiencies were also demonstrated as the genetic etiology of MSMD, although the incidence of *Candida* infections (6.7%) was significantly lower than IL-12Rβ1-deficient patients. Patients with IL-12p40 deficiency suffer from CMC because of impaired IL-23-dependent IL-17 immunity, in a similar way of IL-12Rβ1 deficiency [55].

RAR-related orphan receptor C (RORC), which encodes RORγ, is the master gene controlling Th17 cells differentiation. Homozygous loss-of-function mutations in *RORC* have been described to cause a PID that is predominantly characterized by an increased susceptibility to mycobacterial infection, and *Candida* infections in some cases [78].

3.4.2 CID and CMC

Patients with combined immunodeficiencies (CID), severe combined immunodeficiencies (SCID), and idiopathic CD4 lymphopenia may also develop CMC in infancy due to T-cell deficiency, in addition to multiple other infectious and autoimmune diseases. Biallelic loss-of-function mutations in three components of the CBM complex, including CARD9, CARD11, BCL10, and MALT1, have recently been linked to CID in seven patients [79]. A broad range of clinical manifestations of T- and B-lymphocyte defects including mucosal candidiasis are described in these patients [79].

CD25, encoded by the *IL2RA* gene, is the α-subunit of the IL-2 receptor, which is constitutively expressed on T regulatory cells and involved in the differentiation of effector T cells [80]. In 1995, a patient with a deletion in the *IL2RA* gene was reported to suffer from esophageal candidiasis [80]. Recent studies also found heterozygous mutations of *STAT1* to be associated with progressive CID [81]. Patients display progressive loss of T- and B-lymphocytes number and functions, accompanied by increasing autoimmune features and fatal infections, including mucocutaneous candidiasis [81].

Furthermore, other mutations causing CID (*NEMO, IKBA, MST1/STK4, CRACM1*) [32–34, 82–85], SCID (*JAK3, RAG1, RAG2, ARTEMIS,* and more than 30 genes) [35], and idiopathic CD4 lymphopenia (*UNC119, MAGT1, RAG1*) [86–88] were also reported to precipitate CMC and invasive candidiasis as part of the clinical spectrum, demonstrating the crucial role of CD4 T cells in host defense.

3.4.3 KID and CMC

Keratitis, ichthyosis, and deafness (KID) syndrome is a rare disorder named for the clinical triad of characteristics. It is associated with genetic mutations in the GJB2 gene, which encodes connexin 26, a gap junction protein involved in the formation of intercellular channels with a putative role in epithelial differentiation. CMC and bacterial superinfection are common infectious complications of this disease; however, the exact mechanism remains to be determined [89].

3.5 Polygenic Inheritance of CMC

Besides the monogenic disorders of CMC described above, several studies have suggested a role for polymorphisms in certain PRRs and cytokines causing susceptibility to CMC. A homozygous *Dectin-1* Y238X polymorphism was first described in a family to cause RVVC and onychomycosis, with diminished capacity of β-glucan recognition and Th17 responses [90]. This early stop codon SNP has further been shown to be associated with increased *Candida* colonization in a cohort of hematopoietic stem cell transplant (HSCT) patients [91], but not with systemic candidiasis in a case-control study of candidemia patients [92]. *TLR3* polymorphisms have also been shown to influence susceptibility to CMC due to decreased IFNγ production [36, 93]. Moreover, polymorphisms in the gene encoding the protein PTPN22, which is involved in T-cell and B-cell receptor signaling, was associated with an increased risk of CMC in one study [94].

3.6 Conclusions

In recent years the genetic of CMC has been extensively explored, which has led to novel insights in the pathogenesis of candidiasis. Especially, next-generation sequencing has contributed to the identification of monogenetic disorders with CMC. This approach has identified key pathways in the host defense against *Candida* infections, such as the importance of an optimal IL-17 signaling pathway in preventing mucocutaneous candidiasis. These studies do not only contribute to new insights but will prove to be an essential element to guide the development of future immunotherapeutic strategies.

References

1. Lilic D. New perspectives on the immunology of chronic mucocutaneous candidiasis. Curr Opin Infect Dis. 2002;15(2):143–7.
2. Thorpe ES, Handley H. Chronic tetany and chronic mycelia stomatitis in a child aged four and one half years. Am J Dis Child. 1929;38:228.
3. Puel A, Cypowyj S, Marodi L, Abel L, Picard C, Casanova JL. Inborn errors of human IL-17 immunity underlie chronic mucocutaneous candidiasis. Curr Opin Allergy Clin Immunol. 2012;12(6):616–22. doi:10.1097/ACI.0b013e328358cc0b.
4. Canales L, Middlemas 3rd RO, Louro JM, South MA. Immunological observations in chronic mucocutaneous candidiasis. Lancet. 1969;2(7620):567–71.
5. Depner M, Fuchs S, Raabe J, Frede N, Glocker C, Doffinger R, et al. The extended clinical phenotype of 26 patients with chronic mucocutaneous candidiasis due to gain-of-function mutations in STAT1. J Clin Immunol. 2016;36(1):73–84. doi:10.1007/s10875-015-0214-9.
6. Smeekens SP, Plantinga TS, van de Veerdonk FL, Heinhuis B, Hoischen A, Joosten LA, et al. STAT1 hyperphosphorylation and defective IL12R/IL23R signaling underlie defective immunity in autosomal dominant chronic mucocutaneous candidiasis. PLoS One. 2011;6(12):e29248. doi:10.1371/journal.pone.0029248.
7. Lee PP, Mao H, Yang W, Chan KW, Ho MH, Lee TL, et al. Penicillium marneffei infection and impaired IFN-gamma immunity in humans with autosomal-dominant gain-of-phosphorylation STAT1 mutations. J Allergy Clin Immunol. 2014;133(3):894–6. e5 doi:10.1016/j.jaci.2013.08.051.
8. Aldave JC, Cachay E, Nunez L, Chunga A, Murillo S, Cypowyj S, et al. A 1-year-old girl with a gain-of-function STAT1 mutation treated with hematopoietic stem cell transplantation. J Clin Immunol. 2013;33(8):1273–5. doi:10.1007/s10875-013-9947-5.
9. Wildbaum G, Shahar E, Katz R, Karin N, Etzioni A, Pollack S. Continuous G-CSF therapy for isolated chronic mucocutaneous candidiasis: complete clinical remission with restoration of IL-17 secretion. J Allergy Clin Immunol. 2013;132(3):761–4. doi:10.1016/j.jaci.2013.04.018.
10. Higgins E, Al Shehri T, McAleer MA, Conlon N, Feighery C, Lilic D, et al. Use of ruxolitinib to successfully treat chronic mucocutaneous candidiasis caused by gain-of-function signal transducer and activator of transcription 1 (STAT1) mutation. J Allergy Clin Immunol. 2015;135(2):551–3. doi:10.1016/j.jaci.2014.12.1867.

11. Mossner R, Diering N, Bader O, Forkel S, Overbeck T, Gross U, et al. Ruxolitinib induces interleukin-17 and ameliorates chronic mucocutaneous candidiasis caused by STAT1 gain-of-function mutation. Clinical Infect Dis: Off Publ Infect Dis Soc Am. 2016; doi:10.1093/cid/ciw020.
12. Drummond RA, Saijo S, Iwakura Y, Brown GD. The role of Syk/CARD9 coupled C-type lectins in antifungal immunity. Eur J Immunol. 2011;41(2):276–81. doi:10.1002/eji.201041252.
13. Fellmann F, Angelini F, Wassenberg J, Perreau M, Arenas Ramirez N, Simon G, et al. IL-17 receptor A and adenosine deaminase 2 deficiency in siblings with recurrent infections and chronic inflammation. J Allergy Clin Immunol. 2015; doi:10.1016/j.jaci.2015.07.053.
14. Saito M, Nagasawa M, Takada H, Hara T, Tsuchiya S, Agematsu K, et al. Defective IL-10 signaling in hyper-IgE syndrome results in impaired generation of tolerogenic dendritic cells and induced regulatory T cells. J Exp Med. 2011;208(2):235–49. doi:10.1084/jem.20100799.
15. Engelhardt KR, McGhee S, Winkler S, Sassi A, Woellner C, Lopez-Herrera G, et al. Large deletions and point mutations involving the dedicator of cytokinesis 8 (DOCK8) in the autosomal-recessive form of hyper-IgE syndrome. J Allergy Clin Immunol. 2009;124(6):1289–302. e4 doi:10.1016/j.jaci.2009.10.038.
16. Minegishi Y, Saito M, Tsuchiya S, Tsuge I, Takada H, Hara T, et al. Dominant-negative mutations in the DNA-binding domain of STAT3 cause hyper-IgE syndrome. Nature. 2007;448(7157):1058–62. doi:10.1038/nature06096.
17. Farmand S, Sundin M. Hyper-IgE syndromes: recent advances in pathogenesis, diagnostics and clinical care. Curr Opin Hematol. 2015;22(1):12–22. doi:10.1097/MOH.0000000000000104.
18. Sabry A, Hauk PJ, Jing H, Su HC, Stence NV, Mirsky DM, et al. Vaccine strain varicella-zoster virus-induced central nervous system vasculopathy as the presenting feature of DOCK8 deficiency. J Allergy Clin Immunol. 2014;133(4):1225–7. doi:10.1016/j.jaci.2013.11.031.
19. Aydin SE, Kilic SS, Aytekin C, Kumar A, Porras O, Kainulainen L, et al. DOCK8 deficiency: clinical and immunological phenotype and treatment options – a review of 136 patients. J Clin Immunol. 2015;35(2):189–98. doi:10.1007/s10875-014-0126-0.
20. Engelhardt KR, Gertz ME, Keles S, Schaffer AA, Sigmund EC, Glocker C, et al. The extended clinical phenotype of 64 patients with dedicator of cytokinesis 8 deficiency. J Allergy Clin Immunol. 2015;136(2):402–12. doi:10.1016/j.jaci.2014.12.1945.
21. Su HC. Dedicator of cytokinesis 8 (DOCK8) deficiency. Curr Opin Allergy Clin Immunol. 2010;10(6):515–20. doi:10.1097/ACI.0b013e32833fd718.
22. Bittner TC, Pannicke U, Renner ED, Notheis G, Hoffmann F, Belohradsky BH, et al. Successful long-term correction of autosomal recessive hyper-IgE syndrome due to DOCK8 deficiency by hematopoietic stem cell transplantation. Klin Padiatr. 2010;222(6):351–5. doi:10.1055/s-0030-1265135.
23. McDonald DR, Massaad MJ, Johnston A, Keles S, Chatila T, Geha RS, et al. Successful engraftment of donor marrow after allogeneic hematopoietic cell transplantation in autosomal-recessive hyper-IgE syndrome caused by dedicator of cytokinesis 8 deficiency. J Allergy Clin Immunol. 2010;126(6):1304–5. e3 doi:10.1016/j.jaci.2010.07.034.
24. Gatz SA, Benninghoff U, Schutz C, Schulz A, Honig M, Pannicke U, et al. Curative treatment of autosomal-recessive hyper-IgE syndrome by hematopoietic cell transplantation. Bone Marrow Transplant. 2011;46(4):552–6. doi:10.1038/bmt.2010.169.
25. Metin A, Tavil B, Azik F, Azkur D, Ok-Bozkaya I, Kocabas C, et al. Successful bone marrow transplantation for DOCK8 deficient hyper IgE syndrome. Pediatr Transplant. 2012;16(4):398–9. doi:10.1111/j.1399-3046.2011.01641.x.
26. Kawaguch K, Matsubara K, Uchida Y, Saito A, Miyata K, Hasegawa D, et al. Successful treatment with allogenic hematopoietic stem cell transplantation of a severe congenital neutropenia patient harboring a novel ELANE mutation. [Rinsho Ketsueki] Jpn J Clin Hematol. 2014;55(11):2294–9.

27. Finnish-German AC. An autoimmune disease, APECED, caused by mutations in a novel gene featuring two PHD-type zinc-finger domains. Nat Genet. 1997;17(4):399–403. doi:10.1038/ng1297-399.
28. Puel A, Doffinger R, Natividad A, Chrabieh M, Barcenas-Morales G, Picard C, et al. Autoantibodies against IL-17A, IL-17F, and IL-22 in patients with chronic mucocutaneous candidiasis and autoimmune polyendocrine syndrome type I. J Exp Med. 2010;207(2):291–7. doi:10.1084/jem.20091983.
29. Kisand K, Boe Wolff AS, Podkrajsek KT, Tserel L, Link M, Kisand KV, et al. Chronic mucocutaneous candidiasis in APECED or thymoma patients correlates with autoimmunity to Th17-associated cytokines. J Exp Med. 2010;207(2):299–308. doi:10.1084/jem.20091669.
30. Minegishi Y, Saito M, Morio T, Watanabe K, Agematsu K, Tsuchiya S, et al. Human tyrosine kinase 2 deficiency reveals its requisite roles in multiple cytokine signals involved in innate and acquired immunity. Immunity. 2006;25(5):745–55. doi:10.1016/j.immuni.2006.09.009.
31. Kilic SS, Hacimustafaoglu M, Boisson-Dupuis S, Kreins AY, Grant AV, Abel L, et al. A patient with tyrosine kinase 2 deficiency without hyper-IgE syndrome. J Pediatr. 2012;160(6):1055–7. doi:10.1016/j.jpeds.2012.01.056.
32. Picard C, Casanova JL, Puel A. Infectious diseases in patients with IRAK-4, MyD88, NEMO, or IkappaBalpha deficiency. Clin Microbiol Rev. 2011;24(3):490–7. doi:10.1128/CMR.00001-11.
33. Abdollahpour H, Appaswamy G, Kotlarz D, Diestelhorst J, Beier R, Schaffer AA, et al. The phenotype of human STK4 deficiency. Blood. 2012;119(15):3450–7. doi:10.1182/blood-2011-09-378158.
34. Schimke LF, Rieber N, Rylaarsdam S, Cabral-Marques O, Hubbard N, Puel A, et al. A novel gain-of-function IKBA mutation underlies ectodermal dysplasia with immunodeficiency and polyendocrinopathy. J Clin Immunol. 2013;33(6):1088–99. doi:10.1007/s10875-013-9906-1.
35. Puck JM. Neonatal screening for severe combined immunodeficiency. Curr Opin Pediatr. 2011;23(6):667–73. doi:10.1097/MOP.0b013e32834cb9b0.
36. Nahum A, Dadi H, Bates A, Roifman CM. The L412F variant of Toll-like receptor 3 (TLR3) is associated with cutaneous candidiasis, increased susceptibility to cytomegalovirus, and autoimmunity. J Allergy Clin Immunol. 2011;127(2):528–31. doi:10.1016/j.jaci.2010.09.031.
37. Liu L, Okada S, Kong XF, Kreins AY, Cypowyj S, Abhyankar A, et al. Gain-of-function human STAT1 mutations impair IL-17 immunity and underlie chronic mucocutaneous candidiasis. J Exp Med. 2011;208(8):1635–48. doi:10.1084/jem.20110958.
38. van de Veerdonk FL, Plantinga TS, Hoischen A, Smeekens SP, Joosten LA, Gilissen C, et al. STAT1 mutations in autosomal dominant chronic mucocutaneous candidiasis. N Engl J Med. 2011;365(1):54–61. doi:10.1056/NEJMoa1100102.
39. Hori T, Ohnishi H, Teramoto T, Tsubouchi K, Naiki T, Hirose Y, et al. Autosomal-dominant chronic mucocutaneous candidiasis with STAT1-mutation can be complicated with chronic active hepatitis and hypothyroidism. J Clin Immunol. 2012;32(6):1213–20. doi:10.1007/s10875-012-9744-6.
40. Takezaki S, Yamada M, Kato M, Park MJ, Maruyama K, Yamazaki Y, et al. Chronic mucocutaneous candidiasis caused by a gain-of-function mutation in the STAT1 DNA-binding domain. J Immunol. 2012;189(3):1521–6. doi:10.4049/jimmunol.1200926.
41. Soltesz B, Toth B, Shabashova N, Bondarenko A, Okada S, Cypowyj S, et al. New and recurrent gain-of-function STAT1 mutations in patients with chronic mucocutaneous candidiasis from Eastern and Central Europe. J Med Genet. 2013;50(9):567–78. doi:10.1136/jmedgenet-2013-101570.
42. Mizoguchi Y, Tsumura M, Okada S, Hirata O, Minegishi S, Imai K, et al. Simple diagnosis of STAT1 gain-of-function alleles in patients with chronic mucocutaneous candidiasis. J Leukoc Biol. 2014;95(4):667–76. doi:10.1189/jlb.0513250.
43. Yamazaki Y, Yamada M, Kawai T, Morio T, Onodera M, Ueki M, et al. Two novel gain-of-function mutations of STAT1 responsible for chronic mucocutaneous candidiasis disease:

impaired production of IL-17A and IL-22, and the presence of anti-IL-17F autoantibody. J Immunol. 2014;193(10):4880–7. doi:10.4049/jimmunol.1401467.
44. Dhalla F, Fox H, Davenport EE, Sadler R, Anzilotti C, van Schouwenburg PA, et al. Chronic mucocutaneous candidiasis: characterisation of a family with STAT1 gain-of-function and development of an ex vivo assay for Th17 deficiency of diagnostic utility. Clin Exp Immunol. 2015; doi:10.1111/cei.12746.
45. Dotta L, Scomodon O, Padoan R, Timpano S, Plebani A, Soresina A, et al. Clinical heterogeneity of dominant chronic mucocutaneous candidiasis disease: presenting as treatment-resistant candidiasis and chronic lung disease. Clin Immunol. 2015;164:1–9. doi:10.1016/j.clim.2015.12.010.
46. Giardino G, Somma D, Cirillo E, Ruggiero G, Terrazzano G, Rubino V, et al. Novel STAT1 gain of function mutation and suppurative infections. Pediatr Allergy Immunol: Off Publ Eur Soc Pediatr Allergy Immunol. 2015; doi:10.1111/pai.12496.
47. Martinez-Martinez L, Martinez-Saavedra MT, Fuentes-Prior P, Barnadas M, Rubiales MV, Noda J, et al. A novel gain-of-function STAT1 mutation resulting in basal phosphorylation of STAT1 and increased distal IFN-gamma-mediated responses in chronic mucocutaneous candidiasis. Mol Immunol. 2015;68(2 Pt C):597–605. doi:10.1016/j.molimm.2015.09.014.
48. Nielsen J, Kofod-Olsen E, Spaun E, Larsen CS, Christiansen M, Mogensen TH. A STAT1-gain-of-function mutation causing Th17 deficiency with chronic mucocutaneous candidiasis, psoriasiform hyperkeratosis and dermatophytosis. BMJ Case Rep. 2015;2015 doi:10.1136/bcr-2015-211372.
49. Tanimura M, Dohi K, Hirayama M, Sato Y, Sugiura E, Nakajima H, et al. Recurrent inflammatory aortic aneurysms in chronic mucocutaneous candidiasis with a gain-of-function STAT1 mutation. Int J Cardiol. 2015;196:88–90. doi:10.1016/j.ijcard.2015.05.183.
50. Najjar I, Fagard R. STAT1 and pathogens, not a friendly relationship. Biochimie. 2010;92(5):425–44. doi:10.1016/j.biochi.2010.02.009.
51. Zheng J, van de Veerdonk FL, Crossland KL, Smeekens SP, Chan CM, Al Shehri T, et al. Gain-of-function STAT1 mutations impair STAT3 activity in patients with chronic mucocutaneous candidiasis (CMC). Eur J Immunol. 2015;45(10):2834–46. doi:10.1002/eji.201445344.
52. Sampaio EP, Hsu AP, Pechacek J, Bax HI, Dias DL, Paulson ML, et al. Signal transducer and activator of transcription 1 (STAT1) gain-of-function mutations and disseminated coccidioidomycosis and histoplasmosis. J Allergy Clin Immunol. 2013;131(6):1624–34. doi:10.1016/j.jaci.2013.01.052.
53. Wang X, Lin Z, Gao L, Wang A, Wan Z, Chen W, et al. Exome sequencing reveals a signal transducer and activator of transcription 1 (STAT1) mutation in a child with recalcitrant cutaneous fusariosis. J Allergy Clin Immunol. 2013;131(4):1242–3. doi:10.1016/j.jaci.2012.11.005.
54. Kumar N, Hanks ME, Chandrasekaran P, Davis BC, Hsu AP, Van Wagoner NJ, et al. Gain-of-function signal transducer and activator of transcription 1 (STAT1) mutation-related primary immunodeficiency is associated with disseminated mucormycosis. J Allergy Clin Immunol. 2014;134(1):236–9. doi:10.1016/j.jaci.2014.02.037.
55. Sassi A, Lazaroski S, Wu G, Haslam SM, Fliegauf M, Mellouli F, et al. Hypomorphic homozygous mutations in phosphoglucomutase 3 (PGM3) impair immunity and increase serum IgE levels. J Allergy Clin Immunol. 2014;133(5):1410–9. 9 e1–13 doi:10.1016/j.jaci.2014.02.025.
56. van de Veerdonk FL, Koenen HJ, van der Velden WJ, van der Meer JW, Netea MG. Immunotherapy with G-CSF in patients with chronic mucocutaneous candidiasis. Immunol Lett. 2015;167(1):54–6. doi:10.1016/j.imlet.2015.05.008.
57. Glocker EO, Hennigs A, Nabavi M, Schaffer AA, Woellner C, Salzer U, et al. A homozygous CARD9 mutation in a family with susceptibility to fungal infections. N Engl J Med. 2009;361(18):1727–35. doi:10.1056/NEJMoa0810719.
58. Romani L. Immunity to fungal infections. Nat Rev Immunol. 2011;11(4):275–88. doi:10.1038/nri2939.

59. Drewniak A, Gazendam RP, Tool AT, van Houdt M, Jansen MH, van Hamme JL, et al. Invasive fungal infection and impaired neutrophil killing in human CARD9 deficiency. Blood. 2013;121(13):2385–92. doi:10.1182/blood-2012-08-450551.
60. Gavino C, Cotter A, Lichtenstein D, Lejtenyi D, Fortin C, Legault C, et al. CARD9 deficiency and spontaneous central nervous system candidiasis: complete clinical remission with GM-CSF therapy. Clin Infect Dis: Off Publ Infect Dis Soc Am. 2014;59(1):81–4. doi:10.1093/cid/ciu215.
61. Lanternier F, Mahdaviani SA, Barbati E, Chaussade H, Koumar Y, Levy R, et al. Inherited CARD9 deficiency in otherwise healthy children and adults with Candida species-induced meningoencephalitis, colitis, or both. J Allergy Clin Immunol. 2015;135(6):1558–68. e2 doi:10.1016/j.jaci.2014.12.1930.
62. Lanternier F, Barbati E, Meinzer U, Liu L, Pedergnana V, Migaud M, et al. Inherited CARD9 deficiency in 2 unrelated patients with invasive Exophiala infection. J Infect Dis. 2015;211(8):1241–50. doi:10.1093/infdis/jiu412.
63. Lanternier F, Pathan S, Vincent QB, Liu L, Cypowyj S, Prando C, et al. Deep dermatophytosis and inherited CARD9 deficiency. N Engl J Med. 2013;369(18):1704–14. doi:10.1056/NEJMoa1208487.
64. Wang X, Wang W, Lin Z, Wang X, Li T, Yu J, et al. CARD9 mutations linked to subcutaneous phaeohyphomycosis and TH17 cell deficiencies. J Allergy Clin Immunol. 2014;133(3):905–8. e3 doi:10.1016/j.jaci.2013.09.033.
65. Jachiet M, Lanternier F, Rybojad M, Bagot M, Ibrahim L, Casanova JL, et al. Posaconazole treatment of extensive skin and nail dermatophytosis due to autosomal recessive deficiency of CARD9. JAMA Dermatol. 2015;151(2):192–4. doi:10.1001/jamadermatol.2014.2154.
66. Gu C, Wu L, Li X. IL-17 family: cytokines, receptors and signaling. Cytokine. 2013;64(2):477–85. doi:10.1016/j.cyto.2013.07.022.
67. Puel A, Cypowyj S, Bustamante J, Wright JF, Liu L, Lim HK, et al. Chronic mucocutaneous candidiasis in humans with inborn errors of interleukin-17 immunity. Science. 2011;332(6025):65–8. doi:10.1126/science.1200439.
68. Ling Y, Cypowyj S, Aytekin C, Galicchio M, Camcioglu Y, Nepesov S, et al. Inherited IL-17RC deficiency in patients with chronic mucocutaneous candidiasis. J Exp Med. 2015;212(5):619–31. doi:10.1084/jem.20141065.
69. Boisson B, Wang C, Pedergnana V, Wu L, Cypowyj S, Rybojad M, et al. An ACT1 mutation selectively abolishes interleukin-17 responses in humans with chronic mucocutaneous candidiasis. Immunity. 2013;39(4):676–86. doi:10.1016/j.immuni.2013.09.002.
70. Davis SD, Schaller J, Wedgwood RJ. Job's syndrome. Recurrent, "cold", staphylococcal abscesses. Lancet. 1966;1(7445):1013–5.
71. Holland SM, DeLeo FR, Elloumi HZ, Hsu AP, Uzel G, Brodsky N, et al. STAT3 mutations in the hyper-IgE syndrome. N Engl J Med. 2007;357(16):1608–19. doi:10.1056/NEJMoa073687.
72. Ma CS, Avery DT, Chan A, Batten M, Bustamante J, Boisson-Dupuis S, et al. Functional STAT3 deficiency compromises the generation of human T follicular helper cells. Blood. 2012;119(17):3997–4008. doi:10.1182/blood-2011-11-392985.
73. Zhang Q, Davis JC, Lamborn IT, Freeman AF, Jing H, Favreau AJ, et al. Combined immunodeficiency associated with DOCK8 mutations. N Engl J Med. 2009;361(21):2046–55. doi:10.1056/NEJMoa0905506.
74. Kreins AY, Ciancanelli MJ, Okada S, Kong XF, Ramirez-Alejo N, Kilic SS, et al. Human TYK2 deficiency: mycobacterial and viral infections without hyper-IgE syndrome. J Exp Med. 2015; doi:10.1084/jem.20140280.
75. Fieschi C, Dupuis S, Catherinot E, Feinberg J, Bustamante J, Breiman A, et al. Low penetrance, broad resistance, and favorable outcome of interleukin 12 receptor beta1 deficiency: medical and immunological implications. J Exp Med. 2003;197(4):527–35.
76. Ouederni M, Sanal O, Ikinciogullari A, Tezcan I, Dogu F, Sologuren I, et al. Clinical features of Candidiasis in patients with inherited interleukin 12 receptor beta1 deficiency. Clin Infect Dis:Off Publ Infect Dis Soc Am. 2014;58(2):204–13. doi:10.1093/cid/cit722.

77. de Beaucoudrey L, Samarina A, Bustamante J, Cobat A, Boisson-Dupuis S, Feinberg J, et al. Revisiting human IL-12Rbeta1 deficiency: a survey of 141 patients from 30 countries. Medicine. 2010;89(6):381–402. doi:10.1097/MD.0b013e3181fdd832.
78. Okada S, Markle JG, Deenick EK, Mele F, Averbuch D, Lagos M, et al. IMMUNODEFICIENCIES. Impairment of immunity to Candida and Mycobacterium in humans with bi-allelic RORC mutations. Science. 2015;349(6248):606–13. doi:10.1126/science.aaa4282.
79. Perez de Diego R, Sanchez-Ramon S, Lopez-Collazo E, Martinez-Barricarte R, Cubillos-Zapata C, Ferreira Cerdan A, et al. Genetic errors of the human caspase recruitment domain-B-cell lymphoma 10-mucosa-associated lymphoid tissue lymphoma-translocation gene 1 (CBM) complex: molecular, immunologic, and clinical heterogeneity. J Allergy Clin Immunol. 2015; doi:10.1016/j.jaci.2015.06.031.
80. Sakaguchi S, Sakaguchi N, Asano M, Itoh M, Toda M. Immunologic self-tolerance maintained by activated T cells expressing IL-2 receptor alpha-chains (CD25). Breakdown of a single mechanism of self-tolerance causes various autoimmune diseases. J Immunol. 1995;155(3):1151–64.
81. Sharfe N, Nahum A, Newell A, Dadi H, Ngan B, Pereira SL, et al. Fatal combined immunodeficiency associated with heterozygous mutation in STAT1. J Allergy Clin Immunol. 2014;133(3):807–17. doi:10.1016/j.jaci.2013.09.032.
82. Feske S, Gwack Y, Prakriya M, Srikanth S, Puppel SH, Tanasa B, et al. A mutation in Orai1 causes immune deficiency by abrogating CRAC channel function. Nature. 2006;441(7090):179–85. doi:10.1038/nature04702.
83. Morgan NV, Goddard S, Cardno TS, McDonald D, Rahman F, Barge D, et al. Mutation in the TCRalpha subunit constant gene (TRAC) leads to a human immunodeficiency disorder characterized by a lack of TCRalphabeta+ T cells. J Clin Invest. 2011;121(2):695–702. doi:10.1172/JCI41931.
84. Ouederni M, Vincent QB, Frange P, Touzot F, Scerra S, Bejaoui M, et al. Major histocompatibility complex class II expression deficiency caused by a RFXANK founder mutation: a survey of 35 patients. Blood. 2011;118(19):5108–18. doi:10.1182/blood-2011-05-352716.
85. Nehme NT, Pachlopnik Schmid J, Debeurme F, Andre-Schmutz I, Lim A, Nitschke P, et al. MST1 mutations in autosomal recessive primary immunodeficiency characterized by defective naive T-cell survival. Blood. 2012;119(15):3458–68. doi:10.1182/blood-2011-09-378364.
86. Kuijpers TW, Ijspeert H, van Leeuwen EM, Jansen MH, Hazenberg MD, Weijer KC, et al. Idiopathic CD4+ T lymphopenia without autoimmunity or granulomatous disease in the slipstream of RAG mutations. Blood. 2011;117(22):5892–6. doi:10.1182/blood-2011-01-329052.
87. Li FY, Chaigne-Delalande B, Kanellopoulou C, Davis JC, Matthews HF, Douek DC, et al. Second messenger role for Mg2+ revealed by human T-cell immunodeficiency. Nature. 2011;475(7357):471–6. doi:10.1038/nature10246.
88. Gorska MM, Alam R. A mutation in the human Uncoordinated 119 gene impairs TCR signaling and is associated with CD4 lymphopenia. Blood. 2012;119(6):1399–406. doi:10.1182/blood-2011-04-350686.
89. Coggshall K, Farsani T, Ruben B, McCalmont TH, Berger TG, Fox LP, et al. Keratitis, ichthyosis, and deafness syndrome: a review of infectious and neoplastic complications. J Am Acad Dermatol. 2013;69(1):127–34. doi:10.1016/j.jaad.2012.12.965.
90. Ferwerda B, Ferwerda G, Plantinga TS, Willment JA, van Spriel AB, Venselaar H, et al. Human dectin-1 deficiency and mucocutaneous fungal infections. N Engl J Med. 2009;361(18):1760–7. doi:10.1056/NEJMoa0901053.
91. Plantinga TS, van der Velden WJ, Ferwerda B, van Spriel AB, Adema G, Feuth T, et al. Early stop polymorphism in human DECTIN-1 is associated with increased candida colonization in hematopoietic stem cell transplant recipients. Clin Infect Dis: Off Publ Infect Dis Soc Am. 2009;49(5):724–32. doi:10.1086/604714.

92. Rosentul DC, Plantinga TS, Oosting M, Scott WK, Velez Edwards DR, Smith PB, et al. Genetic variation in the dectin-1/CARD9 recognition pathway and susceptibility to candidemia. J Infect Dis. 2011;204(7):1138–45. doi:10.1093/infdis/jir458.
93. Nahum A, Dadi H, Bates A, Roifman CM. The biological significance of TLR3 variant, L412F, in conferring susceptibility to cutaneous candidiasis, CMV and autoimmunity. Autoimmun Rev. 2012;11(5):341–7. doi:10.1016/j.autrev.2011.10.007.
94. Nahum A, Bates A, Sharfe N, Roifman CM. Association of the lymphoid protein tyrosine phosphatase, R620W variant, with chronic mucocutaneous candidiasis. J Allergy Clin Immunol. 2008;122(6):1220–2. doi:10.1016/j.jaci.2008.10.027.

Chronic Granulomatous Disease and Aspergillosis

4

Melissa J. Grimm and Brahm H. Segal

Abstract

The phagocyte NADPH oxidase is rapidly activated as an emergency response to infection. Activation of the NADPH oxidase requires translocation of cytoplasmic constituents to a membrane-bound flavocytochrome, and results in the conversion of molecular oxygen to superoxide anion and downstream reactive oxidant metabolites. Chronic granulomatous disease (CGD) is an inherited disorder of the NADPH oxidase characterized by recurrent and severe bacterial and fungal infections. Invasive aspergillosis and other filamentous fungi are the major causes of mortality in CGD. CGD is also characterized by inflammatory disorders, including inflammatory bowel disease, obstructive granulomata of the genitourinary tract, and pneumonitis. These findings underscore the dual role of NADPH oxidase as a critical component of host defense and as a modulator of inflammation. Management of CGD patients involves antibacterial and antifungal prophylaxis, recombinant interferon-γ, and early diagnosis and treatment of infections. Hematopoietic stem cell transplantation is a potentially curative treatment for CGD, and is being used with greater frequency. Knowledge gained from CGD patients and engineered mouse models have resulted in important insight regarding host and fungal pathogen interactions that determine control versus progression of infection and pathways that activate and limit inflammatory responses. This knowledge is broadly important to our understanding of innate immunity and for the development of novel immunotherapy approaches.

M.J. Grimm, PhD
Department of Medicine, Roswell Park Cancer Institute, Buffalo, NY, USA

B.H. Segal, MD, FACP, FIDSA (✉)
Departments of Medicine and Immunology, Roswell Park Cancer Institute, and University at Buffalo Jacobs School of Medicine and Biomedical Sciences, Buffalo, NY, USA

Division of Infectious Diseases, Department of Immunology, Roswell Park Cancer Institute, University at Buffalo Jacobs School of Medicine and Biomedical Sciences, Elm & Carlton Streets, Buffalo, NY 14263, USA
e-mail: brahm.segal@roswellpark.org

A. Carvalho (ed.), *Immunogenetics of Fungal Diseases*,
DOI 10.1007/978-3-319-50842-9_4

4.1 Introduction

Chronic granulomatous disease (CGD) is an inherited disorder of NADPH oxidase characterized by life-threatening bacterial and fungal diseases and by abnormally exuberant inflammatory responses (e.g., inflammatory bowel disease, obstructive granulomata of the genitourinary tract) [1]. The phagocyte NADPH oxidase (NOX2) is responsible for the respiratory burst, a rapid consumption of oxygen which generates superoxide anion. NOX2 activation occurs in response to physiologic stimuli such as opsonized particles, integrin-dependent adhesion to the extracellular matrix [2, 3], and ligation of specific pathogen recognition receptors [4, 5, 6]. CGD is both a disease of impaired host defense and dysregulated inflammation. Patients with CGD suffer from recurrent and life-threatening bacterial and fungal infections and from excessive inflammation, including Crohn's-like inflammatory bowel disease, obstructive inflammation of the genitourinary tract, and pneumonitis resembling sarcoidosis [7, 8]. Infections by *Aspergillus* species and other filamentous fungi are the major causes of mortality in CGD. The following chapter will review complications of CGD, including susceptibility to *Aspergillus* species; standard prophylaxis and treatment for CGD, including immunotherapies; and also the role of innate immunity in anti-fungal defense. Allogeneic HSCT is presently the definitive curative treatment for CGD. As a hematopoietic stem cell disorder, gene therapy has been evaluated for decades and remains an active area of research; the major hurdle relates to maintaining a stable long-term population of gene-corrected cells.

4.2 Infectious Complications in CGD

Patients with X-linked CGD typically have a greater risk for infectious complications than autosomal recessive forms of CGD [8]. This increased risk likely reflects complete absence of NOX2 activity with mutations that completely disable gp91*phox* function. Kuhns et al. [12] showed that residual NOX2 activity in neutrophils from CGD patients was associated with less severe illness and a greater likelihood of long-term survival than patients with little or no NOX2 function. This effect on survival was observed in both X-linked and autosomal recessive forms of CGD. These results demonstrate that even low residual levels of NOX2 activity in neutrophils are protective and support the notion that a small proportion of NOX2-competent neutrophils that may be achievable with gene therapy will reduce infection risk in CGD patients.

CGD patients are at high risk for a limited spectrum of pathogens [7, 8], highlighting the fact that pathogens have varying sensitivity to NOX2-dependent host defense. In a US data registry of 368 patients with CGD, pneumonia was the most frequent infection with aspergillosis being the most common pathogen [8]. Other major infections included suppurative adenitis, soft tissue abscesses, and liver abscesses with *Staphylococcus aureus* being the most common cause. *Serratia* infection (commonly manifesting as osteomyelitis), *Burkholderia cepacia* (commonly manifesting as pneumonia and sepsis), *Salmonella* sepsis were also common complications. Nocardiosis typically manifests as pulmonary infection in CGD. In a review of the

NIH experience of 28 episodes of nocardiosis in CGD, 25% had disseminated infection, and one-third had concurrent fungal infections [13]. Analysis of clinical data from 429 European patients with CGD showed that the most frequently cultured pathogens per episode were *Staphylococcus aureus* (30%) and *Aspergillus* spp. (26%); *Aspergillus* species (111 cases) was the most common cause of pneumonia [7]. CGD patients do not appear to be at increased risk for several pathogens that are commonly observed in the general population (e.g., streptococcal infections) or opportunistic pathogens that commonly affect other immunocompromised patients, such as *Pseudomonas aeruginosa* infections in patients with chemotherapy-induced neutropenia, and neutrophil bactericidal studies demonstrate NOX2-independent killing of these pathogens [14, 15]. These results show that NOX2 has a required host defense function to protect against specific pathogens, while NOX2-independent pathways are required to defend against others.

4.3 Clinical Manifestations of Invasive Aspergillosis in CGD

Aspergillosis and other filamentous fungi account for a substantial proportion of infection-related mortality in CGD. In the US data registry, about one-third of the 368 patients had an episode of *Aspergillus* pneumonia [8]. In a French national database, the overall incidence of invasive fungal diseases was 0.040/patient-years, with aspergillosis accounting for 40% [16]. Very rarely, invasive aspergillosis may occur in a female carrier of X-linked CGD in whom the random process of lyonization (X-chromosome inactivation) has led to a skewing of the circulating normal neutrophil population to less than 10% oxidant competent [17].

Aspergillus fumigatus and *Aspergillus nidulans* are the most common *Aspergillus* species in CGD. With the exception of CGD patients, *A. nidulans* is a rare pathogen. We reviewed all cases in which *A. nidulans* was isolated from patients at the National Institutes of Health (Bethesda, MD) between 1976 and 1997 [10]. *A. nidulans* infection occurred in six patients with CGD, but was not a pathogen in any other patient group. *A. fumigatus* was a more common pathogen in CGD (n = 17 cases), but *A. nidulans* was more virulent. *A. nidulans* was significantly more likely to result in death compared with *A. fumigatus* (3 of 6 versus 1 of 17 cases, respectively), to involve adjacent bone, and to cause disseminated disease. Patients with *A. nidulans* received longer courses of amphotericin B therapy than patients with *A. fumigatus* and were treated with surgery more often. In contrast to *A. fumigatus*, *A. nidulans* was generally refractory to intensive antifungal therapy, suggesting that early surgery may be important. However, the need for early resection of pulmonary lesions will need to be reevaluated with the availability of extended spectrum azoles (see Sect. 4.3.1). Kontoyiannis et al. [18] found that *A. nidulans* isolates were frequently resistant to amphotericin B, another potential cause of treatment failure in CGD patients.

CGD patients often do not have typical symptoms and signs of infection [19]. Fever and leukocytosis may be absent, and an elevated sedimentation rate may be the only abnormal laboratory test [19]. In a review of aspergillosis in CGD patients at the NIH, one-third of patients were asymptomatic at diagnosis and only ~20%

were febrile [10]. In many of these patients, a pulmonary infiltrate on routine screening chest x-ray or CT scan was the first indication of an infection. The white blood cell count was ≤10,000/μl in 13/23 cases, and the sedimentation rate was ≤40 mm/hr. in 9/20 cases.

In contrast to patients with chemotherapy-induced neutropenia, hyphal angioinvasion is not a feature of CGD. In CGD mice, pulmonary aspergillosis is characterized by dense pyogranulomatous areas of consolidation in the absence of vascular hyphal invasion [20, 21]. These findings suggest that NADPH oxidase-independent pathways are sufficient to protect against hyphal angioinvasion. Serum galactomannan is not elevated in experimental pulmonary aspergillosis in CGD mice [20] and is an insensitive diagnostic marker of aspergillosis in CGD patients [22].

4.3.1 Antifungal Prophylaxis and Treatment in CGD

Prevention of invasive aspergillosis and other filamentous fungal diseases relies on avoiding environments where high levels of fungal spores are expected (e.g., gardening and building renovations) and mold-active antifungal prophylaxis. Itraconazole prophylaxis has been shown to be safe and effective in patients with CGD [11, 23]. In a French national database study of 29 episodes of invasive mold infections in CGD patients, the first proven fungal infection occurred later in the group that received itraconazole than in the group without (10 versus 4 years of age, respectively), with a higher proportion of *A. nidulans* and other opportunistic molds in itraconazole recipients. The prognosis appeared to improve over time, possibly reflecting improvements in antifungal regimens [24].

Similar to other immunocompromised patients, invasive aspergillosis in CGD most commonly manifests with pulmonary disease [8]. Chest CT imaging is more sensitive than radiography for detecting early fungal disease. Since the differential diagnosis for pulmonary lesions is broad, a tissue-based diagnosis may be required for early diagnosis. Since CGD is a rare disease, there are no randomized trials of antifungal therapy for aspergillosis specifically among CGD patients. Voriconazole was shown to be superior to conventional amphotericin B as primary therapy for aspergillosis [25]. Underlying conditions in enrolled patients were primarily hematologic malignancies and transplantation. Voriconazole has been evaluated in pediatric patients with invasive fungal infections, including CGD patients [26]. Based on this clinical database, the Infectious Diseases Society of America (IDSA) guidelines recommend voriconazole as primary therapy for invasive aspergillosis [27], a recommendation that can be reasonably applied to CGD patients. Lipid formulations of amphotericin B, posaconazole [28], isavuconazole, and echinocandins are additional options for therapy of invasive aspergillosis in patients who are intolerant to voriconazole or who have refractory disease. Similar to other immunocompromised patients with invasive aspergillosis, development of azole resistance is a barrier to treatment of aspergillosis in CGD patients [29, 30]. In addition to antifungal therapy, debridement or resection of infected tissue may be required. This is particularly the case for refractory aspergillosis or extension of fungal disease to vertebrae or chest wall.

4.4 Immunotherapy for Aspergillosis in CGD

4.4.1 Recombinant Interferon-γ

Recombinant interferon-γ has been widely used as prophylaxis in patients with CGD for approximately 25 years. In a randomized trial of CGD patients, prophylactic recombinant interferon-γ significantly reduced the incidence of serious infections and was beneficial regardless of age, the use of prophylactic antibiotics, and the type of CGD (X-linked or autosomal recessive) [31]. Although prior studies showed that interferon-γ could augment superoxide production in phagocytes from CGD patients, there were no significant changes in the measures of superoxide production by phagocytes in the randomized trial. Thus, the benefit of prophylactic recombinant interferon-γ likely results from augmentation of oxidant-independent pathways. Although there are case reports of use of recombinant interferon-γ as adjunctive therapy in CGD patients with severe infections, the value of interferon-γ in this setting is unclear.

4.4.2 Granulocyte Transfusions

Adjunctive granulocyte transfusions have been used for severe or refractory infections in CGD patients. The principle of granulocyte transfusions in CGD patients (who have normal circulating neutrophil numbers) is that a small proportion of normal neutrophils can augment host defense in CGD neutrophils by providing a source of ROIs. Hydrogen peroxide generated by normal neutrophils can diffuse into CGD neutrophils and provide the necessary substrate to generate hypohalous acid and hydroxyl anion in vitro [32]. In addition, mixtures of small numbers of normal neutrophils with larger numbers of CGD neutrophils damaged *A. fumigatus* hyphae more efficiently than either population of cells alone [33]. These results support the notion of diffusible reactive oxidants generated by NOX2-competent neutrophils at least in part rescuing the impaired host defense in CGD neutrophils. Transfused granulocytes retain respiratory burst activity and appear to traffic normally based on their recovery from sites of infection. A recent randomized trial of granulocyte transfusions in neutropenic patients with severe bacterial or fungal infections failed to show a benefit [34]. The benefit of granulocyte transfusions in CGD remains unclear and is unlikely to ever be definitively evaluated.

4.4.3 Hematopoietic Stem Cell Transplantation

Allogeneic hematopoietic stem cell transplantation is usually curative in CGD and is becoming accepted as a standard of care. The major risk is graft-versus-host disease [35, 36]. Gene therapy is another promising experimental option. However, major obstacles are maintenance of a stable long-term population of gene-corrected myeloid cells and malignancies from insertional mutagenesis [37]. There are limited data regarding the use of allogeneic stem cell transplantation and gene therapy as salvage treatment in CGD patients with refractory aspergillosis [24, 38, 39].

4.5 Aspergillosis in CGD: A Disorder of Impaired Host Defense and Excessive Inflammation

The lung is an interface where inhaled microbes and microbial products (e.g., bacterial and fungal cell wall constituents) interact with host defense cells. The ability of the mammalian host to evolve in the context of continual exposure to fungi requires a well-calibrated immune response. First, the immune system must kill or at least control the growth of inhaled pathogens, such as fungal spores. Second, counter-regulatory mechanisms must be active to limit the inflammatory response to avert tissue injury and allergy. There is strong evidence that NOX2 is critical for both antimicrobial function and regulation of inflammation.

In addition to recurrent infections, CGD is also characterized by abnormally exuberant inflammatory responses leading to granuloma formation, such as granulomatous enteritis resembling Crohn's disease [1] and genitourinary obstruction. "Mulch pneumonitis" is a life-threatening fungal pneumonia in CGD patients characterized by an acute fulminant pneumonitis, which is treated with both antifungals and corticosteroids to dampen uncontrolled inflammation [40]. Mulch pneumonitis underscores the critical role for NOX2 in dampening inflammatory responses.

Dectin-1 is a receptor and immunomodulator of beta-glucans, which are ubiquitous cell wall constituents of fungi and plants [41, 42]. Dectin-1 signals through the tyrosine kinase Syk and the caspase recruitment domain, CARD9 [43–45]. Activation of dectin-1 by beta-glucans can stimulate NOX2 activation [4]. Data in mice support the notion that dectin-1 and NOX2 have coordinated effects in regulating antifungal host defense and the inflammatory response to inhaled fungi. Dectin-1 induces pro-inflammatory cytokines and chemokines, including IL-17 [44, 46–50]. In contrast, while the immediate effects of NOX2 activation are to produce injurious reactive oxidants that target microbes, the overall effect of NOX2 can be to dampen the inflammatory response through intracellular and paracrine signaling pathways.

Mouse models of CGD support the notion of NOX2 restricting excessive inflammation to pro-inflammatory fungal constituents. Morgenstern et al. [51] showed that intratracheal administration of heat-killed *A. fumigatus* hyphae elicited mild self-limited inflammation in wild-type mice but robust and persistent inflammation in CGD mice. Romani et al. [52] linked impaired antifungal host defense and excessive inflammation in CGD mice to defective activation of tryptophan catabolism and generation of regulatory T-cell responses. Results showing defective tryptophan metabolism were not confirmed in CGD patients [53]. Segal et al. [54] showed that NOX2 limited innate immune responses in the lung following zymosan (a fungal cell wall preparation enriched for particulate beta-glucan) challenge through modulation of NF-kB and Nrf2 signaling.

Although there are limitations in extrapolating results from murine aspergillosis to humans, these results support the dual functions of NOX2 in aspergillosis. The principal role of NOX2 is to defend against fungi. In addition, NOX2 appears to play a key role in calibrating the inflammatory response to inhaled molds to avoid excessive lung inflammation and injury.

4.6 Roles of Macrophage and Neutrophil NOX2 in Antifungal Defense

Alveolar macrophages ingest and kill *Aspergillus* spores, whereas neutrophils principally target the hyphal stage [55]. Alveolar macrophages are the first-line phagocytes that respond to inhaled pathogens. They phagocytose and kill microbes and also coordinate the inflammatory response. Although it is well established that NOX2 is critical for neutrophil-mediated host defense, the importance of NOX2 in macrophages is less established. The strongest evidence for the role of macrophage NOX2 in host defense is from the finding that mutations in gp91*phox* that selectively affect macrophages lead to increased susceptibility to mycobacterial diseases [56]. There have been conflicting results as to the role of macrophage NOX2 in controlling the growth of *A. fumigatus* spores [57, 58]. Using knock-in transgenic mice with NOX2 selectively reconstituted in the monocyte/macrophage and dendritic cell lineages, Grimm et al. [59] showed that macrophage NOX2 was protective against pulmonary challenge with *A. fumigatus* and limited the germination of phagocytosed spores in isolated alveolar macrophages. Additional results using these knock-in mice pointed to macrophage NOX2 also limiting the inflammatory response to zymosan [59]. Together, results from these murine models point to a key role for macrophage NOX2 restricting fungal growth and limiting the inflammatory response to *Aspergillus*. Recent additional studies show that NOX2 has broad roles in phagosomal maturation including autophagy required for antibacterial and antifungal host defense and control of inflammation [60–64].

Under conditions in which fungal escape from lung macrophages occurs, rapid recruitment of neutrophils is required to target hyphae to prevent tissue invasion [65]. NOX2 embedded in the plasma membrane releases ROIs into the extracellular environment, while NOX2 in neutrophil secondary granules targets phagocytosed pathogens. While neutrophils inhibit *A. fumigatus* conidial growth by lactoferrin-mediated iron depletion, inhibition of growth of hyphae requires NOX2 [66]. These findings underscore that NOX2-dependent killing of *Aspergillus* is fungal stage specific.

How does neutrophil NOX2 inhibit hyphal growth and invasion? There are a number of mechanisms. First, and the most obvious, is the direct antimicrobial effects of ROIs generated by the NOX2/MPO system. NOX2 is required for phagocyte phagosomal alkalinization, and defective alkalinization is linked to impaired bactericidal activity [67]. The acidotropic, antimalarial drug chloroquine increased the antifungal activity of CGD neutrophils against *Aspergillus*, thereby demonstrating the importance of phagosomal pH in host defense and the potential for chloroquine as a therapeutic approach in CGD [68]. Another putative mechanism relates to the signaling functions of NOX2 resulting in activation of granular serine proteases and generation of neutrophil extracellular traps. Reeves et al. [69] showed that activation of the NOX2 in neutrophils results in the release of neutrophil serine proteases from an anionic proteoglycan matrix within primary granules of neutrophils [69]. The released granular constituents can target phagocytosed microbes.

In a landmark study, Brinkmann et al. [70] showed that neutrophils are capable of releasing extracellular traps that target extracellular bacteria. (NET; Neutrophil Extracellular Traps) NETosis is triggered as an emergency response to infection and to conditions mimicking sepsis [71, 72]. NETs are characterized by extracellular stretches of chromatin that co-localize with cytosolic and granular proteins [73–75].

NOX2 was required for NET generation in murine aspergillosis (Fig. 4.1) [75]. In addition, neutrophils from CGD patients are defective in NETosis, and gene therapy results in restored NETosis in NOX2-competent neutrophils in vitro [73, 76].

These results point to the potential for NOX2 to target pathogens through a multistep process: direct antimicrobial effect of reactive oxidants, the intracellular activation of sequestered proteases that can target phagocytosed pathogens, and

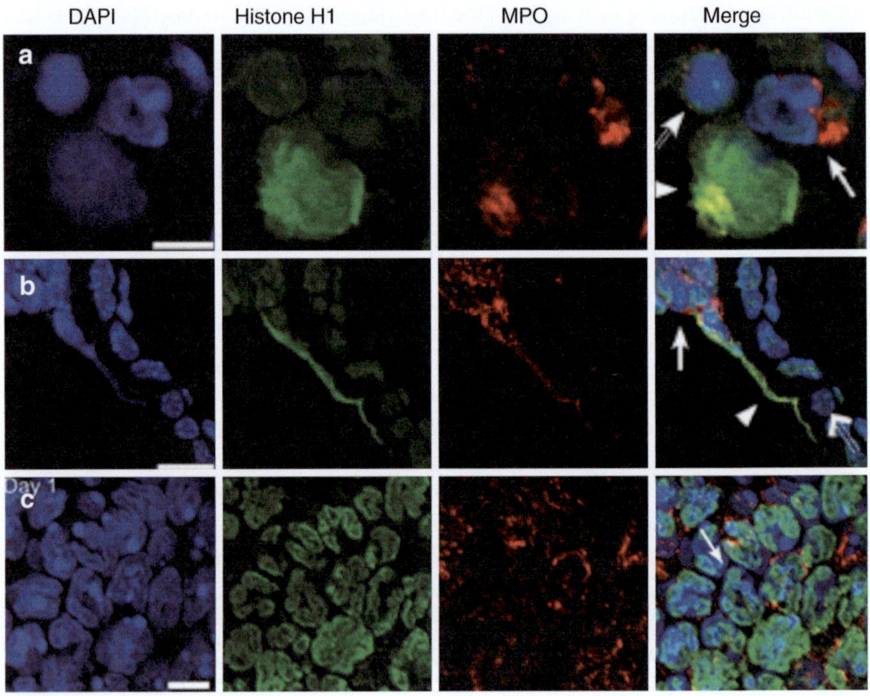

Fig. 4.1 Detection of neutrophil extracellular traps (NETs) by immunofluorescence. Neutrophils in the lungs of WT mice showed evidence of NETosis after oropharyngeal instillation of A. fumigatus hyphae (*n* _ 3 per genotype per time point). Using representative samples, NETs were visualized by indirect immunofluorescence in sections of lung tissue using primary antibodies against histone H1 and neutrophil myeloperoxidase (MPO). Alexa Fluor 488- and 568-conjugated secondary antibodies were used for visualization of histone H1 (*green channel*) and MPO (*red channel*), respectively. (**a**) NETs exhibiting rounded morphology, ~3-fold the size of an intact neutrophil, were prominent in alveoli at day 1 post-infection. Three adjacent neutrophils show different stages of NET formation: (i) a non-NETotic neutrophil with intact nucleus showing typical lobulated morphology and clear separation of euchromatin and heterochromatin visualized by DAPI staining (*solid arrow*); (ii) a neutrophil at an early stage of NETosis characterized by loss of nuclear integrity resulting in decondensed chromatin, identified based on diffuse DAPI and anti-histone staining, but intact azurophilic granules containing MPO (*hollow arrow*); and (iii) a bona fide NET, identified by laminar extracellular DNA (DAPI positive) that colocalized with histone and MPO immunostaining (*arrowhead*). (**b**) NET formation by intrabronchiolar neutrophils (solid arrow), resulting in stretches of laminar DNA (*arrowhead*) identified by colocalization of DAPI-stained DNA, histone, and MPO. Adjacent bronchial epithelia cells (*hollow arrow*) are MPO negative. (**c**) Three-dimensional view of panel B, assembled by Z-stacking of captured images showing elongated NET structure in close proximity to the epithelial surface. The image is turned slightly counter clockwise, with the Z-axis tilted backward (bird's-eye view). Pictures were taken with a Nikon C1 confocal microscope at X100 magnification. Scale bars, 5 μm (**a**) and 10 μm (**b**)

generation of NETs that can attack extracellular pathogens [73]. A gap in knowledge persists regarding the relative roles of direct ROI attack from the NOX2/MPO system versus the downstream activation of neutrophil granular constituents and NETosis in host defense [77]. In this regard, engineered mice with deficiencies or reconstitution of specific pathways are likely to yield important mechanistic knowledge about how NOX2 defends against microbes.

4.7 NETosis in Antifungal Defense

NETs can mediate host defense through a number of pathways, including binding to microbes preventing dissemination, degrading pathogen virulence factors, and killing of pathogens [70, 76, 78]. A number of NET constituents (e.g., histones, serine proteases) have antimicrobial activity. MPO, following release with NET formation, can generate hypohalous acid directed at extracellular microbes [79]. In addition, calprotectin is a NET constituent that mediates nutritional immunity by sequestering divalent metal ions and targets *Candida* and *Aspergillus* species [80, 81].

How NETosis is triggered is incompletely understood. The stimuli for NETosis are encountered during acute infection or conditions mimicking sepsis. NETosis can be triggered by exposure of neutrophils to bacteria, bacterial products, activation of specific Toll-like receptors, and complement-mediated opsonization [71, 82]. Activated platelets can induce NETosis in neutrophils during bacterial sepsis, thereby capturing microbes and promoting their clearance [83–85]. Interferon-gamma produced by neutrophils can stimulate NETosis through an autocrine/paracrine process [86]. In murine pulmonary aspergillosis, NOX2 was required for NET generation [75], but depending on the stimulus, NETs can also be induced by NOX2 independent pathways. Douda et al. [87] showed that NETosis can be activated by mitochondrial ROIs independently of NOX2, through a pathway dependent on calcium-induced activation of SK3 (small conductance potassium channels) and Akt.

NETosis is dependent on complex intracellular signaling, including activation of the Raf-MEK-ERK pathway and potentially anti-apoptotic pathways [88]. Autophagy pathways may stimulate NETosis [89]. Mammalian target of rapamycin (mTOR) may be required for LPS-stimulated NET formation by posttranscriptional control of expression of hypoxia-inducible factor-1α (HIF-1α) [90]. Histone citrullination can stimulate chromatin decondensation and generation of NETs [91]. In addition, specific NET constituents are required for NET generation. Neutrophil elastase (NE) is required for NET generation in pneumonia in mice [92]. In this model, NE traffics from azurophilic granules to the nucleus where, together with myeloperoxidase, it degrades histones and promotes chromatin decondensation.

4.8 Model for NOX2 Modulating Antifungal Host Defense and Inflammation

Based on recent studies, a model for NOX2 modulation of host defense and inflammation can be made. In this model, alveolar macrophages are the first-line phagocytes that sense and defend against inhaled pathogens, including filamentous fungi.

Macrophage NOX2 is the central modulator of both antifungal host defense and the inflammatory response to inhaled filamentous fungi. Dectin-1 in lung macrophages recognizes fungal cell wall β-glucans which activates NOX2 and NF-κB. After translocating to the nucleus, NF-κB stimulates production of IL-17A and other cytokine and chemokines that recruit neutrophils. NOX2 activation in macrophage disables growth of phagocytosed conidia and limits inflammatory and injurious responses through downstream signaling functions that include activation of Nrf2, a transcription factor that controls the expression of several antioxidants and anti-inflammatory proteins. If fungal escape from macrophages occurs, recruitment and activation of neutrophils and NOX2-dependent NETosis are required to target hyphae and avert tissue invasion.

4.9 Future Directions for Preventing and Treating Aspergillosis in CGD

Allogeneic HSCT is being used more widely as the definitive curative treatment for CGD. As a hematopoietic stem cell disorder, gene therapy has been evaluated for decades in CGD [93] and remains an active area of research; the major hurdle relates to maintaining a stable long-term population of gene-corrected cells. While these approaches offer the potential for cure of CGD, knowledge gained about mechanisms by which NOX2 mediates host defense and regulates inflammation also have the potential to lead to therapeutic advances that prevent or reduce infection-related morbidity in CGD. There are a number of examples that are relevant to aspergillosis in CGD. Activation of Nrf2 has the potential to dampen inflammatory responses to pro-inflammatory fungal cell wall products. NOX2 plays a key role in phagosomal maturation, and IL-1 receptor blockade restored autophagy and was protective against aspergillosis in CGD mice [61]. A CD4+ T-cell vaccine-based strategy led to enhanced cross-presentation of fungal antigens and resulted in long-term protection against aspergillosis in CGD mice [94]. Yet another therapeutic approach that merits evaluation in murine CGD is the use of agents that can stimulate NOX2-independent NET generation in neutrophils [87]. Finally, long-lived alveolar macrophages are also a promising target for therapeutic intervention in CGD, including inhalation of antimicrobial drugs, cytokine modulation, and gene correction approaches.

References

1. Marciano BE, Rosenzweig SD, Kleiner DE, Anderson VL, Darnell DN, Anaya-O'Brien S, Hilligoss DM, Malech HL, Gallin JI, Holland SM. Gastrointestinal involvement in chronic granulomatous disease. Pediatrics. 2004;114(2):462–8.
2. Graham DB, Stephenson LM, Lam SK, Brim K, Lee HM, Bautista J, Gilfillan S, Akilesh S, Fujikawa K, Swat W. An ITAM-signaling pathway controls cross-presentation of particulate but not soluble antigens in dendritic cells. J Exp Med. 2007;204(12):2889–97.
3. Mocsai A, Abram CL, Jakus Z, Hu Y, Lanier LL, Lowell CA. Integrin signaling in neutrophils and macrophages uses adaptors containing immunoreceptor tyrosine-based activation motifs. Nat Immunol. 2006;7(12):1326–33.

4. Gantner BN, Simmons RM, Canavera SJ, Akira S, Underhill DM. Collaborative induction of inflammatory responses by dectin-1 and Toll-like receptor 2. J Exp Med. 2003;197(9):1107–17.
5. Abo A, Pick E, Hall A, Totty N, Teahan CG, Segal AW. Activation of the NADPH oxidase involves the small GTP-binding protein p21rac1. Nature. 1991;353(6345):668–70.
6. Knaus UG, Heyworth PG, Evans T, Curnutte JT, Bokoch GM. Regulation of phagocyte oxygen radical production by the GTP-binding protein Rac 2. Science. 1991;254(5037):1512–5.
7. van den Berg JM, van Koppen E, Ahlin A, Belohradsky BH, Bernatowska E, Corbeel L, Espanol T, Fischer A, Kurenko-Deptuch M, Mouy R, et al. Chronic granulomatous disease: the European experience. PLoS ONE. 2009;4(4):e5234.
8. Winkelstein JA, Marino MC, Johnston Jr RB, Boyle J, Curnutte J, Gallin JI, Malech HL, Holland SM, Ochs H, Quie P, et al. Chronic granulomatous disease. Report on a national registry of 368 patients. Medicine. 2000;79(3):155–69.
9. De Ravin SS, Naumann N, Robinson MR, Barron KS, Kleiner DE, Ulrick J, Friend J, Anderson VL, Darnell D, Kang EM, et al. Sarcoidosis in chronic granulomatous disease. Pediatrics. 2006;117(3):e590–5.
10. Segal BH, DeCarlo ES, Kwon-Chung KJ, Malech HL, Gallin JI, Holland SM. Aspergillus nidulans infection in chronic granulomatous disease. Medicine. 1998;77(5):345–54.
11. Gallin JI, Alling DW, Malech HL, Wesley R, Koziol D, Marciano B, Eisenstein EM, Turner ML, DeCarlo ES, Starling JM, et al. Itraconazole to prevent fungal infections in chronic granulomatous disease. N Engl J Med. 2003;348(24):2416–22.
12. Kuhns DB, Alvord WG, Heller T, Feld JJ, Pike KM, Marciano BE, Uzel G, DeRavin SS, Priel DA, Soule BP, et al. Residual NADPH oxidase and survival in chronic granulomatous disease. N Engl J Med. 2010;363(27):2600–10.
13. Dorman SE, Guide SV, Conville PS, DeCarlo ES, Malech HL, Gallin JI, Witebsky FG, Holland SM. Nocardia infection in chronic granulomatous disease. Clin Infect Dis : Off Publ Infect Dis Soc Am. 2002;35(4):390–4.
14. Standish AJ, Weiser JN. Human neutrophils kill Streptococcus pneumoniae via serine proteases. J Immunol. 2009;183(4):2602–9.
15. Speert DP, Bond M, Woodman RC, Curnutte JT. Infection with Pseudomonas cepacia in chronic granulomatous disease: role of nonoxidative killing by neutrophils in host defense. J Infect Dis. 1994;170(6):1524–31.
16. Beaute J, Obenga G, Le Mignot L, Mahlaoui N, Bougnoux ME, Mouy R, Gougerot-Pocidalo MA, Barlogis V, Suarez F, Lanternier F, et al. Epidemiology and outcome of invasive fungal diseases in patients with chronic granulomatous disease: a multicenter study in France. Pediatr Infect Dis J. 2011;30(1):57–62.
17. Rosen-Wolff A, Soldan W, Heyne K, Bickhardt J, Gahr M, Roesler J. Increased susceptibility of a carrier of X-linked chronic granulomatous disease (CGD) to Aspergillus fumigatus infection associated with age- related skewing of lyonization. Ann Hematol. 2001;80(2):113–5.
18. Kontoyiannis DP, Lewis RE, May GS, Osherov N, Rinaldi MG. Aspergillus nidulans is frequently resistant to amphotericin B. Mycoses. 2002;45(9–10):406–7.
19. Gallin JI, Buescher ES, Seligmann BE, Nath J, Gaither T, Katz P. NIH conference. Recent advances in chronic granulomatous disease. Ann Intern Med. 1983;99(5):657–74.
20. Dennis CG, Greco WR, Brun Y, Youn R, Slocum HK, Bernacki RJ, Lewis R, Wiederhold N, Holland SM, Petraitiene R, et al. Effect of amphotericin B and micafungin combination on survival, histopathology, and fungal burden in experimental aspergillosis in the p47phox−/− mouse model of chronic granulomatous disease. Antimicrob Agents Chemother. 2006;50(2):422–7.
21. Chang YC, Segal BH, Holland SM, Miller GF, Kwon-Chung KJ. Virulence of catalase-deficient aspergillus nidulans in p47(phox) −/− mice. Implications for fungal pathogenicity and host defense in chronic granulomatous disease. J Clin Invest. 1998;101(9):1843–50.
22. Verweij PE, Weemaes CM, Curfs JH, Bretagne S, Meis JF. Failure to detect circulating Aspergillus markers in a patient with chronic granulomatous disease and invasive aspergillosis. J Clin Microbiol. 2000;38(10):3900–1.

23. Mouy R, Veber F, Blanche S, Donadieu J, Brauner R, Levron JC, Griscelli C, Fischer A. Long-term itraconazole prophylaxis against Aspergillus infections in thirty-two patients with chronic granulomatous disease. J Pediatr. 1994;125(6 Pt 1):998–1003.
24. Blumental S, Mouy R, Mahlaoui N, Bougnoux ME, Debre M, Beaute J, Lortholary O, Blanche S, Fischer A. Invasive mold infections in chronic granulomatous disease: a 25-year retrospective survey. Clin Infect Dis: Off Publ Infect Dis Soc Am. 2011;53(12):e159–69.
25. Herbrecht R, Denning DW, Patterson TF, Bennett JE, Greene RE, Oestmann JW, Kern WV, Marr KA, Ribaud P, Lortholary O, et al. Voriconazole versus amphotericin B for primary therapy of invasive aspergillosis. N Engl J Med. 2002;347(6):408–15.
26. Walsh TJ, Lutsar I, Driscoll T, Dupont B, Roden M, Ghahramani P, Hodges M, Groll AH, Perfect JR. Voriconazole in the treatment of aspergillosis, scedosporiosis and other invasive fungal infections in children. Pediatr Infect Dis J. 2002;21(3):240–8.
27. Patterson TF, Thompson 3rd GR, Denning DW, Fishman JA, Hadley S, Herbrecht R, Kontoyiannis DP, Marr KA, Morrison VA, Nguyen MH, et al. Practice guidelines for the diagnosis and management of aspergillosis: 2016 update by the infectious diseases society of America. Clin Infect Dis: Off Publ Infect Dis Soc Am. 2016;63(4):e1–e60.
28. Segal BH, Barnhart LA, Anderson VL, Walsh TJ, Malech HL, Holland SM. Posaconazole as salvage therapy in patients with chronic granulomatous disease and invasive filamentous fungal infection. Clin Infect Dis: Off Publ Infect Dis Soc Am. 2005;40(11):1684–8.
29. Arendrup MC, Mavridou E, Mortensen KL, Snelders E, Frimodt-Moller N, Khan H, Melchers WJ, Verweij PE. Development of azole resistance in Aspergillus fumigatus during azole therapy associated with change in virulence. PLoS ONE. 2010;5(4):e10080.
30. Hodiamont CJ, Dolman KM, Ten Berge IJ, Melchers WJ, Verweij PE, Pajkrt D. Multiple-azole-resistant Aspergillus fumigatus osteomyelitis in a patient with chronic granulomatous disease successfully treated with long-term oral posaconazole and surgery. Med Mycol : Off Publ Int Soc Hum Anim Mycol. 2009;47(2):217–20.
31. International. A controlled trial of interferon gamma to prevent infection in chronic granulomatous disease. The International Chronic Granulomatous Disease Cooperative Study Group [see comments]. N Engl J Med. 1991;324(8):509–16.
32. Ohno Y, Gallin JI. Diffusion of extracellular hydrogen peroxide into intracellular compartments of human neutrophils. Studies utilizing the inactivation of myeloperoxidase by hydrogen peroxide and azide. J Biol Chem. 1985;260(14):8438–46.
33. Rex JH, Bennett JE, Gallin JI, Malech HL, Melnick DA. Normal and deficient neutrophils can cooperate to damage Aspergillus fumigatus hyphae. J Infect Dis. 1990;162(2):523–8.
34. Price TH, Boeckh M, Harrison RW, McCullough J, Ness PM, Strauss RG, Nichols WG, Hamza TH, Cushing MM, King KE, et al. Efficacy of transfusion with granulocytes from G-CSF/dexamethasone-treated donors in neutropenic patients with infection. Blood. 2015;126(18):2153–61.
35. Gungor T, Teira P, Slatter M, Stussi G, Stepensky P, Moshous D, Vermont C, Ahmad I, Shaw PJ, Telles da Cunha JM, et al. Reduced-intensity conditioning and HLA-matched haemopoietic stem-cell transplantation in patients with chronic granulomatous disease: a prospective multicentre study. Lancet. 2014;383(9915):436–48.
36. Martinez CA, Shah S, Shearer WT, Rosenblatt HM, Paul ME, Chinen J, Leung KS, Kennedy-Nasser A, Brenner MK, Heslop HE, et al. Excellent survival after sibling or unrelated donor stem cell transplantation for chronic granulomatous disease. J Allergy Clin Immunol. 2012;129(1):176–83.
37. Stein S, Ott MG, Schultze-Strasser S, Jauch A, Burwinkel B, Kinner A, Schmidt M, Kramer A, Schwable J, Glimm H, et al. Genomic instability and myelodysplasia with monosomy 7 consequent to EVI1 activation after gene therapy for chronic granulomatous disease. Nat Med. 2010;16(2):198–204.
38. Shigemura T, Nakazawa Y, Yoshikawa K, Hirabayashi K, Saito S, Kobayashi N, Sakashita K, Shiohara M, Wada T, Shimodaira S, et al. Successful cord blood transplantation after repeated transfusions of unmobilized neutrophils in addition to antifungal treatment in an infant with chronic granulomatous disease complicated by invasive pulmonary aspergillosis. Transfusion. 2013.

39. Siler U, Paruzynski A, Holtgreve-Grez H, Kuzmenko E, Koehl U, Renner ED, Alhan C, de Loosdrecht AA, Schwable J, Pfluger T, et al. Successful combination of sequential gene therapy and rescue Allo-HSCT in two children with X-CGD – importance of timing. Curr Gene Ther. 2015;15(4):416–27.
40. Siddiqui S, Anderson VL, Hilligoss DM, Abinun M, Kuijpers TW, Masur H, Witebsky FG, Shea YR, Gallin JI, Malech HL, et al. Fulminant mulch pneumonitis: an emergency presentation of chronic granulomatous disease. Clin Infect Dis: Off Publ Infect Dis Soc Am. 2007;45(6):673–81.
41. Brown GD, Gordon S. Immune recognition. A new receptor for beta-glucans. Nature. 2001;413(6851):36–7.
42. Netea MG, Gow NA, Munro CA, Bates S, Collins C, Ferwerda G, Hobson RP, Bertram G, Hughes HB, Jansen T, et al. Immune sensing of *Candida albicans* requires cooperative recognition of mannans and glucans by lectin and Toll-like receptors. J Clin Invest. 2006;116(6):1642–50.
43. Gross O, Gewies A, Finger K, Schafer M, Sparwasser T, Peschel C, Forster I, Ruland J. Card9 controls a non-TLR signalling pathway for innate anti-fungal immunity. Nature. 2006;442(7103):651–6.
44. LeibundGut-Landmann S, Gross O, Robinson MJ, Osorio F, Slack EC, Tsoni SV, Schweighoffer E, Tybulewicz V, Brown GD, Ruland J, et al. Syk- and CARD9-dependent coupling of innate immunity to the induction of T helper cells that produce interleukin 17. Nat Immunol. 2007;8(6):630–8.
45. Rogers NC, Slack EC, Edwards AD, Nolte MA, Schulz O, Schweighoffer E, Williams DL, Gordon S, Tybulewicz VL, Brown GD, et al. Syk-dependent cytokine induction by Dectin-1 reveals a novel pattern recognition pathway for C type lectins. Immunity. 2005;22(4): 507–17.
46. Zenaro E, Donini M, Dusi S. Induction of Th1/Th17 immune response by Mycobacterium tuberculosis: role of dectin-1, mannose receptor, and DC-SIGN. J Leukoc Biol. 2009;86(6):1393–401.
47. Werner JL, Metz AE, Horn D, Schoeb TR, Hewitt MM, Schwiebert LM, Faro-Trindade I, Brown GD, Steele C. Requisite role for the dectin-1 beta-glucan receptor in pulmonary defense against Aspergillus fumigatus. J Immunol. 2009;182(8):4938–46.
48. Manicassamy S, Ravindran R, Deng J, Oluoch H, Denning TL, Kasturi SP, Rosenthal KM, Evavold BD, Pulendran B. Toll-like receptor 2-dependent induction of vitamin A-metabolizing enzymes in dendritic cells promotes T regulatory responses and inhibits autoimmunity. Nat Med. 2009;15(4):401–9.
49. Glocker EO, Hennigs A, Nabavi M, Schaffer AA, Woellner C, Salzer U, Pfeifer D, Veelken H, Warnatz K, Tahami F, et al. A homozygous CARD9 mutation in a family with susceptibility to fungal infections. N Engl J Med. 2009;361(18):1727–35.
50. Ferwerda B, Ferwerda G, Plantinga TS, Willment JA, van Spriel AB, Venselaar H, Elbers CC, Johnson MD, Cambi A, Huysamen C, et al. Human dectin-1 deficiency and mucocutaneous fungal infections. N Engl J Med. 2009;361(18):1760–7.
51. Morgenstern DE, Gifford MA, Li LL, Doerschuk CM, Dinauer MC. Absence of respiratory burst in X-linked chronic granulomatous disease mice leads to abnormalities in both host defense and inflammatory response to Aspergillus fumigatus. J Exp Med. 1997;185(2):207–18.
52. Romani L, Fallarino F, De Luca A, Montagnoli C, D'Angelo C, Zelante T, Vacca C, Bistoni F, Fioretti MC, Grohmann U, et al. Defective tryptophan catabolism underlies inflammation in mouse chronic granulomatous disease. Nature. 2008;451(7175):211–5.
53. De Ravin SS, Zarember KA, Long-Priel D, Chan KC, Fox SD, Gallin JI, Kuhns DB, Malech HL. Tryptophan/kynurenine metabolism in human leukocytes is independent of superoxide and is fully maintained in chronic granulomatous disease. Blood. 2010;116(10):1755–60.
54. Segal BH, Han W, Bushey JJ, Joo M, Bhatti Z, Feminella J, Dennis CG, Vethanayagam RR, Yull FE, Capitano M, et al. NADPH oxidase limits innate immune responses in the lungs in mice. PLoS ONE. 2010;5(3):e9631.

55. Schaffner A, Douglas H, Braude A. Selective protection against conidia by mononuclear and against mycelia by polymorphonuclear phagocytes in resistance to Aspergillus. Observations on these two lines of defense in vivo and in vitro with human and mouse phagocytes. J Clin Invest. 1982;69(3):617–31.
56. Bustamante J, Arias AA, Vogt G, Picard C, Galicia LB, Prando C, Grant AV, Marchal CC, Hubeau M, Chapgier A, et al. Germline CYBB mutations that selectively affect macrophages in kindreds with X-linked predisposition to tuberculous mycobacterial disease. Nat Immunol. 2011;12(3):213–21.
57. Philippe B, Ibrahim-Granet O, Prevost MC, Gougerot-Pocidalo MA, Sanchez Perez M, Van der Meeren A, Latge JP. Killing of Aspergillus fumigatus by alveolar macrophages is mediated by reactive oxidant intermediates. Infect Immun. 2003;71(6):3034–42.
58. Cornish EJ, Hurtgen BJ, McInnerney K, Burritt NL, Taylor RM, Jarvis JN, Wang SY, Burritt JB. Reduced nicotinamide adenine dinucleotide phosphate oxidase-independent resistance to Aspergillus fumigatus in alveolar macrophages. J Immunol. 2008;180(10):6854–67.
59. Grimm MJ, Vethanayagam RR, Almyroudis NG, Dennis CG, Khan AN, D'Auria AC, Singel KL, Davidson BA, Knight PR, Blackwell TS, et al. Monocyte- and macrophage-targeted NADPH oxidase mediates antifungal host defense and regulation of acute inflammation in mice. J Immunol. 2013;190(8):4175–84.
60. Tam JM, Mansour MK, Khan NS, Seward M, Puranam S, Tanne A, Sokolovska A, Becker CE, Acharya M, Baird MA, et al. Dectin-1 dependent LC3 recruitment to phagosomes enhances fungicidal activity in macrophages. J Infect Dis. 2014;210:1844–54.
61. de Luca A, Smeekens SP, Casagrande A, Iannitti R, Conway KL, Gresnigt MS, Begun J, Plantinga TS, Joosten LA, van der Meer JW, et al. IL-1 receptor blockade restores autophagy and reduces inflammation in chronic granulomatous disease in mice and in humans. Proc Natl Acad Sci U S A. 2014;111(9):3526–31.
62. Ma J, Becker C, Lowell CA, Underhill DM. Dectin-1 triggered recruitment of LC3 to phagosomes facilitates MHC class II presentation of fungal-derived antigens. J Biol Chem. 2012;287:34149–56.
63. Huang J, Canadien V, Lam GY, Steinberg BE, Dinauer MC, Magalhaes MA, Glogauer M, Grinstein S, Brumell JH. Activation of antibacterial autophagy by NADPH oxidases. Proc Natl Acad Sci U S A. 2009;106(15):6226–31.
64. Martinez J, Malireddi RK, Lu Q, Cunha LD, Pelletier S, Gingras S, Orchard R, Guan JL, Tan H, Peng J, et al. Molecular characterization of LC3-associated phagocytosis reveals distinct roles for Rubicon, NOX2 and autophagy proteins. Nat Cell Biol. 2015;17(7):893–906.
65. Jhingran A, Kasahara S, Shepardson KM, Junecko BA, Heung LJ, Kumasaka DK, Knoblaugh SE, Lin X, Kazmierczak BI, Reinhart TA, et al. Compartment-specific and sequential role of MyD88 and CARD9 in chemokine induction and innate defense during respiratory fungal infection. PLoS Pathog. 2015;11(1):e1004589.
66. Zarember KA, Sugui JA, Chang YC, Kwon-Chung KJ, Gallin JI. Human polymorphonuclear leukocytes inhibit Aspergillus fumigatus conidial growth by lactoferrin-mediated iron depletion. J Immunol. 2007;178(10):6367–73.
67. Segal AW, Geisow M, Garcia R, Harper A, Miller R. The respiratory burst of phagocytic cells is associated with a rise in vacuolar pH. Nature. 1981;290(5805):406–9.
68. Henriet SS, Jans J, Simonetti E, Kwon-Chung KJ, Rijs AJ, Hermans PW, Holland SM, de Jonge MI, Warris A. Chloroquine modulates the fungal immune response in phagocytic cells from patients with chronic granulomatous disease. J Infect Dis. 2013;207(12):1932–9.
69. Reeves EP, Lu H, Jacobs HL, Messina CG, Bolsover S, Gabella G, Potma EO, Warley A, Roes J, Segal AW. Killing activity of neutrophils is mediated through activation of proteases by K+ flux. Nature. 2002;416(6878):291–7.
70. Brinkmann V, Reichard U, Goosmann C, Fauler B, Uhlemann Y, Weiss DS, Weinrauch Y, Zychlinsky A. Neutrophil extracellular traps kill bacteria. Science. 2004;303(5663):1532–5.
71. Yipp BG, Petri B, Salina D, Jenne CN, Scott BN, Zbytnuik LD, Pittman K, Asaduzzaman M, Wu K, Meijndert HC, et al. Infection-induced NETosis is a dynamic process involving neutrophil multitasking in vivo. Nat Med. 2012;18(9):1386–93.

72. Caudrillier A, Kessenbrock K, Gilliss BM, Nguyen JX, Marques MB, Monestier M, Toy P, Werb Z, Looney MR. Platelets induce neutrophil extracellular traps in transfusion-related acute lung injury. J Clin Invest. 2012;122(7):2661–71.
73. Fuchs TA, Abed U, Goosmann C, Hurwitz R, Schulze I, Wahn V, Weinrauch Y, Brinkmann V, Zychlinsky A. Novel cell death program leads to neutrophil extracellular traps. J Cell Biol. 2007;176(2):231–41.
74. Brinkmann V, Laube B, Abu Abed U, Goosmann C, Zychlinsky A. Neutrophil extracellular traps: how to generate and visualize them. J Vis Exp JoVE. 201036.
75. Rohm M, Grimm MJ, D'Auria AC, Almyroudis NG, Segal BH, Urban CF. NADPH oxidase promotes neutrophil extracellular trap formation in pulmonary aspergillosis. Infect Immun. 2014;82(5):1766–77.
76. Bianchi M, Hakkim A, Brinkmann V, Siler U, Seger RA, Zychlinsky A, Reichenbach J. Restoration of NET formation by gene therapy in CGD controls aspergillosis. Blood. 2009;114(13):2619–22.
77. Nauseef WM. Editorial: Nyet to NETs? A pause for healthy skepticism. J Leukoc Biol. 2012;91(3):353–5.
78. Urban CF, Lourido S, Zychlinsky A. How do microbes evade neutrophil killing? Cell Microbiol. 2006;8(11):1687–96.
79. Metzler KD, Fuchs TA, Nauseef WM, Reumaux D, Roesler J, Schulze I, Wahn V, Papayannopoulos V, Zychlinsky A. Myeloperoxidase is required for neutrophil extracellular trap formation: implications for innate immunity. Blood. 2011;117(3):953–9.
80. Urban CF, Ermert D, Schmid M, Abu-Abed U, Goosmann C, Nacken W, Brinkmann V, Jungblut PR, Zychlinsky A. Neutrophil extracellular traps contain calprotectin, a cytosolic protein complex involved in host defense against *Candida albicans*. PLoS Pathog. 2009;5(10):e1000639.
81. Bianchi M, Niemiec MJ, Siler U, Urban CF, Reichenbach J. Restoration of anti-Aspergillus defense by neutrophil extracellular traps in human chronic granulomatous disease after gene therapy is calprotectin-dependent. J Allergy Clin Immunol. 2011;127:1243–52.e7.
82. Saitoh T, Komano J, Saitoh Y, Misawa T, Takahama M, Kozaki T, Uehata T, Iwasaki H, Omori H, Yamaoka S, et al. Neutrophil extracellular traps mediate a host defense response to human immunodeficiency virus-1. Cell Host Microbe. 2012;12(1):109–16.
83. Phillipson M, Kubes P. The neutrophil in vascular inflammation. Nat Med. 2011;17(11):1381–90.
84. Clark SR, Ma AC, Tavener SA, McDonald B, Goodarzi Z, Kelly MM, Patel KD, Chakrabarti S, McAvoy E, Sinclair GD, et al. Platelet TLR4 activates neutrophil extracellular traps to ensnare bacteria in septic blood. Nat Med. 2007;13(4):463–9.
85. McDonald B, Urrutia R, Yipp BG, Jenne CN, Kubes P. Intravascular neutrophil extracellular traps capture bacteria from the bloodstream during sepsis. Cell Host Microbe. 2012;12(3):324–33.
86. Yamada M, Gomez JC, Chugh PE, Lowell CA, Dinauer MC, Dittmer DP, Doerschuk CM. Interferon-gamma production by neutrophils during bacterial pneumonia in mice. Am J Respir Crit Care Med. 2011;183(10):1391–401.
87. Douda DN, Khan MA, Grasemann H, Palaniyar N. SK3 channel and mitochondrial ROS mediate NADPH oxidase-independent NETosis induced by calcium influx. Proc Natl Acad Sci U S A. 2015;112(9):2817–22.
88. Hakkim A, Fuchs TA, Martinez NE, Hess S, Prinz H, Zychlinsky A, Waldmann H. Activation of the Raf-MEK-ERK pathway is required for neutrophil extracellular trap formation. Nat Chem Biol. 2011;7(2):75–7.
89. Remijsen Q, Vanden Berghe T, Wirawan E, Asselbergh B, Parthoens E, De Rycke R, Noppen S, Delforge M, Willems J, Vandenabeele P. Neutrophil extracellular trap cell death requires both autophagy and superoxide generation. Cell Res. 2011;21(2):290–304.
90. McInturff AM, Cody MJ, Elliott EA, Glenn JW, Rowley JW, Rondina MT, Yost CC. Mammalian target of rapamycin regulates neutrophil extracellular trap formation via induction of hypoxia-inducible factor 1 alpha. Blood. 2012;120(15):3118–25.

91. Wang Y, Li M, Stadler S, Correll S, Li P, Wang D, Hayama R, Leonelli L, Han H, Grigoryev SA, et al. Histone hypercitrullination mediates chromatin decondensation and neutrophil extracellular trap formation. J Cell Biol. 2009;184(2):205–13.
92. Papayannopoulos V, Metzler KD, Hakkim A, Zychlinsky A. Neutrophil elastase and myeloperoxidase regulate the formation of neutrophil extracellular traps. J Cell Biol. 2010;191(3):677–91.
93. Malech HL, Maples PB, Whiting-Theobald N, Linton GF, Sekhsaria S, Vowells SJ, Li F, Miller JA, DeCarlo E, Holland SM, et al. Prolonged production of NADPH oxidase-corrected granulocytes after gene therapy of chronic granulomatous disease. Proc Natl Acad Sci U S A. 1997;94(22):12133–8.
94. De Luca A, Iannitti RG, Bozza S, Beau R, Casagrande A, D'Angelo C, Moretti S, Cunha C, Giovannini G, Massi-Benedetti C, et al. CD4(+) T cell vaccination overcomes defective cross-presentation of fungal antigens in a mouse model of chronic granulomatous disease. J Clin Invest. 2012;122(5):1816–31.

Primary Immunodeficiencies and Dermatophytosis

5

Claire Rouzaud, Fanny Lanternier, and Anne Puel

Abstract

Dermatophytes are keratinophilic fungi responsible for benign and common infections worldwide. Severe forms including extensive or invasive dermatophytosis are reported in immunocompromised hosts including with primary immunodeficiencies. We describe the clinical presentation and outcome of severe dermatophytosis occuring in primary immunodeficiencies such as autosomal recessive CARD9 deficiency, autosomal dominant STAT1 gain of function, autosomal dominant STAT3 deficiency, or the Keratitis-Ichthyosis-Deafness syndrome. There is no consensus regarding the treatment of severe dermatophytosis, which depends on the site and the extent of the infection as well as the nature of the underlying immunodeficiency. Long life anti-dermatophytic systemic treatment is probably necessary in CARD9 deficient patients.

C. Rouzaud
Paris Descartes University, Sorbonne Paris Cité, Infectious Diseases Unit, Necker-Enfants Malades Universitary Hospital, APHP, Imagine Institute, Paris, France
e-mail: claire.rouzaud@aphp.fr

F. Lanternier
Paris Descartes University, Sorbonne Paris Cité, Infectious Diseases Unit, Necker-Enfants Malades Universitary Hospital, APHP, Imagine Institute, Paris, France

Institut Pasteur, Centre National de Référence Mycoses invasives et Antifongiques, Paris, France

Institut Pasteur, Unité de Mycologie Moléculaire, CNRS URA3012, Paris, France

A. Puel (✉)
Laboratory of Human Genetics of Infectious Diseases, Necker Branch, INSERM UMR1163, Paris, France

Paris Descartes University – Sorbonne Paris Cité, Imagine Institute, Paris, France
e-mail: anne.puel@inserm.fr

A. Carvalho (ed.), *Immunogenetics of Fungal Diseases*,
DOI 10.1007/978-3-319-50842-9_5

5.1 Dermatophytosis

5.1.1 Mycological Data and Epidemiology

Dermatophytes are cosmopolite filamentous fungi classified into geophilic, zoophilic, and anthropophilic species according to their development in soil, animals, or humans, respectively. They are divided in three genera, *Trichophyton*, *Microsporum*, and *Epidermophyton*. Many dermatophyte species are responsible for human infections; however, *Trichophyton rubrum* is the most frequent species responsible of these infections. Dermatophyte species vary according to the geographical area as well as the site of infection. Rare sporadic epidemics with unusual species have been reported (e.g., *T. tonsurans* in student wrestlers [1]). Interhuman transmission is the most frequent mode of contamination, due to close contact with soil or objects contaminated with infected tissues. In case of zoophilic dermatophytosis, animals (cat, dog), either symptomatic or asymptomatic, are the source of infection.

Superficial dermatophytosis is known to be related to lifestyle: contact with animals, activities, or local factors such as heat, moisture, and maceration. The presence of saturated fatty acids in sebum due to hormonal factors reduces *tinea capitis* frequency after puberty [2]. Dermatophytosis is a frequent and worldwide infection. Its prevalence is difficult to evaluate precisely due to its benign presentation. Fungal infections of the skin and nails are reported to affect 20–25% of the world's population [3, 4]. In a multicenter Canadian study, onychomycosis was reported in 6.7% of patients, half due to dermatophytes [5]. Dermatophytosis is the fourth most prevalent human infectious disease and therefore a public health concern [6]. Superficial dermatophytosis is frequent in the general population but usually benign and therefore often neglected.

5.1.2 Physiopathology

Dermatophytes are keratinophilic fungi. Their growth depends on keratin substrates; thereby infection can involve the skin (tinea corporis, tinea pedis, tinea cruris), nails (onychomycosis), and scalp (tinea capitis). Dermatophyte arthrospores are present on the ground and are responsible for inoculation. Geophilic dermatophyte species survive in the environment in contact with keratinized material, anthropophilic dermatophytes only infect humans, and zoophilic dermatophytes infect animals and occasionally, humans. The arthrospores adhere to the keratinocytes [7]. Virulence factors such as proteases, sulfites, and reducing agents responsible of keratin degradation allow fungus to invade keratinized structures such as stratum corneum, hair, nails, or claws [8]. Environmental factors (trauma, humidity) are predisposing factors for stratum corneum dermatophyte penetration, while locally secreted substances (β defensins, unsaturated transferrin contained in sweat and sebum) are limiting factors. Dermatophytes survive in contact with keratinized material;

stratum corneum and hair follicular ostium provide dermatophyte's nutritional and pH requirements and represent the most frequent localizations of infection.

A murine model of *Trichophyton mentagrophytes* subcutaneous inoculation showed lymph nodes, liver, and spleen dissemination before fungus clearance [9]. In this model, dermatophyte infection caused inflammation and granulomatous reaction. The lymph nodes were often infected. Apart from these animal models, clinical data support evidence that, under certain circumstances, dermatophytes can invade the dermis, survive, and spread to lymph nodes and internal organs. Proximal white subungual onychomycosis with nail lunula infection may indicate endogenous reactivation or autoreinfection from a deep site (lymph node) [10]. Dermatophyte frequent dissemination to lymph node and possible dissemination to other organs were reported in deep dermatophytosis [11].

5.1.3 Clinical Presentation and Diagnosis

The classical clinical presentation of dermatophytosis is characterized by superficial infections, limited to stratum corneum. Tinea pedis starts with crack and peeling between the last toes. Lesions then spread to other spaces, side edges, and back of the foot and can spread to nails. Hand injury is rare and often limited to one hand. Onychomycosis is classified in distal and lateral subungual, superficial white, endonyx, proximal subungual, and totally dystrophic forms [12]. Dermatophytes infect others sites: inguinal, axillary, and sub-mammary area. Tinea capitis involves the scalp. Lesions are often itchy and lead to single or multiple squamous scalp area with erythema, inflammation, broken hair, or alopecia. Folliculitis can develop from hair follicles of other sites than the scalp (except axillary and pubic). Tinea corporis affects the skin at any body part. The lesions are erythematous, sometimes with small blisters, with centrifugal evolution.

By contrast with these classical presentations of dermatophyte infections, severe dermatophytoses are rare manifestations of dermatophytosis. They include extensive and invasive forms (deep dermatophytosis and Majocchi granuloma) of infection. Extensive dermatophytosis is confined to stratum corneum but with unusually extensive or numerous lesions at different sites. Majocchi granuloma is a nodular dermatophyte perifolliculitis with localized perifollicular dermal infection. Deep dermatophytosis is defined by dermatophytic dermis invasion, not confined to the perifollicular area in the dermis, which can disseminate to extra-cutaneous sites as lymph nodes, bones, or central nervous system [11]. No specific dermatophyte species appear to be associated with the severe forms. As for common dermatophytosis, *T. rubrum* is most frequently found [13, 14].

Majocchi granulomas appear as nodules or papules on the lower limb or head. Histology evidences granuloma and dermatophyte hyphae into the dermis around hair follicle.

Deep dermatophytosis lesions appear as ill-defined infiltrated plaques, nodules, and papules sometimes associated with itching, pain, and discharge. The number

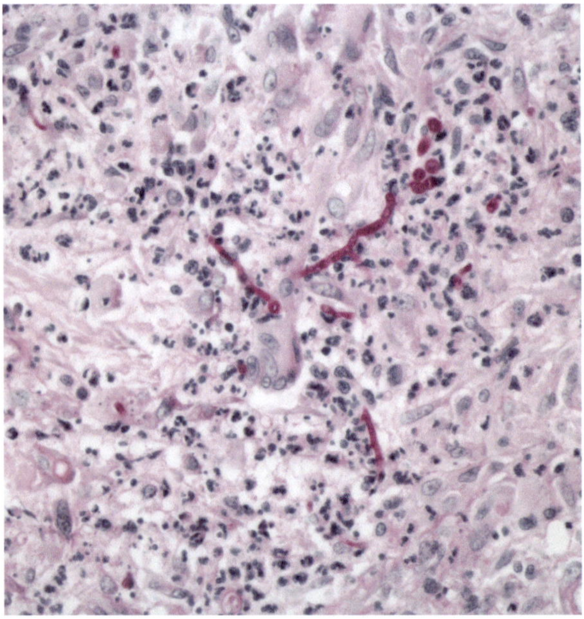

Fig. 5.1 Histopathological presentation of severe dermatophytosis [16]

and location of lesions vary. Infection can spread to lymph nodes or other organs either by contiguity (e.g., bone) or through vascular or lymphatic spread (e.g., central nervous system). Dermatophytosis dissemination has only been reported in patients with a primary immunodeficiency (see below). In patients with deep dermatophytosis, skin histological examination reveals granulomatous dermatitis with dermal extension out of hair follicle (Fig. 5.1), frequent necrosis, and eosinophilic infiltration. Hyphae are found in granuloma center and sometimes in the cytoplasm of giant cells [11]. Diagnosis of invasive forms is based on positive culture for dermatophytes and histological results of skin biopsy. In a French cohort of severe dermatophytosis among solid organ recipient patients [15], beta-D-glucans in blood samples were found positive at diagnosis.

Severe dermatophytosis may occur in different groups of patients, mostly patients with acquired immunodeficiency as HIV-infected patients, solid organ transplant, and other predisposing conditions such as systemic corticosteroid treatment, topical steroid, myelodysplastic syndrome, leukemia or lymphoma, atopic dermatitis and eczema, diabetes mellitus, cirrhosis and hemodialysis for renal failure, Cushing disease, and congenital adrenal hyperplasia [16]. Some patients had been receiving immunosuppressive drugs: azathioprine, cyclosporine, cyclophosphamide, methotrexate, infliximab, tacrolimus, and topical tacrolimus mainly for autoimmune disease (myasthenia, autoimmune hepatitis, lupus, rheumatoid arthritis and Behçet's disease). In case of severe dermatophytosis without predisposing factor, a primary immunodeficiency described below has to be ruled out.

5.1.4 Anti-dermatophyte Immunity

The skin is the first barrier against dermatophytes. Both innate and adaptive immunities play a role in human dermatophyte antifungal defense. Beta-D-glucans present in dermatophyte cell wall are recognized by the C-type lectin receptors (CLR) (e.g., Dectin-1, Dectin-2, MINCLE, or DC-SIGN) [17, 18]. It has been shown that Dectin-2 preferentially recognizes *T. rubrum* hyphae, while Dectin-1 mainly recognizes conidia [19, 20]. DC-SIGN is a major phagocytosis dermatophyte receptor, expressed on human monocyte-derived dendritic cells (MDDC) and monocyte-derived macrophages (MDM) [21]. MDDC but not MDM from patients with dermatophytosis inhibits *T. rubrum* growth. By contrast *T. rubrum* conidia phagocytosis by MDM results in IL-10 production [21]. DC therefore seems to have a key role in anti-dermatophyte immunity. Increased levels of IL-22 and β-defensin-2 were found in serum of patients with superficial dermatophytosis. Levels were inversely correlated with DEFB4 copy number evaluated with qPCR [22]. An experimental mouse model of dermatophyte (*Arthroderma benhamiae* and *A. vanbreuseghemii*) skin inoculation showed that dermal inflammatory cellular infiltrate contained macrophages, dendritic cells, and polymorphonuclear neutrophils (PMN) [23]. The in situ cytokine profile was characterized by the overexpression of transforming growth factor-b (TGF-β), interleukin (IL)-1β, and IL-6 mRNA during infection suggesting a role of the T-helper 17 pathway in the establishment of immunity [23]. In vitro studies showed that peritoneal mice macrophages could ingest *T. rubrum* conidia within 4 hours and in turn produce TNF-α and IL-10. However, after 8 hours of infection, macrophage viability decreased due to development of hyphae inside macrophages [24]. The role of T lymphocytes in anti-dermatophyte immunity has been studied in in vivo mouse models: the transfer of mouse cells from regional lymph node infected by *T. quinckeanum* in sublethally irradiated mice protected them from dermatophyte infection [25]. In human Treg CD4+CD25+ expression was higher in peripheral blood of patients with onychomycosis compared with healthy patients [26].

Table 5.1 Primary immunodeficiencies associated with dermatophytosis, clinical involvement, and associated infection

Primary immunodeficiencies associated with dermatophytosis	AR CARD9 deficiency	AD STAT1 gain of function	AD STAT3 deficiency
Clinical involvement	Deep and persistent dermatophytosis with lymph node involvement	Rare severe dermatophytosis and superficial forms	Rare superficial dermatophytosis
Others infections	Mucocutaneous candidiasis, phaeohyphomycosis; central nervous system candidiasis; *Candida* colitis	*Staphylococcus* sp., respiratory tract and skin infections, viral infections (Herpesviridae)	*Staphylococcus* sp., *Candida* sp., cutaneous infections; pulmonary infections with secondary bronchiectasis and pneumatocele

5.2 Primary Immunodeficiencies and Susceptibility to Dermatophytosis (Table 5.1)

5.2.1 Autosomal Recessive CARD9 Deficiency

Caspase recruitment domain-containing protein 9 (CARD9) is a central adaptor in antifungal innate immunity expressed predominantly by myeloid cells located downstream CLRs, such as Dectin-1, Dectin-2, and MINCLE but also CR3 [27, 28]. In North Africa, severe forms of dermatophytosis (deep dermatophytosis) in patients without any known immunodeficiency were described by physicians as "maladie dermatophytique." A genetic origin was long suspected to predispose to this disease. From 2013 onward, 21 patients (15 males) with severe dermatophytosis and autosomal recessive CARD9 deficiency were reported [11, 29–37]. Most patients were born to known consanguineous unions and originated from Tunisia (4 patients), Algeria (11 patients), Iran (2 patients), Morocco (2 patients), Egypt (1 patient), and Italy (1 patient). Clinically, the lesions started in childhood with recurrent and extensive superficial lesions. In early adulthood, the patients developed extensive erythematous scaly lesions, subcutaneous nodules, or infiltrated ulcerated lesions and fistulae. Lesions were refractory to antifungal treatment and recurrent (Fig. 5.2). Histology evidenced deep dermatophytosis in most patients with dermal invasion by granuloma and hyphae. Numerous eosinophils were present in granuloma. Elevated IgE level and peripheral hypereosinophilia were also reported in most patients [11]. Patients (17/21) displayed typical lesions of tinea corporis (ringworm) and onychomycosis (15/21). Chronic

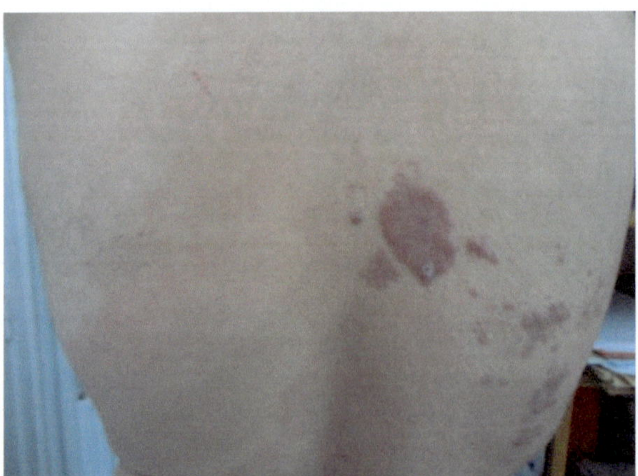

Fig. 5.2 Deep dermatophytosis in a patient with autosomal recessive CARD9 deficiency (On the courtesy of Dr. Boussofara Lobna ép Hadda Service de Dermatologie CHU Farhat Hached Sousse Tunisie)

mucocutaneous candidiasis was associated in 40% of patients. The most frequently isolated dermatophyte species were *T. violaceum* and *T. rubrum.* Lymph node involvement was present in 10 patients, organ involvement by contiguity in 2 patients, and central nervous system (CNS) dermatophytosis in one. Lesions relapsed after discontinuation of antifungal treatment. Median age at first symptoms was 8 (2–21) years [38]. Patients required lifelong anti-dermatophyte maintenance therapy with antifungal treatment. Mortality rate was high (23.5%); four patients with clinically active deep dermatophytosis died at the ages of 28, 29, 37, and 39 years. Bacterial, viral, and mycobacterial infections were not reported in CARD9-deficient patients. However, other invasive fungal infections were reported in AR CARD9-deficient patients as phaeohyphomycosis [39–41], CNS candidiasis [42–44], and *Candida* colitis [45]. Autosomal recessive CARD9 deficiency is therefore associated with a susceptibility to persistent and/or severe fungal infections, with frequent CNS involvement. These clinical data led to evidence that CARD9 has a major role in neutrophil trafficking into CNS after *Candida* infection [46].

5.2.2 AD STAT1 Gain of Function

Signal transducer and activator of transcription (STAT) are a family protein from which *STAT1* is a key transcription factor mediating IFN signaling. *STAT1* deficiency and autosomal dominant gain of *STAT1* activity predispose to different infectious profile [47, 48].

Autosomal dominant *STAT1* gain of functions (GOF) is the most common genetic cause of inherited chronic mucocutaneous candidiasis due to an inhibition of the development of IL-17-producing T cells and is not restricted to a specific group of population [47, 49]. These mutations underlie a variety of infectious manifestations. Most patients display mucocutaneous candidiasis. They also suffer from bacterial infections of the respiratory tract and the skin, mostly due to *Staphylococcus aureus* and viral infections of the skin, mostly due to Herpesviridae [50].

Dermatophytosis was reported in 14% of patients with *STAT1* GOF mutations [51]. In an international cohort of 274 patients with genetically and biochemically confirmed *STAT1* GOF mutations [50], superficial dermatophytosis (skin mainly or scalp or nails) was suspected in 44 (16%) patients (28 males and 16 women) and microbiologically confirmed in 52% of these patients, with *T. rubrum* (major species), *T. interdigitale*, *T. mentagrophytes*, or *Microsporum* spp. Three cases of severe dermatophytosis were reported in patients with *STAT1* GOF mutations [49, 52].

5.2.3 AD STAT3 Deficiency

Autosomal dominant deficiency of signal transducer and activator of transcription 3 (STAT3) is the main genetic etiology of hyper-immunoglobulin (Ig) E syndrome, a complex primary immunodeficiency [53]. In a French cohort of 60 patients [54], mucocutaneous infections (*Staphylococcus* sp., *Candida* sp.) were the most frequent. Patients had chronic mucocutaneous candidiasis of various mucosal sites and nails. Superficial dermatophytosis was only reported in two patients and due to *Trichophyton rubrum* and *T. mentagrophytes* (identified in one patient each).

5.2.4 Keratitis-Ichthyosis-Deafness Syndrome

Keratitis-ichthyosis-deafness (KID) syndrome is a rare hereditary cornification disorder resulting from mutations in connexin 26, a protein important for intercellular communication. This disorder is characterized by vascularizing keratitis, hyperkeratotic skin lesions, and hearing loss. Less than 100 cases have been described so far. The cutaneous manifestations include erythrokeratoderma present at birth, and complications are recurrent infections, sometimes with fatal septicemia and an increased risk of mucosal carcinomas. Some patients were reported to develop extensive dermatophytosis [55].

To our knowledge, no cases of severe dermatophytosis were reported in other primary immunodeficiencies.

5.3 Severe Dermatophytosis Treatment in Primary Immunodeficiency

Systemic antifungals with an in vitro activity against dermatophytes are griseofulvin, terbinafine, ketoconazole, fluconazole, itraconazole, posaconazole, voriconazole, ravuconazole, and isavuconazole [56, 57]. Terbinafine has advantage of good penetration in stratum corneum [58].

The first choice for superficial dermatophytosis treatment is an antifungal topical treatment such as azole or terbinafine in a suitable galenic form according to the infected site (nails, scalp, foot, or skin). In case of proximal subungual, dystrophic onychomycosis, failure, or relapse, a systemic treatment is recommended. In case of superficial dermatophytosis in immunocompromised patients, systemic treatment can be discussed; however, drug interaction with azoles can be an issue [59]. Topical treatment must always be associated with oral antifungals.

Severe dermatophytosis is rare and poorly described; therefore, scarce data on their treatment are available, only based on case reports [11, 16, 35]. In reported cases, first-line treatment was either terbinafine or triazoles such as posaconazole or itraconazole. In patients with severe dermatophytosis without PID, systemic treatment resulted in resolution in few months, and recurrences or relapses were rare [14].

By contrast, severe dermatophytosis associated with AR CARD9 deficiency responded slowly to antifungal treatment and frequently relapsed. Therefore, antifungal anti-dermatophyte therapy should be maintained throughout life.

Moreover, rebound effect upon discontinuation of antifungal therapy has been observed [11]. In the series reporting 17 patients with AR CARD9 deficiency, patients received griseofulvin, itraconazole, voriconazole, posaconazole, or fluconazole, and four patients died [11]. Dermatophytic lesions rarely completely disappeared, even when patients were treated with new azoles. None of the four patients who died received new azole treatment. One recent report described failure of systemic itraconazole, ketoconazole, terbinafine hydrochloride, topical ketoconazole, and ciclopirox olamine, in an Egyptian CARD9-deficient patient with *Trichophyton rubrum* extensive infection (abdomen, back, gluteal region, lower limbs and nails). Only posaconazole during 8 months allowed a complete clinical remission [35]. Terbinafine, itraconazole or posaconazole alone or in combination seem the best options to treat dermatophytosis in CARD9-deficient patients. Lifelong treatment is mandatory to prevent relapses.

5.4 Conclusion

In conclusion, dermatophytes are responsible of worldwide common and frequent superficial benign infections in the general population. In contrast, severe infections (extensive or invasive dermatophytosis) are rare, with unusually extensive lesions or dermis invasion, occurring in immunocompromised patients. However, benign and even severe forms of dermatophytosis are probably still neglected and underdiagnosed. The identification and the molecular, cellular, and clinical description of patients with inborn errors of immunity and susceptibility to dermatophytosis should help in better understanding the physiopathological mechanisms underlying dermatophytosis. An increasing number of cases with severe dermatophytosis are reported in the literature. Indeed, patients receiving immunosuppressive therapies, treated with long-term corticosteroids and infected with HIV or organ transplant recipients, develop severe dermatophytosis with dermis invasion or extensive form. However, the disease is not as serious or difficult to treat as in patients with autosomal recessive CARD9 deficiency. Severe dermatophytosis in a patient without underlying disease must lead to screen the patient for CARD9 deficiency.

Acknowledgment The authors would like to acknowledge Lobna Boussofara and Mohamed Denguezli, Service de Dermatologie, CHU Farhat Hached, Sousse, Tunisie, for providing pictures, and Gregory Jouvion and Fabrice Chretien, Institut Pasteur, Unité d'histopathologie humaine et modèles animaux, Paris, France, for histopathology analysis.

This research is supported by grants from Institut National de la Santé et de la Recherche Médicale (INSERM), University Paris Descartes, PRES Sorbonne Paris Cité, DGOS (Direction Générale de l'Offre de Soins), the French National Research Agency (ANR) ((grant n°ANR-14-CE15-0006-HGDIFD) under the "Investissement d'avenir" program (grant n°ANR-10-IAHU-01)) and Laboratoire d'Excellence Integrative Biology of Emerging Infectious Diseases (ANR-10-LABX-62-IBEID).

References

1. Stiller M, Klein W, Dorman R, Rosenthal S. Tinea corporis gladiatorum: an epidemic of trichophyton tonsurans in student wrestlers. J Am Acad Dermatol. 1992;27:632–3.
2. Wagner D, Sohnle P. Cutaneous defenses against dermatophytes and yeasts. Clin Microbiol Rev. 1995;8:317–35.
3. Havlickova B, Czaika V, Friedrich M. Epidemiological trends in skin mycoses worldwide. Mycoses. 2008;51:2–15.
4. Ameen M. Epidemiology of superficial fungal infections. Clin Dermatol. 2010;28:197–201.
5. Gupta A, Gupta G, Jain H, Lynde C, Foley K, Daigle D, Cooper E, Summerbell R. The prevalence of unsuspected onychomycosis and its causative organisms in a multicentre canadian sample of 30 000 patients visiting physicians' offices. *J Eur Acad Dermatol Venereol.* 2016;30:1567.
6. Hay R, Johns N, Williams H, Bolliger I, Dellavalle R, Margolis D, Marks R, Naldi L, Weinstock M, Wulf S, et al. The global burden of skin disease in 2010: an analysis of the prevalence and impact of skin conditions. J Invest Dermatol. 2014;134:1527–34.
7. Zurita J, Hay R. Adherence of dermatophyte microconidia and arthroconidia to human keratinocytes in vitro. J Invest Dermatol. 1987;89:529–34.
8. Baldo A, Monod M, Mathy A, Cambier L, Bagut E, Defaweux V, Symoens F, Antoine N, Mignon B. Mechanisms of skin adherence and invasion by dermatophytes. Mycoses. 2012;55:218–23.
9. Venturini J, Alvares A, Camargo M, Marchetti C, Fraga-Silva T, Luchini A, Arruda M. Dermatophyte-host relationship of a murine model of experimental invasive dermatophytosis. Microbes Infect. 2012;14:1144–51.
10. Hay R, Baran R. Deep dermatophytosis: rare infections or common, but unrecognised, complications of lymphatic spread? Curr Opin Infect Dis. 2004;17:77–9.
11. Lanternier F, Pathan S, Vincent Q, Liu L, Cypowyj S, Prando C, Migaud M, Taibi L, Ammar-Khodja A, Boudghene Stambouli O, et al. Deep dermatophytosis and inherited card9 deficiency. N Engl J Med. 2013;369:1704–14.
12. Hay R, Baran R. Onychomycosis: a proposed revision of the clinical classification. J Am Acad Dermatol. 2011;65:1219–27.
13. Inaoki M, Nishijima C, Miyake M, Asaka T, Hasegawa Y, Anzawa K, Mochizuki T. Case of dermatophyte abscess caused by trichophyton rubrum: a case report and review of the literature. Mycoses. 2015;58:318–23.
14. Marconi V, Kradin R, Marty F, Hospenthal D, Kotton C. Disseminated dermatophytosis in a patient with hereditary hemochromatosis and hepatic cirrhosis: case report and review of the literature. Med Mycol. 2010;48:518–27.
15. Rouzaud C, Scemla A, Anglicheau D, Fraitag S, Dupin N, Chosidow O, Bouaziz J, Longvert C, Hantz V, Bougnoux M, et al. Severe dermatophytoses in solid organ transplant recipients: about 6 cases and literature review. ECMID 2015.
16. Rouzaud C, Hay R, Chosidow O, Dupin N, Puel A, Lortholary O, Lanternier F. Severe dermatophytosis and acquired or innate immunodeficiency: a review. J Fungi. 2016;2:4.
17. Engelhardt K, Grimbacher B. Mendelian traits causing susceptibility to mucocutaneous fungal infections in human subjects. J Allergy Clin Immunol. 2012;129:294–305.
18. García-Romero M, Arenas R. New insights into genes, immunity, and the occurrence of dermatophytosis. J Invest Dermatol. 2015;135:655–7.
19. Nakamura T, Nishibu A, Yasoshima M, Tanoue C, Yoshida N, Hatta J, Miyamoto T, Nishii M, Yanagibashi T, Nagai Y, et al. Analysis of trichophyton antigen-induced contact hypersensitivity in mouse. J Dermatol Sci. 2012;66:144–53.
20. Sato K, Yang X, Yudate T, Chung J, Wu J, Luby-Phelps K, Kimberly R, Underhill D, Cruz PJ, Ariizumi K. Dectin-2 is a pattern recognition receptor for fungi that couples with the fc

receptor gamma chain to induce innate immune responses. J Biol Chem. 2006;281:38854–66.
21. Santiago K, Bomfim G, Criado P, Almeida S. Monocyte-derived dendritic cells from patients with dermatophytosis restrict the growth of trichophyton rubrum and induce cd4-t cell activation. PloS One. 2014;9(11):e110879.
22. Jaradat S, Cubillos S, Krieg N, Lehmann K, Issa B, Piehler S, Wehner-Diab S, Hipler U, Norgauer J. Low defb4 copy number and high systemic hbd-2 and il-22 levels are associated with dermatophytosis. J Invest Dermatol. 2015;135:750–8.
23. Cambier L, Weatherspoon A, Defaweux V, Bagut E, Heinen M, Antoine N, Mignon B. Assessment of the cutaneous immune response during arthroderma benhamiae and a. Vanbreuseghemii infection using an experimental mouse model. Br J Dermatol. 2014;170:625–33.
24. Campos M, Russo M, Gomes E, Almeida S. Stimulation, inhibition and death of macrophages infected with trichophyton rubrum. Microbes Infect. 2006;8:372–9.
25. Calderon R, Hay R. Cell-mediated immunity in experimental murine dermatophytosis. Ii. Adoptive transfer of immunity to dermatophyte infection by lymphoid cells from donors with acute or chronic infections. Immunology. 1984;53:465–72.
26. Kaya T, Eskandari G, Guvenc U, Gunes G, Tursen U, Burak Cimen M, Ikizoglu G. Cd4+cd25+ treg cells in patients with toenail onychomycosis. Arch Dermatol Res. 2009;301:725–9.
27. Gazendam R, van Hamme J, Tool A, van Houdt M, Verkuijlen P, Herbst M, Liese J, van de Veerdonk F, Roos D, van den Berg T, et al. Two independent killing mechanisms of *Candida albicans* by human neutrophils: evidence from innate immunity defects. Blood. 2014;124:590–7.
28. Yamamoto H, Nakamura Y, Sato K, Takahashi Y, Nomura T, Miyasaka T, Ishii K, Hara H, Yamamoto N, Kanno E, et al. Defect of card9 leads to impaired accumulation of gamma interferon-producing memory phenotype t cells in lungs and increased susceptibility to pulmonary infection with *Cryptococcus neoformans*. Infect Immun. 2014;82:1606–15.
29. Boudghène-Stambouli O, Mérad-Boudia A, Allal M. Cerebral injury in dermatophytic disease. J Mycol Med. 1992;2:106–8.
30. Boudghène-Stambouli O, Mérad- Boudia A. Trichophyton rubrum dermatophytic disease: a new case. Ann Dermatol Venereol. 1989;116:725–7.
31. Boudghène-Stambouli O, Mérad- Boudia A. Antifungal agents in dermato-phytic disease: failure of griseofulvin, ketoconazole and itraconazole. Bull Soc Pathol Exot. 1990;83:170–6.
32. Boudghène-Stambouli O, Mérad- Boudia A. Dermatophytic disease in algeria: a new case and review of the literature. Ann Dermatol Venereol. 1991;118:17–21.
33. Boudghène-Stambouli O, Mérad- Boudia A. Dermatophytic disease: exuberant hyperkeratosis with cutaneous horns. Ann Dermatol Venereol. 1998;125:705–7.
34. Grumach A, de Queiroz-Telles F, Migaud M, Lanternier F, Filho NR, Palma S, Constantino-Silva R, Casanova J, Puel A. A homozygous card9 mutation in a brazilian patient with deep dermatophytosis. J Clin Immunol. 2015;35:486–90.
35. Jachiet M, Lanternier F, Rybojad M, Bagot M, Ibrahim L, Casanova J, Puel A, Bouaziz J. Extensive skin and nail dermatophytosis due to autosomal recessive card9 deficiency in an egyptian patient cured with posaconazole. J Am Acad Dermatol. 2015;151:192–4.
36. Pruszkowski A, Bourgault Villada I, Cremer G, Ammar-Khodja A, Emilie D, Revuz J. Dermatophytic disease: role of type tc2 cd8 lymphocytes. Ann Dermatol Venereol. 1995;122:1–55.
37. Glocker E, Hennigs A, Nabavi M, Schäffer A, Woellner C, Salzer U, Pfeifer D, Veelken H, Warnatz K, Tahami F, et al. A homozygous card9 mutation in a family with susceptibility to fungal infections. N Engl J Med. 2009;361:1727–35.

38. Pilmis B, Puel A, Lortholary O, Lanternier F. New clinical phenotypes of fungal infections in special hosts. Clin Microbiol Infect. 2016;22:681.
39. Wang X, Wang W, Lin Z, Wang X, Li T, Yu J, Liu W, Tong Z, Xu Y, Zhang J, et al. Card9 mutations linked to subcutaneous phaeohyphomycosis and th17 cell deficiencies. J Allergy Clin Immunol. 2014;133:905–8.
40. Yan X, Yu C, Fu X, Bao F, Du D, Wang C, Wang N, Wang S, Shi Z, Zhou G, et al. Card9 mutation linked to corynespora cassiicola infection in a chinese patient. Br J Dermatol. 2016;174:174–9.
41. Lanternier F, Barbati E, Meinzer U, Liu L, Pedergnana V, Migaud M, Héritier S, Chomton M, Frémond M, Gonzales E, et al. Inherited card9 deficiency in 2 unrelated patients with invasive exophiala infection. J Infect Dis. 2015;211:1241–50.
42. Fernandez M, Moylett E, Noyola D, Baker C. Candidal meningitis in neonates: a 10-year review. Clin Infect Dis. 2000;31:458–63.
43. Chaussade H, Chandenier J, Bernard L, Cazals X, Gruson B, Bougnoux M, Jouvion G, Lortholary O, Lanternier F. Étude rétrospective nationale sur les infections du système nerveux central à Candida. Med Mal Infect. 2016;46(4 Suppl 1):68.
44. Gavino C, Hamel N, Zeng J, Legault C, Guiot M, Chankowsky J, Lejtenyi D, Lemire M, Alarie I, Dufresne S, et al. Impaired rasgrf1/erk-mediated gm-csf response characterizes card9 deficiency in french-canadians. J Allergy Clin Immunol. 2016;137:1178–88.
45. Lanternier F, Mahdaviani S, Barbati E, Chaussade H, Koumar Y, Levy R, Denis B, Brunel A, Martin S, Loop M, et al. Inherited card9 deficiency in otherwise healthy children and adults with candida species-induced meningoencephalitis, colitis, or both. J Allergy Clin Immunol. 2015;135:1558–68.
46. Drummond R, Collar A, Swamydas M, Rodriguez C, Lim J, Mendez L, Fink D, Hsu A, Zhai B, Karauzum H, et al. Card9-dependent neutrophil recruitment protects against fungal invasion of the central nervous system. PLoS Pathol. 2015;11:12.
47. Liu L, Okada S, Kong X, Kreins A, Cypowyj S, Abhyankar A, Toubiana J, Itan Y, Audry M, Nitschke P, et al. Gain-of-function human stat1 mutations impair il-17 immunity and underlie chronic mucocutaneous candidiasis. J Exp Med. 1635-1648;2011:208.
48. Boisson-Dupuis S, Kong X, Okada S, Cypowyj S, Puel A, Abel L, Casanova J. Inborn errors of human stat1: allelic heterogeneity governs the diversity of immunological and infectious phenotypes. Curr Opin Immunol. 2012;24:364–78.
49. van de Veerdonk F, Plantinga T, Hoischen A, Smeekens S, Joosten L, Gilissen C, Arts P, Rosentul D, Carmichael A, Smits-van der Graaf C, et al. Stat1 mutations in autosomal dominant chronic mucocutaneous candidiasis. N Engl J Med. 2011;365:54–61.
50. Toubiana J, Okada S, Hiller J, Oleastro M, Lagos Gomez M, Aldave Becerra J, Ouachée-Chardin M, Fouyssac F, Girisha K, Etzioni A, et al. Heterozygous stat1 gain-of-function mutations underlie an unexpectedly broad clinical phenotype: an international survey of 274 patients from 167 kindreds. *Blood.* 2016;127:3154.
51. Depner M, Fuchs S, Raabe J, Frede N, Glocker C, Doffinger R, Gkrania-Klotsas E, Kumararatne D, Atkinson T, Schroeder HJ, et al. The extended clinical phenotype of 26 patients with chronic mucocutaneous candidiasis due to gain-of-function mutations in stat1. J Clin Immunol. 2016;36:73–84.
52. Nielsen J, Kofod-Olsen E, Spaun E, Larsen C, Christiansen M, Mogensen T. A stat1-gain-of-function mutation causing th17 deficiency with chronic mucocutaneous candidiasis, psoriasiform hyperkeratosis and dermatophytosis. BMJ Case Rep 2015;22. doi:10.1136/bcr-2015-211372.
53. Holland S, DeLeo F, Elloumi H, Hsu A, Uzel G, Brodsky N, Freeman A, Demidowich A, Davis J, Turner M, et al. Stat3 mutations in the hyper-ige syndrome. N Engl J Med. 2007;357:1608–19.
54. Chandesris M, Melki I, Natividad A, Puel A, Fieschi C, Yun L, Thumerelle C, Oksenhendler E, Boutboul D, Thomas C, et al. Autosomal dominant stat3 deficiency and hyper-ige syndrome: molecular, cellular, and clinical features from a french national survey. Medicine (Baltimore). 2012;91:1–19.

55. Machan M, Kestenbaum T, Fraga G. Diffuse hyperkeratosis in a deaf and blind 48-year-old woman – quiz case. Diagnosis: keratitis-ichthyosis-deafness (kid) syndrome with secondary dermatophytosis. Arch Dermatol. 2012;148:1199–200.
56. Badali H, Mohammadi R, Mashedi O, de Hoog G, Meis J. In vitro susceptibility patterns of clinically important trichophyton and epidermophyton species against nine antifungal drugs. Mycoses. 2015;58:303–7.
57. Gupta A, Kohli Y, Batra R. In vitro activities of posaconazole, ravuconazole, terbinafine, itraconazole and fluconazole against dermatophyte, yeast and non-dermatophyte species. Med Mycol. 2005;43:179–85.
58. Gupta A, Prussick R, Sibbald R, Knowles S. Terbinafine in the treatment of majocchi's granuloma. Int J Dermatol. 1995;34:489.
59. Virgili A, Zampino M, Mantovani L. Fungal skin infections in organ transplant recipients. Am J Clin Dermatol. 2002;3:19–35.

Genetic Determinants of Host Susceptibility to Fungal Diseases in Solid Organ Transplantation and Hematological Patients

6

Agnieszka Wójtowicz, Frédéric Lamoth, and Pierre-Yves Bochud

Abstract

Invasive fungal infections caused by Aspergillus and Candida species represent a major threat in oncohematological patients as well as hematopoietic stem cell and solid organ transplant recipient. Novel strategies are needed to identify patients who are most likely to develop such infections and would benefit the most from targeted antifungal prophylaxis. After initial studies revealed that polymorphisms in immune genes can influence susceptibility to invasive aspergillosis among immunocompromised patients, the concept emerged that the risk to develop invasive aspergillosis could be stratified according to individual genetic risk profiles. Such genetic polymorphisms may be used in the future as part of a scoring system of risk that would include a combination of demographic, clinical and biological indicators.

A. Wójtowicz • P.-Y. Bochud (✉)
Infectious Diseases Service, Department of Medicine, University Hospital (CHUV) and University of Lausanne, Lausanne, Switzerland
e-mail: Agnieszka.Wojtowicz@chuv.ch; Pierre-Yves.Bochud@chuv.ch

F. Lamoth
Infectious Diseases Service, Department of Medicine, University Hospital (CHUV) and University of Lausanne, Lausanne, Switzerland

Institute of Microbiology, University Hospital (CHUV) and University of Lausanne, Lausanne, Switzerland
e-mail: Frederic.Lamoth@chuv.ch

A. Carvalho (ed.), *Immunogenetics of Fungal Diseases*,
DOI 10.1007/978-3-319-50842-9_6

6.1 Introduction

Invasive fungal infections (IFIs) caused by *Aspergillus* and *Candida* species represent a major threat in onco-hematological patients as well as hematopoietic stem cell (HSCT) and solid organ transplant (SOT) recipient.

Aspergillus fumigatus and other *Aspergillus* spp. (*A. flavus*, *A. terreus*, *A. niger*) are ubiquitous molds that are responsible for invasive opportunistic infections in severely immunocompromised patients. The incidence of invasive aspergillosis (IA) is estimated 1–10% in SOT recipient, acute leukemia patients, and HSCT recipients [21, 37, 44, 51, 55], but incidence rates can differ among centers due to the use of different conditioning regimen, antifungal prophylaxis, and other management strategies. The overall mortality of patients with IA has slightly declined over the last decades, probably due to improvement in the diagnostic and treatment, but remains unacceptably high (estimated 20–40%) [3, 42, 64, 69].

Candida albicans and other *Candida* spp. (*C. tropicalis*, *C. glabrata*, *C. krusei*, *C. parapsilosis*) represent a genus of yeast that usually causes only superficial infections among immunocompetent patients. Invasive infections mainly occur in patients hospitalized for extended periods of time and are favored by the use of antibacterial agents and central venous catheters. The most common forms of invasive candidiasis (IC) include candidemia, peritonitis (patients with complicated abdominal surgery and/or pancreatitis), and hepatosplenic candidiasis (onco-hematological patients with prolonged neutropenia).

Three antifungal drug classes are currently available for the treatment of IFI, the polyenes (amphotericin B), the azoles (fluconazole, itraconazole, voriconazole, posaconazole, and isavuconazole), and the echinocandins (caspofungin, micafungin, anidulafungin). Amphotericin B has broad-spectrum fungicidal activity, but its use is limited by toxicity, although new lipid formulations are better tolerated. Voriconazole has become the first-line treatment of IA [38]. However, emergence of pan-azole resistance among *Aspergillus fumigatus* isolates as a consequence of the widespread use of fungicides in agriculture and industry is a concern [73]. Echinocandins have limited antifungal activity against *Aspergillus* spp. but have become the first-line treatment of IC with possibility to step down to fluconazole after a few days [19]. However, emergence of resistance to echinocandins among *Candida* spp. is increasingly reported [2], and a shift of the epidemiology of IC toward yeasts other than *C. albicans* with decreased susceptibility to fluconazole and/or echinocandins is also observed [54, 56].

In order to prevent the occurrence of IFI, antifungal prophylaxis, such as daily posaconazole in high-risk onco-hematological patients or fluconazole in ICU patients, has become a common approach [19, 20, 70]. While such strategies have been associated with reduction in the incidence of IFIs, they are not selective and unnecessarily expose a large number of patients to antifungals, with associated toxicity and important costs. Furthermore, there is concern about the possible emergence of fungal pathogens with decreased antifungal susceptibility profile. More selective strategies, such as empiric or preemptive treatments, have been proposed and still need further validation to demonstrate their efficacy [10, 18].

A novel approach would consist in targeted antifungal prophylaxis based on the individual host susceptibility profile. A number of risk factors have been identified, such as the duration and severity of neutropenia, the number and type of immunosuppressive drugs, the type of induction therapy for leukemia and/or hematopoietic cell transplantation, and the type of HSCT (HLA mismatch, presence/absence of T cell depletion) and concomitant infections due to CMV and/or other viruses [31, 51, 72, 67]. Yet, most patients are exposed to several risk factors at the same time, so that it is virtually impossible to individually stratify the risk of IFIs. Novel strategies are needed to refine our understanding of individual immunosuppression profiles and identify patients who are most likely to develop such infections.

6.2 Genetic Association Studies: Focus on Candidate Gene Approach

Over the last decades, an increasing number of investigators have suggested that host genetic polymorphism influences susceptibility to infections in immunocompromised patients. Susceptibility to infectious diseases is often considered to result from two types of inheritance, i.e., monogenic (Mendelian) or polygenic (complex) inheritance. Primary immunodeficiencies are classically considered to result from "monogenic inheritance," as they are often due to a single, rare mutation (point mutation, deletion, insertion, inversion, duplication, translocation, amplifications) in genes that have a strong impact on immunity, leading to a clear-cut phenotype. These include difficult-to-treat forms of infections caused by a common fungal pathogen (i.e., chronic mucocutaneous candidiasis, Chap. 3) or infections due to an opportunistic pathogen (i.e., invasive aspergillosis due to chronic granulomatous diseases, Chap. 4).

Susceptibility to common infections in the general population is usually considered as a complex phenomenon involving both host and environmental factors, including exposure to a specific pathogen. Invasive fungal infections usually occur in previously healthy individuals who are immunosuppressed at a specific time of their life. Yet, despite similar immunosuppression patterns, some individuals rapidly develop IFIs, while others do not. These differences may result from the presence of several polymorphisms in immune genes (complex inheritance). Because of the implication of numerous environmental risk factors, the identification of polymorphisms influencing susceptibility to infections in immunosuppressed patients requires an exhaustive and refined analysis of all clinical risk factors that can influence the phenotype. Otherwise immunocompetent individuals can become immunosuppressed as a result from intensive chemotherapy (e.g., for the treatment of onco-hematological diseases) or from the use of immunomodulatory drugs (e.g., to prevent organ rejection after transplantation or graft versus host disease). Such immunosuppressive states are iatrogenic and may not have been mimicked by environmental conditions during human evolution. Therefore, immunocompromised patients represent a particularly interesting group for immunogenetic studies of susceptibility to infections.

Complex genetic traits can be studied by performing linkage analysis or association studies, such as candidate gene and genome-wide association (GWA) approaches [4, 5]. A candidate gene approach is widely used to study the correlation between single nucleotide polymorphisms (SNPs) and common disease phenotypes. It is based on the "a priori" hypothesis that the gene and its polymorphisms are implicated in disease pathogenesis. SNPs in candidate genes are anticipated to influence the gene function (may lead to gene transcription, RNA splicing, mRNA stability, mRNA translation, protein change, folding, or gene deletion) or to tag another SNP or phased combination of SNPs (haplotype) that exert this function. This approach gives a higher plausibility to discover markers that have some impact on disease phenotype. However it is often restricted by low reproducibility and possibility to miss biologically relevant variants. On the contrary, the GWAS approach is designed to study thousands of SNPs at the genome-wide level and to determine their impact on disease phenotypes, without an "a priori" hypothesis [4] (see Chap. 8).

Over the past 10 years, we identified around 30 candidate gene studies assessing the risk of IFI in immunocompromised patients (Table 6.1). Genes were mostly selected within the innate immune system and include pattern recognition receptors (PRRs), downstream signaling molecules, cytokines and chemokines released by effector cells, antimicrobial peptides, as well as other molecules (see Chap. 2) [76]. The studies reporting associations with polymorphisms in these genes are heterogeneous in terms of patients (onco-hematological patients, hematopoietic stem cell, and solid organ transplant recipients), ethnic groups (not always defined), case definitions, type of controls (not always undergoing the same risk pattern as cases), sample size (dozens to hundreds cases and controls), and statistical approaches (case-control, Kaplan-Meier cumulative incidence/survival models). A major issue results from the lack of a clear list of polymorphisms that have been tested, pretest power to detect an association (based on the number of patients and allele frequencies), and lack of correction for multiple testing. The heterogeneity of studies together with their limitations has complicated the interpretation of results, so that genetic polymorphisms have not been used so far in the clinical practice for individual risk stratification. Yet, some studies are more promising, because their results have been validated and/or are supported by convincing evidence for a functional role in antifungal immunity (Table 6.2).

The first immunogenetic studies of susceptibility to IA were performed among allogenic HSCT recipients. Allogenic HSCT represents an unusual situation, because recipients are chimerical individuals carrying circulating immune cells from the donor, while other cells possibly involved in the immune response against the pathogen, such as lung epithelial cells, are issued from recipient. Therefore, it can be questioned whether polymorphisms conferring susceptibility to IFIs are issued from the donor or the recipient. In fact, some studies reported evidence that polymorphisms in immune genes from the donor and/or the recipient can influence susceptibility to IA in the recipients (Table 6.1).

Table 6.1 Polymorphisms associated with invasive aspergillosis in onco-hematological or transplant patients

Gene	HSCT donor		HSCT recipient		SOT recipient		Acute leukemia	
	Variant	Studies	Variant	Studies	Variant	Studies	Variant	Studies
Pattern recognition receptor genes								
PTX3	rs2305619	[22]			rs2305619	[25, 78]		
	rs3816527				rs3816527			
CLEC7A (dectin-1)	rs16910526	[15, 23]	rs16910526	[23]			rs7309123	[60]
							rs3901533	
TLR4	rs4986790	[6, 26, 43]	rs4986790	[11]				
	rs4986791		rs4986791					
TLR1			rs5743611	[41]				
			rs4833095					
TLR6			rs5743810	[41]				
TLR3	rs3775296	[13]						
TLR5			rs5744168	[36]				
DC-SIGN (CD209)							rs4804800	[60]
							rs11465384	
							rs7248637	
							rs7252229	
MBL	rs5030737	[34]	rs5030737	[50]				
	rs1800450		rs1800450					
	rs1800451		rs1800451					
			rs11003125					
			rs7095891					
			rs7096206					

(continued)

Table 6.1 (continued)

Gene	HSCT donor		HSCT recipient		SOT recipient		Acute leukemia	
	Variant	Studies	Variant	Studies	Variant	Studies	Variant	Studies
Cytokine/chemokine, their receptors or natural antagonist genes								
IL1B					rs16944	[77]	rs1143627	[61]
IL1RN					rs419598	[77]	VNTR2	[61]
IL1A							rs1800587	[61]
IL10			rs1800896	[66]			rs1800896	[59]
			rs1800871				rs1800871	
			rs1800872				rs1800872	
IL4							rs2243250	[17]
							rs2070874	
							rs2243248	
IL4R			rs2107356	[45]				
IL23R	rs11209026	[12]						
IFNG			rs2069705	[45]				
TNFR1							rs4149570	[63]
TNFR2							VNTR at −322	[62]
CXCL10	rs3921	[48]						
	rs1554013							
	rs4257674							
Other genes								
MASP2			rs72550870	[34]				
RAGE	rs1800624	[24]	rs1800624	[24]				
S100B	rs9722	[24]						

Gene	HSCT donor		HSCT recipient		SOT recipient		Acute leukemia	
	Variant	Studies	Variant	Studies	Variant	Studies	Variant	Studies
PLG			rs4252125	[79]				
DEFB1					rs1800972	[77]		
VEGFA			rs3024994	[45]				

CLEC7A C-type lectin domain 7 (known as dectin-1), *CXCL10* CXC-chemokine ligand-10, *DC-SIGN* dendritic cell-specific intercellular adhesion molecule-3-grabbing non-integrin (known as CD209), *DEFB1* β-defensin 1, *HSCT* hematopoietic stem cell transplant, *IL* interleukin, *IL1RN* interleukin-1 receptor antagonist, *IL4R* interleukin-4 receptor, *IL23R* interleukin-23 receptor, *IFNG* interferon gamma, *MASP2* mannan-binding lectin serine peptidase 2, *MBL* mannose-binding lectin, *PLG* plasminogen, *PTX3* pentraxin 3, *RAGE* advanced glycosylation end product-specific receptor (known as AGER), *S100B* S100 calcium-binding protein B, *SOT* solid organ transplant, *TNFR* tumor necrosis factor receptor, *TLR* toll-like receptor, *VEGFA* vascular endothelial growth factor A, *VNTR* variable number of tandem repeats

Table 6.2 Role of significant genes in immunity to invasive fungal infections

	Role in immunity to invasive fungal infections			Role of significant polymorphisms	
Protein	Function	Ligand	In vivo and ex vivo evidence	Risk allele(s)	In vitro or ex vivo effect of risk allele
Dectin-1 (CLEC7A)	PRR	β-glucan	Dectin-1 KO mice are susceptible to IA	238X	Leads to production of a truncated protein
	Promote innate and adaptive immune responses to fungi		Dectin-1 silencing in respiratory epithelial cells is associated with impaired *Aspergillus* driven pro-inflammatory responses		Associated with reduced dectin-1 expression on monocytes cell surface
					Associated with diminished production of IL-1β, IL-6, IFN-γ, IL-10, and IL-17A cytokines by PBMCs upon stimulation with *A. fumigatus*
TLR4	PRR	O-linked mannan	TLR4 KO showed increased fungal burden	299D[a]	Associated with hyporesponsiveness to endotoxin and impaired LPS-mediated signal transduction in monocytes
	Promote innate immune responses to fungi			399 T	
PTX3	Soluble PRR	Galactomannan	PTX3 KO mice are susceptible to IA	h2/h2	Associated with lower expression of PTX3 by neutrophil precursors upon exposure to *Aspergillus* most likely due to changes in mRNA folding
	Promote fungal		Administration of PTX3 helps to cure IA in vivo	Haplotype	Associated with reduced ability to phagocyte and kill *Aspergillus* conidia by neutrophils from IA patients
					Associated with reduced PTX3 levels in BAL and lung biopsies from patients with IA

	Role in immunity to invasive fungal infections			Role of significant polymorphisms	
Protein	Function	Ligand	In vivo and ex vivo evidence	Risk allele(s)	In vitro or ex vivo effect of risk allele
IL-1β	Key pro-inflammatory cytokine		Production of IL-1β upon recognizing *Aspergillus* results in the induction of T_H17 responses leading to an increased recruitment of neutrophils and monocytes, which is controlled by its natural receptor antagonist, IL1RA	−511T[a]	Associated with decreased production of IL-1β, TNF-α, and IL-22 by PBMCs upon stimulation with *Aspergillus*
	Involved in promoting both innate and adaptive responses to fungi			−33C	
			IL1RA KO mice are protected from IA		
			IL1R KO mice are highly susceptible to IA		

BAL bronchoalveolar lavage fluid, *CLEC7A* C-type lectin domain 7, *IA* invasive aspergillosis, *IL* interleukin, *IL1R* interleukin-1 receptor, *ILRA* interleukin-1 receptor antagonist, *IFN* interferon, *KO* knockout, *LPS* lipopolysaccharide, *PBMC* peripheral blood mononuclear cells, *PTX3* pentraxin 3, *PRR* pattern recognition receptor, *TLR* toll-like receptor, *TNF* tumor necrosis factor

[a]Both polymorphisms are in almost complete linkage disequilibrium

In a study of 336 HSCT patients [6], two SNPs in toll-like receptor 4 (TLR4, D299G, and T399I, both in strong linkage disequilibrium) in HSCT donors were associated with an increased risk of IA in the corresponding recipient [6]. These observations were confirmed by two groups of investigators [6, 26, 43]. However, they were not confirmed in two small studies of HSCT patient [11, 41]. TLR4 is a PRR that detects O-linked mannan, an important component of the fungal cell wall. The D299G TLR4 SNP has been associated with hyporesponsiveness to endotoxin and impaired lipopolysaccharide-mediated signal transduction in monocytes [1, 65]. While TLR4 has been clearly involved in host defense mechanisms against *Aspergillus* [8, 16, 47, 52, 53], the exact mechanism by which D299G and T399I polymorphisms influence immune response to *Aspergillus* has not been fully understood [71].

A polymorphism in dectin-1 (Y238X) present either in the donor or the recipient was associated with the risk to develop IA after HSCT [23]. Dectin-1 is a PRR that recognizes β-glucan [33, 68, 75] and is expressed at the surface of immune cells, including dendritic cells, macrophages and neutrophils, as well as epithelial cells. Dectin-1 plays a role in fungal phagocytosis and killing as well as in mediating inflammatory response to the fungi. Experiments using peripheral blood monocytes and lung alveolar cells suggest that dectin-1 can probably contribute to achieve protection against IA through cells of both the donor and recipient lineage [23]. In CD14+ monocytes, the risk allele (238X) is associated with a decline of surface dectin-1 expression [23]. In peripheral blood mononuclear cells (PBMCs) stimulated with *A. fumigatus* or β-glucan, the risk allele is associated with an impaired production of cytokines (IL-1β, IL-6, IFN-γ, IL-10, and IL-17A) compared to the wild-type allele [23]. Airway epithelial cells, stimulated with β-glucan or *A. fumigatus* conidia where dectin-1 is knocked down, show an impaired inflammatory cytokine production [23]. Further experimental evidence coming from mice models of IA supports a role of dectin-1 in both the donor and recipient of HSCT in immunity against *Aspergillus*. Recipient mice deficient in dectin-1 transplanted with hematopoietic cells from wild-type donor mice or dectin-1-deficient mice have expanded fungal growth and IL-17 production and reduced IFN-γ/IL-10 cytokine production after infection with *Aspergillus* [23]. The stop codon variant of dectin-1 (Y238X) was also associated with mucocutaneous *Candida* infection [28], but not disseminated candidiasis [57], suggesting that this PRR may be specific for mucosal anti-*Candida* defense rather than systemic infection [14].

Only a few studies investigated the role of genetic polymorphisms in patients other than HSCT recipients. Polymorphisms in the interleukin-1 (IL-1) cluster genes, in particular IL-1β -31T/C and/or -511C/T (which are in strong linkage disequilibrium), have been reported to increase susceptibility to IA in SOT recipients [77]. Similar results were reported in a study of acute leukemia patients [61]. The presence of -511T/C IL-1β SNP in HSCT recipients was however not associated with IA, but this study did not genotype the donors [26]. IL-1β is a key proinflammatory cytokine implicated in innate and adaptive antifungal immunity [9, 40, 74]. IL-1β produced by macrophages is crucial for recruitments of neutrophils and monocytes to the lungs during infection and clearing *Aspergillus* [49]. IL-1β induces T_H17 responses that are characterized by the production of IL-17, leading to an increased recruitment of neutrophils. Additionally, the activated T-helper cells induce IL-22 responses that will stimulate production of defensins by epithelial cells [35, 58]. Functionally, the presence of the minor allele -511C is associated with reduced *Aspergillus*-induced IL-1β production as well as TNF-α release by PBMCs, thereby leading to defective anti-*Aspergillus* immune responses [77]. The exact mechanism on how -31T/C and -511C/T polymorphisms regulate IL-1β levels is unknown. As both are located within promoter region of IL-1β gene, they could have an effect on promoter activity leading to decreased expression of IL-1β [27].

Finally, a haplotype within long pentraxin 3 (PTX3), a soluble PRR, recently emerged as particularly promising marker, because it was shown to influence susceptibility to IA in both HSCT and SOT recipients, two population that are exposed to different risks and environmental conditions. The haplotype at risk originates from the donor in HSCT [22] and from the recipient in SOT [25, 78]. Long PTX3 can exert different immune functions, including pathogen recognition, opsonization, phagocytosis, classical pathway of complement activation, and clearance of apoptotic cells [7, 29, 46]. Circulating PTX3 is able to bind *Aspergillus* conidia most likely by detecting galactomannan, thereby facilitating fungal recognition and phagocytosis by macrophages [30]. While PTX3 can be produced by several cells, such as dendritic cells, mononuclear phagocyte endothelial cells, and lung alveolar epithelial cells, neutrophils have the unique ability to store the molecule within granules that can be rapidly released in the circulation upon infection. Therefore, neutrophils probably represent an important source of PTX3 during IA. This may explain why the association in HSCT recipient was observed with the polymorphism in the donor, but not the recipient. The association of PTX3 haplotypes with IA is further supported by several experiments. The h2/h2 haplotype associated with increased susceptibility to IA carries two 281G and 734A SNPs that were shown to reduce PTX3 expression or production, possibly due to changes in mRNA folding [22]. The haplotype was associated with reduced phagocytic activity of neutrophils and their ability to kill *Aspergillus* conidia [22]. The role of PTX3 was confirmed in two models of IA (immunocompetent and neutropenic) using PTX3-deficient versus WT mice [30], as well as IA models of neutropenic or HSCT mice with/without complementation with soluble PTX3 [30] or PTX3-competent/deficient neutrophils [39], respectively. Besides, in vivo pharmacological studies revealed that administration of PTX3 is able to cure infection with *A. fumigatus,* revealing possibility to use it as potential mold-active therapeutic drug [32].

6.3 Conclusion

After initial studies revealed that polymorphisms in immune genes can influence susceptibility to IA among immunocompromised patients, the concept emerged that the risk to develop IA could be stratified according to individual genetic risk profiles. However, this concept has been challenged by several issues, including insufficient statistical power, heterogeneity among studies in terms of case definition, assessment of relevant co-variables and management strategies, and lack of replication and/or functional testing supporting reported associations. Even for those polymorphisms that have been largely validated, the predictive value alone will remain too low, as they only explain a small proportion of the susceptibility to IFIs. So far, PTX3 polymorphisms represent the most promising genetic markers for the risk of IA, because of their high frequency (thereby facilitating replication), the strong functional evidence supporting the association, and the fact that the genetic effect seems to overcome environmental factors, as suggested by an association replicated in patients presenting different types of immunosuppression. Altogether, genetic polymorphisms may be used in the future as part of a scoring system of risk that would include a combination of demographic, clinical, and biological indicators.

References

1. Arbour NC, Lorenz E, Schutte BC, Zabner J, Kline JN, Jones M, et al. TLR4 mutations are associated with endotoxin hyporesponsiveness in humans. Nat Genet. 2000;25(2):187–91. doi:10.1038/76048.
2. Arendrup MC, Perlin DS. Echinocandin resistance: an emerging clinical problem? Curr Opin Infect Dis. 2014;27(6):484–92. doi:10.1097/QCO.0000000000000111.
3. Baddley JW, Andes DR, Marr KA, Kontoyiannis DP, Alexander BD, Kauffman CA, et al. Factors associated with mortality in transplant patients with invasive aspergillosis. Clin Infect Dis: Off Publ Infect Dis Soc Am. 2010;50(12):1559–67. doi:10.1086/652768.
4. Bochud M. Genetics for clinicians: from candidate genes to whole genome scans (technological advances). Best Pract Res Clin Endocrinol Metab. 2012;26(2):119–32. doi:10.1016/j.beem.2011.09.001.
5. Bochud PY, Bochud M, Telenti A, Calandra T. Innate immunogenetics: a tool for exploring new frontiers of host defence. Lancet Infect Dis. 2007;7(8):531–42. doi:10.1016/S1473-3099(07)70185-8.
6. Bochud PY, Chien JW, Marr KA, Leisenring WM, Upton A, Janer M, et al. Toll-like receptor 4 polymorphisms and aspergillosis in stem-cell transplantation. N Engl J Med. 2008;359(17):1766–77. doi:10.1056/NEJMoa0802629.
7. Bottazzi B, Bastone A, Doni A, Garlanda C, Valentino S, Deban L, et al. The long pentraxin PTX3 as a link among innate immunity, inflammation, and female fertility. J Leukoc Biol. 2006;79(5):909–12. doi:10.1189/jlb.1005557.
8. Braedel S, Radsak M, Einsele H, Latge JP, Michan A, Loeffler J, et al. Aspergillus fumigatus antigens activate innate immune cells via toll-like receptors 2 and 4. Br J Haematol. 2004;125(3):392–9. doi:10.1111/j.1365-2141.2004.04922.x.
9. Caffrey AK, Lehmann MM, Zickovich JM, Espinosa V, Shepardson KM, Watschke CP, et al. IL-1alpha signaling is critical for leukocyte recruitment after pulmonary Aspergillus fumigatus challenge. PLoS Pathog. 2015;11(1):e1004625. doi:10.1371/journal.ppat.1004625.
10. Calandra T, Roberts JA, Antonelli M, Bassetti M, Vincent JL. Diagnosis and management of invasive candidiasis in the ICU: an updated approach to an old enemy. Crit Care. 2016;20(1):125. doi:10.1186/s13054-016-1313-6.
11. Carvalho A, Cunha C, Carotti A, Aloisi T, Guarrera O, Di Ianni M, et al. Polymorphisms in Toll-like receptor genes and susceptibility to infections in allogeneic stem cell transplantation. Exp Hematol. 2009;37(9):1022–9. doi:10.1016/j.exphem.2009.06.004.

12. Carvalho A, Cunha C, Di Ianni M, Pitzurra L, Aloisi T, Falzetti F, et al. Prognostic significance of genetic variants in the IL-23/Th17 pathway for the outcome of T cell-depleted allogeneic stem cell transplantation. Bone Marrow Transplant. 2010;45(11):1645–52. doi:10.1038/bmt.2010.28.
13. Carvalho A, De Luca A, Bozza S, Cunha C, D'Angelo C, Moretti S, et al. TLR3 essentially promotes protective class I-restricted memory CD8(+) T-cell responses to Aspergillus fumigatus in hematopoietic transplanted patients. Blood. 2012a;119(4):967–77. doi:10.1182/blood-2011-06-362582.
14. Carvalho A, Giovannini G, De Luca A, D'Angelo C, Casagrande A, Iannitti RG, et al. Dectin-1 isoforms contribute to distinct Th1/Th17 cell activation in mucosal candidiasis. Cell Mol Immunol. 2012b;9(3):276–86. doi:10.1038/cmi.2012.1.
15. Chai LY, de Boer MG, van der Velden WJ, Plantinga TS, van Spriel AB, Jacobs C, et al. The Y238X stop codon polymorphism in the human beta-glucan receptor dectin-1 and susceptibility to invasive aspergillosis. J Infect Dis. 2011;203(5):736–43. doi:10.1093/infdis/jiq102.
16. Chai LY, Kullberg BJ, Vonk AG, Warris A, Cambi A, Latge JP, et al. Modulation of Toll-like receptor 2 (TLR2) and TLR4 responses by Aspergillus fumigatus. Infect Immun. 2009;77(5):2184–92. doi:10.1128/IAI.01455-08.
17. Choi EH, Foster CB, Taylor JG, Erichsen HC, Chen RA, Walsh TJ, et al. Association between chronic disseminated candidiasis in adult acute leukemia and common IL4 promoter haplotypes. J Infect Dis. 2003;187(7):1153–6. doi:10.1086/368345.
18. Cordonnier C, Pautas C, Maury S, Vekhoff A, Farhat H, Suarez F, et al. Empirical versus preemptive antifungal therapy for high-risk, febrile, neutropenic patients: a randomized, controlled trial. Clin Infect Dis: Off Publ Infect Dis Soc Am. 2009;48(8):1042–51. doi:10.1086/597395.
19. Cornely OA, Bassetti M, Calandra T, Garbino J, Kullberg BJ, Lortholary O, et al. ESCMID* guideline for the diagnosis and management of Candida diseases 2012: non-neutropenic adult patients. Clin Microbiol Infect: Off Publ Eur Soc Clin Microbiol Infect Dis. 2012;18(Suppl 7):19–37. doi:10.1111/1469-0691.12039.
20. Cornely OA, Maertens J, Winston DJ, Perfect J, Ullmann AJ, Walsh TJ, et al. Posaconazole vs. fluconazole or itraconazole prophylaxis in patients with neutropenia. N Engl J Med. 2007;356(4):348–59. doi:10.1056/NEJMoa061094.
21. Corzo-Leon DE, Satlin MJ, Soave R, Shore TB, Schuetz AN, Jacobs SE, et al. Epidemiology and outcomes of invasive fungal infections in allogeneic haematopoietic stem cell transplant recipients in the era of antifungal prophylaxis: a single-centre study with focus on emerging pathogens. Mycoses. 2015;58(6):325–36. doi:10.1111/myc.12318.
22. Cunha C, Aversa F, Lacerda JF, Busca A, Kurzai O, Grube M, et al. Genetic PTX3 deficiency and aspergillosis in stem-cell transplantation. N Engl J Med. 2014;370(5):421–32. doi:10.1056/NEJMoa1211161.
23. Cunha C, Di Ianni M, Bozza S, Giovannini G, Zagarella S, Zelante T, et al. Dectin-1 Y238X polymorphism associates with susceptibility to invasive aspergillosis in hematopoietic transplantation through impairment of both recipient- and donor-dependent mechanisms of antifungal immunity. Blood. 2010;116(24):5394–402. doi:10.1182/blood-2010-04-279307.
24. Cunha C, Giovannini G, Pierini A, Bell AS, Sorci G, Riuzzi F, et al. Genetically-determined hyperfunction of the S100B/RAGE axis is a risk factor for aspergillosis in stem cell transplant recipients. PLoS ONE. 2011;6(11):e27962. doi:10.1371/journal.pone.0027962.
25. Cunha C, Monteiro AA, Oliveira-Coelho A, Kuhne J, Rodrigues F, Sasaki SD, et al. PTX3-based genetic testing for risk of aspergillosis after lung transplant. Clin Infect Dis: Off Publ Infect Dis Soc Am. 2015; doi:10.1093/cid/civ679.
26. de Boer MG, Jolink H, Halkes CJ, van der Heiden PL, Kremer D, Falkenburg JH, et al. Influence of polymorphisms in innate immunity genes on susceptibility to invasive aspergillosis after stem cell transplantation. PLoS ONE. 2011;6(4):e18403. doi:10.1371/journal.pone.0018403.

27. El-Omar EM, Carrington M, Chow WH, McColl KE, Bream JH, Young HA, et al. Interleukin-1 polymorphisms associated with increased risk of gastric cancer. Nature. 2000;404(6776):398–402. doi:10.1038/35006081.
28. Ferwerda B, Ferwerda G, Plantinga TS, Willment JA, van Spriel AB, Venselaar H, et al. Human dectin-1 deficiency and mucocutaneous fungal infections. N Engl J Med. 2009;361(18):1760–7. doi:10.1056/NEJMoa0901053.
29. Garlanda C, Bottazzi B, Salvatori G, De Santis R, Cotena A, Deban L, et al. Pentraxins in innate immunity and inflammation. Novartis Found Symp. 2006;279:80–6. discussion 6-91, 216-9
30. Garlanda C, Hirsch E, Bozza S, Salustri A, De Acetis M, Nota R, et al. Non-redundant role of the long pentraxin PTX3 in anti-fungal innate immune response. Nature. 2002;420(6912):182–6. doi:10.1038/nature01195.
31. Gavalda J, Meije Y, Fortun J, Roilides E, Saliba F, Lortholary O et al. Invasive fungal infections in solid organ transplant recipients. Clinical microbiology and infection : the official publication of the European Society of Clinical Microbiology and Infectious Diseases. 2014;20 Suppl 7:27–48. doi:10.1111/1469-0691.12660.
32. Gaziano R, Bozza S, Bellocchio S, Perruccio K, Montagnoli C, Pitzurra L, et al. Anti-Aspergillus fumigatus efficacy of pentraxin 3 alone and in combination with antifungals. Antimicrob Agents Chemother. 2004;48(11):4414–21. doi:10.1128/AAC.48.11.4414-4421.2004.
33. Gessner MA, Werner JL, Lilly LM, Nelson MP, Metz AE, Dunaway CW, et al. Dectin-1-dependent interleukin-22 contributes to early innate lung defense against Aspergillus fumigatus. Infect Immun. 2012;80(1):410–7. doi:10.1128/IAI.05939-11.
34. Granell M, Urbano-Ispizua A, Suarez B, Rovira M, Fernandez-Aviles F, Martinez C, et al. Mannan-binding lectin pathway deficiencies and invasive fungal infections following allogeneic stem cell transplantation. Exp Hematol. 2006;34(10):1435–41. doi:10.1016/j.exphem.2006.06.005.
35. Gresnigt MS, Becker KL, Smeekens SP, Jacobs CW, Joosten LA, van der Meer JW, et al. Aspergillus fumigatus-induced IL-22 is not restricted to a specific Th cell subset and is dependent on complement receptor 3. J Immunol. 2013;190(11):5629–39. doi:10.4049/jimmunol.1202601.
36. Grube M, Loeffler J, Mezger M, Kruger B, Echtenacher B, Hoffmann P, et al. TLR5 stop codon polymorphism is associated with invasive aspergillosis after allogeneic stem cell transplantation. Med Mycol. 2013;51(8):818–25. doi:10.3109/13693786.2013.809630.
37. Harrison N, Mitterbauer M, Tobudic S, Kalhs P, Rabitsch W, Greinix H, et al. Incidence and characteristics of invasive fungal diseases in allogeneic hematopoietic stem cell transplant recipients: a retrospective cohort study. BMC Infect Dis. 2015;15(1):584. doi:10.1186/s12879-015-1329-6.
38. Herbrecht R, Denning DW, Patterson TF, Bennett JE, Greene RE, Oestmann JW, et al. Voriconazole versus amphotericin B for primary therapy of invasive aspergillosis. N Engl J Med. 2002;347(6):408–15. doi:10.1056/NEJMoa020191.
39. Jaillon S, Peri G, Delneste Y, Fremaux I, Doni A, Moalli F, et al. The humoral pattern recognition receptor PTX3 is stored in neutrophil granules and localizes in extracellular traps. J Exp Med. 2007;204(4):793–804. doi:10.1084/jem.20061301.
40. Jhingran A, Kasahara S, Shepardson KM, Junecko BA, Heung LJ, Kumasaka DK, et al. Compartment-specific and sequential role of MyD88 and CARD9 in chemokine induction and innate defense during respiratory fungal infection. PLoS Pathog. 2015;11(1):e1004589. doi:10.1371/journal.ppat.1004589.
41. Kesh S, Mensah NY, Peterlongo P, Jaffe D, Hsu K, Vanden Brink M, et al. TLR1 and TLR6 polymorphisms are associated with susceptibility to invasive aspergillosis after allogeneic stem cell transplantation. Ann N Y Acad Sci. 2005;1062:95–103. doi:10.1196/annals.1358.012.
42. Klingspor L, Saaedi B, Ljungman P, Szakos A. Epidemiology and outcomes of patients with invasive mould infections: a retrospective observational study from a single centre (2005-2009). Mycoses. 2015;58(8):470–7. doi:10.1111/myc.12344.

43. Koldehoff M, Beelen DW, Elmaagacli AH. Increased susceptibility for aspergillosis and post-transplant immune deficiency in patients with gene variants of TLR4 after stem cell transplantation. Transplant Infect Dis: Off J Transplant Soc. 2013;15(5):533–9. doi:10.1111/tid.12115.
44. Kontoyiannis DP, Marr KA, Park BJ, Alexander BD, Anaissie EJ, Walsh TJ, et al. Prospective surveillance for invasive fungal infections in hematopoietic stem cell transplant recipients, 2001–2006: overview of the Transplant-Associated Infection Surveillance Network (TRANSNET) Database. Clin Infect Dis: Off Publ Infect Dis Soc Am. 2010;50(8):1091–100. doi:10.1086/651263.
45. Lupianez CB, Canet LM, Carvalho A, Alcazar-Fuoli L, Springer J, Lackner M, et al. Polymorphisms in host immunity-modulating genes and risk of invasive aspergillosis: results from the AspBIOmics consortium. Infect Immun. 2015;84(3):643–57. doi:10.1128/IAI.01359-15.
46. Mantovani A, Garlanda C, Doni A, Bottazzi B. Pentraxins in innate immunity: from C-reactive protein to the long pentraxin PTX3. J Clin Immunol. 2008;28(1):1–13. doi:10.1007/s10875-007-9126-7.
47. Meier A, Kirschning CJ, Nikolaus T, Wagner H, Heesemann J, Ebel F. Toll-like receptor (TLR) 2 and TLR4 are essential for Aspergillus-induced activation of murine macrophages. Cell Microbiol. 2003;5(8):561–70.
48. Mezger M, Steffens M, Beyer M, Manger C, Eberle J, Toliat MR, et al. Polymorphisms in the chemokine (C-X-C motif) ligand 10 are associated with invasive aspergillosis after allogeneic stem-cell transplantation and influence CXCL10 expression in monocyte-derived dendritic cells. Blood. 2008;111(2):534–6. doi:10.1182/blood-2007-05-090928.
49. Mircescu MM, Lipuma L, van Rooijen N, Pamer EG, Hohl TM. Essential role for neutrophils but not alveolar macrophages at early time points following Aspergillus fumigatus infection. J Infect Dis. 2009;200(4):647–56. doi:10.1086/600380.
50. Moreto A, Farinas-Alvarez C, Puente M, Ocejo-Vinyals JG, Sanchez-Velasco P, Horcajada JP, et al. Mannose-binding lectin gene variants and infections in patients receiving autologous stem cell transplantation. BMC Immunol. 2014;15:17. doi:10.1186/1471-2172-15-17.
51. Neofytos D, Treadway S, Ostrander D, Alonso CD, Dierberg KL, Nussenblatt V, et al. Epidemiology, outcomes, and mortality predictors of invasive mold infections among transplant recipients: a 10-year, single-center experience. Transplant Infect Dis: Off J Transplant Soc. 2013;15(3):233–42. doi:10.1111/tid.12060.
52. Netea MG, Van Der Graaf CA, Vonk AG, Verschueren I, Van Der Meer JW, Kullberg BJ. The role of toll-like receptor (TLR) 2 and TLR4 in the host defense against disseminated candidiasis. J Infect Dis. 2002;185(10):1483–9. doi:10.1086/340511.
53. Netea MG, Warris A, Van der Meer JW, Fenton MJ, Verver-Janssen TJ, Jacobs LE, et al. Aspergillus fumigatus evades immune recognition during germination through loss of toll-like receptor-4-mediated signal transduction. J Infect Dis. 2003;188(2):320–6. doi:10.1086/376456.
54. Orasch C, Marchetti O, Garbino J, Schrenzel J, Zimmerli S, Muhlethaler K, et al. Candida species distribution and antifungal susceptibility testing according to European Committee on Antimicrobial Susceptibility Testing and new vs. old Clinical and Laboratory Standards Institute clinical breakpoints: a 6-year prospective candidaemia survey from the fungal infection network of Switzerland. Clin Microbiol Infect: Off Publ Eur Soc Clin Microbiol Infect Dis. 2014;20(7):698–705. doi:10.1111/1469-0691.12440.
55. Pappas PG, Alexander BD, Andes DR, Hadley S, Kauffman CA, Freifeld A, et al. Invasive fungal infections among organ transplant recipients: results of the Transplant-Associated Infection Surveillance Network (TRANSNET). Clin Infect Dis: Off Publ Infect Dis Soc Am. 2010;50(8):1101–11. doi:10.1086/651262.
56. Pfaller MA, Diekema DJ, Gibbs DL, Newell VA, Ellis D, Tullio V, et al. Results from the ARTEMIS DISK Global Antifungal Surveillance Study, 1997 to 2007: a 10.5-year analysis of susceptibilities of Candida Species to fluconazole and voriconazole as determined by CLSI

standardized disk diffusion. J Clin Microbiol. 2010;48(4):1366–77. doi:10.1128/JCM.02117-09.
57. Plantinga TS, van der Velden WJ, Ferwerda B, van Spriel AB, Adema G, Feuth T, et al. Early stop polymorphism in human DECTIN-1 is associated with increased candida colonization in hematopoietic stem cell transplant recipients. Clin Infect Dis: Off Publ Infect Dis Soc Am. 2009;49(5):724–32.
58. Romani L. Immunity to fungal infections. Nat Rev Immunol. 2011;11(4):275–88. doi:10.1038/nri2939.
59. Sainz J, Hassan L, Perez E, Romero A, Moratalla A, Lopez-Fernandez E, et al. Interleukin-10 promoter polymorphism as risk factor to develop invasive pulmonary aspergillosis. Immunol Lett. 2007a;109(1):76–82. doi:10.1016/j.imlet.2007.01.005.
60. Sainz J, Lupianez CB, Segura-Catena J, Vazquez L, Rios R, Oyonarte S, et al. Dectin-1 and DC-SIGN polymorphisms associated with invasive pulmonary Aspergillosis infection. PLoS ONE. 2012;7(2):e32273. doi:10.1371/journal.pone.0032273.
61. Sainz J, Perez E, Gomez-Lopera S, Jurado M. IL1 gene cluster polymorphisms and its haplotypes may predict the risk to develop invasive pulmonary aspergillosis and modulate C-reactive protein level. J Clin Immunol. 2008;28(5):473–85. doi:10.1007/s10875-008-9197-0.
62. Sainz J, Perez E, Hassan L, Moratalla A, Romero A, Collado MD, et al. Variable number of tandem repeats of TNF receptor type 2 promoter as genetic biomarker of susceptibility to develop invasive pulmonary aspergillosis. Hum Immunol. 2007b;68(1):41–50. doi:10.1016/j.humimm.2006.10.011.
63. Sainz J, Salas-Alvarado I, Lopez-Fernandez E, Olmedo C, Comino A, Garcia F, et al. TNFR1 mRNA expression level and TNFR1 gene polymorphisms are predictive markers for susceptibility to develop invasive pulmonary aspergillosis. Int J Immunopathol Pharmacol. 2010;23(2):423–36.
64. Santos T, Aguiar B, Santos L, Romaozinho C, Tome R, Macario F, et al. Invasive fungal infections after kidney transplantation: a single-center experience. Transplant Proc. 2015;47(4):971–5. doi:10.1016/j.transproceed.2015.03.040.
65. Schwartz DA. The role of TLR4 in endotoxin responsiveness in humans. J Endotoxin Res. 2001;7(5):389–93.
66. Seo KW, Kim DH, Sohn SK, Lee NY, Chang HH, Kim SW, et al. Protective role of interleukin-10 promoter gene polymorphism in the pathogenesis of invasive pulmonary aspergillosis after allogeneic stem cell transplantation. Bone Marrow Transplant. 2005;36(12):1089–95. doi:10.1038/sj.bmt.1705181.
67. Silveira FP, Husain S. Fungal infections in solid organ transplantation. Medical mycology. 2007;45(4):305–20. doi:10.1080/13693780701200372.
68. Steele C, Rapaka RR, Metz A, Pop SM, Williams DL, Gordon S, et al. The beta-glucan receptor dectin-1 recognizes specific morphologies of Aspergillus fumigatus. PLoS Pathog. 2005;1(4):e42. doi:10.1371/journal.ppat.0010042.
69. Steinbach WJ, Marr KA, Anaissie EJ, Azie N, Quan SP, Meier-Kriesche HU, et al. Clinical epidemiology of 960 patients with invasive aspergillosis from the PATH Alliance registry. J Infect. 2012;65(5):453–64. doi:10.1016/j.jinf.2012.08.003.
70. Ullmann AJ, Lipton JH, Vesole DH, Chandrasekar P, Langston A, Tarantolo SR, et al. Posaconazole or fluconazole for prophylaxis in severe graft-versus-host disease. N Engl J Med. 2007;356(4):335–47. doi:10.1056/NEJMoa061098.
71. van der Graaf C, Kullberg BJ, Joosten L, Verver-Jansen T, Jacobs L, Van der Meer JW, et al. Functional consequences of the Asp299Gly Toll-like receptor-4 polymorphism. Cytokine. 2005;30(5):264–8. doi:10.1016/j.cyto.2005.02.001.
72. Vazquez JA, Miceli MH, Alangaden G. Invasive fungal infections in transplant recipients. Therapeutic advances in infectious disease. 2013;1(3):85–105. doi:10.1177/2049936113491936.
73. Vermeulen E, Lagrou K, Verweij PE. Azole resistance in Aspergillus fumigatus: a growing public health concern. Curr Opin Infect Dis. 2013;26(6):493–500. doi:10.1097/QCO.0000000000000005.

74. Vonk AG, Netea MG, van Krieken JH, Iwakura Y, van der Meer JW, Kullberg BJ. Endogenous interleukin (IL)-1 alpha and IL-1 beta are crucial for host defense against disseminated candidiasis. J Infect Dis. 2006;193(10):1419–26. doi:10.1086/503363.
75. Werner JL, Metz AE, Horn D, Schoeb TR, Hewitt MM, Schwiebert LM, et al. Requisite role for the dectin-1 beta-glucan receptor in pulmonary defense against Aspergillus fumigatus. J Immunol. 2009;182(8):4938–46. doi:10.4049/jimmunol.0804250.
76. Wojtowicz A, Bochud PY. Host genetics of invasive Aspergillus and Candida infections. Semin Immunopathol. 2015;37(2):173–86. doi:10.1007/s00281-014-0468-y.
77. Wojtowicz A, Gresnigt MS, Lecompte T, Bibert S, Manuel O, Joosten LA, et al. IL1B and DEFB1 polymorphisms increase susceptibility to invasive mold infection after solid-organ transplantation. J Infect Dis. 2015a;211(10):1646–57. doi:10.1093/infdis/jiu636.
78. Wojtowicz A, Lecompte TD, Bibert S, Manuel O, Rueger S, Berger C, et al. PTX3 polymorphisms and invasive mold infections after solid organ transplant. Clin Infect Dis: Off Publ Infect Dis Soc Am. 2015b;61(4):619–22. doi:10.1093/cid/civ386.
79. Zaas AK, Liao G, Chien JW, Weinberg C, Shore D, Giles SS, et al. Plasminogen alleles influence susceptibility to invasive aspergillosis. PLoS Genet. 2008;4(6):e1000101. doi:10.1371/journal.pgen.1000101.

Immunogenetics of Chronic and Allergic Aspergillosis

7

Nicola Overton, Sara Gago, and Paul Bowyer

Abstract

Although invasive fungal diseases are often assumed to be the only form of fungal disease, fungi more commonly cause chronic disease in individuals with ostensibly normal immune systems, or allergic disease in those with hyperactive immune systems, such as atopic asthmatics. Invasive fungal diseases affect individuals with an underlying defect in the immune system and are rapid in onset with high mortality, whereas chronic and allergic diseases primarily affect individuals with normal immune systems and are long-term, even lifelong, conditions.

7.1 Introduction

Although invasive fungal diseases are often assumed to be the only form of fungal disease, fungi more commonly cause chronic disease in individuals with ostensibly normal immune systems, or allergic disease in those with hyperactive immune systems, such as atopic asthmatics. Invasive fungal diseases affect individuals with an underlying defect in the immune system and are rapid in onset with high mortality, whereas chronic and allergic diseases primarily affect individuals with normal immune systems and are long-term, even lifelong, conditions.

Chronic aspergillosis is a long-term disease occurring in those with a prior or underlying lung-damaging condition. At-risk individuals commonly have prior or current tuberculosis, COPD or sarcoidosis. The course of the disease can range from

N. Overton • S. Gago • P. Bowyer (✉)
Manchester Fungal Infection Group, Division of Infection, Immunity and Respiratory Medicine, School of Biological Sciences, Faculty of Biology, Medicine and Health, Manchester Academic Health Science Centre, The University of Manchester and University Hospital of South Manchester NHS Foundation Trust, Manchester, UK
e-mail: paul.bowyer@manchester.ac.uk

A. Carvalho (ed.), *Immunogenetics of Fungal Diseases*,
DOI 10.1007/978-3-319-50842-9_7

months to many years and is associated with significant mortality. Allergic forms of aspergillosis affect individuals with atopic asthma or severe asthma or may affect atopic individuals in the context of primary allergy or rhinitis.

Allergic and chronic forms of fungal disease are far more common than invasive disease, and it is therefore important to understand the immunology of these diseases and the potential defects in host defence against fungal infection that may lead to them. There is an increasing global awareness of these conditions, and since individuals with chronic or allergic fungal disease require long-term antifungal therapy, this results in a rapidly increasing healthcare cost. The issue of antifungal drug resistance is acute in these individuals as resistance frequently arises during their long-term therapy. This chapter will outline the features of allergic and chronic fungal diseases and our knowledge of the underlying immunology.

7.2 Disease Frequency

Allergic and chronic forms of fungal disease are far more common than invasive disease. This arises from the fact that these diseases are complications or sequelae of common underlying conditions such as asthma or tuberculosis, whereas the underlying condition for invasive disease and immune dysfunction is limited to small numbers of individuals with active HIV or those clinically immunocompromised for transplant or by chemotherapy. Complications of atopic asthma by fungal colonisation, such as allergic bronchopulmonary aspergillosis (ABPA) and severe asthma with fungal sensitisation (SAFS), represent the most severe and debilitating forms of asthma [1–3]. More than 4.8 million adult asthmatics have ABPA worldwide [4]; however, the disease is rare in children [5]. The exact numbers affected by ABPA is unclear, but ABPA is identified in 1–8% of asthmatics seen in hospital referral clinics [6, 7].

7.3 Description of Allergic and Chronic Fungal Disease Types

Several forms of allergic fungal disease have been described. These include fungal rhinosinusitis, allergic bronchopulmonary aspergillosis (ABPA), allergic bronchopulmonary mycosis (ABPM) and severe asthma with fungal sensitisation (SAFS). ABPA is the best studied disease in this group, and it is not known whether the other diseases are separate entities or form part of a disease continuum resulting from fungal persistence in the airway interacting with different underlying inflammatory diseases such as asthma or severe asthma.

Allergic bronchopulmonary aspergillosis (ABPA) is a hypersensitivity lung disease associated to airway colonisation by the pathogenic mould *A. fumigatus* [2, 8]. When other fungi are found to cause this condition, it is referred to as ABPM. Exposure to fungi is universal; every day we inhale litres of air that contains thousands of *Aspergillus* spores [9]. Due to the small size of spores, they can rapidly be deposited into the lower bronchial airways. In the healthy human host, spores are recognised and cleared by the innate immune system via a Th1 immune response. ABPA is caused by an exuberant and distinctive host response to *Aspergillus* antigens [10–12]. It is frequently seen in asthma (2.5%) and cystic fibrosis patients (15%) [13, 14], who develop ABPA following inhalation and airway colonisation of *A. fumigatus* [14, 15]. In these patients, an allergic Th2 response develops on exposure to *A. fumigatus*.

Studies have attempted to elucidate the underlying mechanism for this Th2 response in ABPA. Some have focused on the response of the bronchial epithelium, while others have focussed on specific cells such as macrophages [16–21]. The numerous *A. fumigatus* antigens promote an IgE-mediated and eosinophilic response, which is thought to be responsible for the disease features and symptoms. IgG and cellular responses are implicated as well, but tissue invasion does not occur [22]. This unusual reaction induces the production of Th2 pro-inflammatory cytokines responsible for IgE production, mast cell degranulation and allergic airway response activation [10, 11, 23]. Stimulation of PBMCs with *Aspergillus* results in production of Th2 cytokines IL5 and IL13, and ABPA patients show increased *Aspergillus*-induced IL5 and IL13, and decreased IFNγ production, compared to healthy controls [24]. IgE production, eosinophil recruitment and production of an abnormal host inflammatory response in the bronchi and bronchioles of the lungs is observed [25]. This is followed by excessive mucin production, eosinophil infiltration of the bronchial mucin and development of the features of ABPA [15]. Moreover, certain secreted *Aspergillus* proteins can induce toxicity in the bronchial epithelium causing cell detachment and death.

7.4 Clinical Symptoms of ABPA

Although ABPA caused by *A. fumigatus* is the most common form of allergic bronchopulmonary mycosis, other fungi can cause the disease [4]. Patients have poorly controlled asthma, wheezing, haemoptysis and expectoration of mucus plugs [22]. Other symptoms include fever, malaise and fatigue. Recurrent pulmonary infiltrates with or without bronchiectasis is frequent [4]. Elevated total blood IgE levels and IgE reactivity to *A. fumigatus* is observed in patients, and *A. fumigatus* is often isolated from sputum. Often central bronchiectasis and mucoid impaction of bronchi with distal atelectasis occurs. Untreated ABPA can result in pulmonary fibrosis and eventually respiratory failure [22].

Differential diagnosis of ABPA used to be difficult as clinical signs are unspecific and frequently misdiagnosed as pulmonary tuberculosis. However, in 2013, the ABPA complicating asthma group, from the International Society for Human and Animal Mycology (ISHAM), proposed the new diagnostic and classification criteria for ABPA [22]. They agreed on the need for one of the predisposing conditions of bronchial asthma and cystic fibrosis and two obligatory criteria. Patients should have a Type I *Aspergillus* skin test positive or elevated IgE levels specific against *A. fumigatus*, and the total IgE levels should be >1000 IU/ml. Moreover, at least two out three of the next criteria should be met: the presence of precipitating of IgG antibodies against *A. fumigatus* in serum, radiographic pulmonary opacities consistent with ABPA or total eosinophil counts >500 cells/ml in patients that have never been treated with steroids before [22].

Severe asthma with fungal sensitisation (SAFS) (also known as fungal-associated severe asthma) is a complication of severe asthma caused by sensitisation to one or many fungi including *A. fumigatus, Penicillium chrysogenum, Cladosporium herbarum, Alternaria alternata, Candida albicans* and *Trichophyton* spp. The underlying condition, severe asthma, is defined by the 2009 ATS/ERS guidelines or earlier BTS guidelines. In practice this means a low FEV1 or peak flow (usually persistently), high-dose inhaled steroids and/or frequent courses of oral steroids. SAFS is indicated when total IgE to fungi is <1000 KIU/L or when skin test or specific IgE test is positive for any fungus. Severe asthma affects 5–20% of those with asthma; of these, 35–50% have SAFS, depending on how extensively they are tested. It is conservatively estimated that SAFS might affect 6 million people worldwide. Treatments for SAFS include treatment for severe asthma with additional antifungal treatment for asthma. Itraconazole treatment benefits ~60% patients in terms of quality of life, although not necessarily improved lung function. Severe asthma is a very debilitating disorder, with frequent medical contacts and multiple treatments. Poor or late treatment of severe asthma results in a number of intensive care admissions or deaths each year, but it is not known how many of these are in SAFS patients.

7.5 Fungal Sinusitis

The terms allergic fungal rhinosinusitis (AFRS), eosinophilic fungal rhinosinusitis (EFRS), allergic *Aspergillus* sinusitis and eosinophilic mucin rhinosinusitis encompass several disease entities, with unclear boundaries between them. The predominant fungus responsible varies geographically but includes *A. fumigatus, A. flavus, Bipolaris spicifera, Curvularia lunata* and *Alternaria alternata. Alternaria alternata* is the most common causative agent in the USA, while *A. flavus* is the most common in the Middle East, India and Pakistan. Fungal sinusitis is usually a chronic condition causing nasal obstruction, loss of smell, nasal discharge (productive sneezing and/or postnasal mucus) and a pressure sensation over the sinus area. Patients often have asthma. AFRS and EFRS are estimated to affect ~12 million people at any time.

7.6 Chronic Pulmonary Aspergillosis (CPA, Aspergilloma, Chronic Necrotising Pulmonary Aspergillosis, Chronic Cavitary Aspergillosis)

The term chronic pulmonary aspergillosis embraces several closely related disease entities including simple aspergilloma, chronic cavitary pulmonary aspergillosis and chronic fibrosing pulmonary aspergillosis. CPA is a slowly progressive and destructive disease of the lungs, usually of one or both upper lobes, with cavity formation the most common radiological feature. It is arbitrarily defined as being present for at least 3 months. It occurs in non-immunocompromised or minimally immunocompromised patients. Some patients have nodules, which probably represent early disease, may be mistaken for lung cancer and have a positive PET scan. Common symptoms are fatigue, weight loss, breathlessness, productive cough and haemoptysis (coughing up blood). The disease is often mistaken for pulmonary tuberculosis and both diseases can coexist. About 25% of patients have an aspergilloma (fungal ball) present; the remainder have one or more cavities and/or nodules. Chronic pulmonary aspergillosis is estimated to affect over 3 million people worldwide, of whom ~1.2 million have had tuberculosis.

7.7 Clinical Symptoms of Chronic Pulmonary Aspergillosis

7.7.1 Aspergilloma

Aspergillomas (or fungal balls) are a gelatinous mass of fungus, usually *A. fumigatus*. Diagnosis is normally from an x-ray or CT scan showing an approximately spherical shadow with surrounding air in a pulmonary cavity, with serological or microbiological evidence that *Aspergillus* spp. is present in the material. Patients are normally not immunocompromised, and aspergillomas can remain stable for many months without progression or obvious symptoms. Multiple aspergillomas or those that are complicated by cavities may be known as complex aspergillomas [26].

7.7.2 Chronic Cavitary Pulmonary Aspergillosis (CCPA)

CCPA is defined as the presence of one or more pulmonary cavities, which may or may not contain a fungal ball, with serological or microbiological evidence implicating *Aspergillus* spp. in a non-immunocompromised patient (or one whose immunocompromising condition has remitted or is trivial) with significant pulmonary or systemic symptoms and overt radiological progression (new cavities, increasing pericavity infiltrates or increasing fibrosis) over at least 3 months of observation [27]. If untreated, cavities can continue to form and/or expand over a period of months or years, with progressive lung fibrosis and chronic inflammation [27]. *Aspergillus* growth on the cavity surface, without tissue invasion, may lead to fungal balls (aspergillomas). The mechanisms underlying the observed pathology are largely unknown, but development of aspergilloma(s) represents a later phase of CCPA [28]. If biopsy of the affected area is performed, it demonstrates hyphae with surrounding chronic inflammation and fibrosis but not tissue invasion.

7.7.3 Chronic Fibrosing Pulmonary Aspergillosis (CFPA)

CFPA patients have severe fibrotic destruction of at least two lobes of lung complicating chronic cavitary pulmonary aspergillosis, leading to a major loss of lung function. Usually the fibrosis is in the form of consolidation, but it may be large cavities with surrounding fibrosis. Severe fibrotic destruction of one lobe with a cavity is simply referred to as chronic cavitary pulmonary aspergillosis affecting that lobe.

7.7.4 Subacute Invasive Aspergillosis or Chronic Necrotising Pulmonary Aspergillosis (CNPA)

More mild than true invasive aspergillosis, subacute invasive aspergillosis usually occurs in mildly immunocompromised patients, occurring over 1–3 months, with marked pleiotropic radiological features (cavitation, nodules and progressive consolidation with "abscess formation") and hyphae visible in destroyed lung tissue or inferred from microbiological investigations (i.e. positive *Aspergillus* antigen).

7.8 Predisposing Conditions for CPA

Individuals affected with chronic cavitary pulmonary aspergillosis (CCPA) almost invariably have some prior lung disease (e.g. chronic obstructive pulmonary disorder [COPD] or pulmonary tuberculosis [TB]) but are overtly immunocompetent and do not generally have clinical history of recurrent infection [29, 30]. The commonest underlying lung diseases are tuberculosis, chronic obstructive pulmonary disease, sarcoidosis, ABPA, prior pneumothorax, prior lung cancer (sometimes with lung radiotherapy or surgery) and asthma (including SAFS). Most patients are not taking corticosteroids or other immunosuppressant drugs, but many are on inhaled corticosteroids or take small doses of oral corticosteroid. Many patients have low IFNγ responses to standard stimuli.

7.8.1 Tuberculosis

A recent study identified tuberculosis (either classical TB or non-tuberculous mycobacterial infection, atypical TB) as an underlying condition in 32.5% (41/126) of patients [30]. This finding is lower than in other earlier studies, which identified tuberculosis as an underlying condition in 50–72% of CPA patients [27, 31, 32]. The importance of tuberculosis in the development of aspergillosis is supported by various studies of tuberculosis patients. Of 544 patients who had cured tuberculosis but who had been left with a residual cavity of ≥2.5 cm 1 year after recovery, 36% were found to have positive *Aspergillus* antibodies, and 22% were found to have radiological aspergillomas after 3 years [33, 34]. As these reports are historical and are from a time when the various forms of CPA were not recognised as separate entities, they are likely to contain cases of what we now recognise as CCPA, SAIA and CFPA, as well as simple aspergilloma cases. As 21–35% of patients who survive pulmonary tuberculosis have residual cavities [35, 36], it is likely that 8–12%

patients who recover from classical tuberculosis develop CPA over 4 years. In addition, CPA can occur simultaneously to tuberculosis; one study has identified *Aspergillus* coinfection in 14/136 (10%) cases of *Mycobacterium xenopi* pulmonary infection [37], while another found that in 4% of 302 patients with *Mycobacterium kansasii* infections developed aspergillosis [38].

7.8.2 ABPA, SAFS and Asthma

Case reports of coexistent ABPA and CPA exist, and studies of aspergilloma and CPA patients have identified ABPA as an underlying condition in 12–14% (10/85) of the cases [30, 39–42]. In one recent study, ABPA was found to be the most common primary underlying condition [30]. Additionally, this study identified SAFS [43] as an underlying condition in 2.4% of CPA patients, and SAFS was found to be the primary underlying condition for 1.6% of cases [30]. Asthma has also been identified in 6–12% of CPA patients [27, 30, 31, 42].

7.8.3 COPD and/or Emphysema

COPD and/or emphysema is one of the most common underlying conditions in CPA, identified in over a third of patients in various studies [27, 30, 31, 42]. In addition, recent data indicates a substantial rise in acute invasive pulmonary aspergillosis (IPA) diagnosed in COPD patients, and this disease has a 95% mortality [44, 45]. It is possible that transformation from CPA to acute IPA can occur following an exacerbation of COPD and treatment with corticosteroids.

7.8.4 Pneumonia

Various studies have identified pneumonia as a predisposing factor for aspergilloma and CPA. One identified *Pneumocystis carinii* pneumonia in 12% of aspergilloma cases, while another identified pneumonia and lung abscess in 9.4% of aspergilloma cases [32, 41]. A more recent study found that 22.2% (28/126) of the CPA patients analysed have pneumonia as an underlying condition [30].

7.8.5 Sarcoidosis

Sarcoidosis has been identified as a predisposing factor for CPA, in a number of published case reports and studies [30, 46, 47]. Cohort studies have identified sarcoidosis as an underlying condition in 11.8–17% of CPA patients [31, 32, 41]. In addition, a study that followed 100 sarcoidosis patients over a 10 year period found that 10% (10/100) developed aspergillomas [48].

7.8.6 Pneumothorax

History of pneumothorax has been identified by various studies, in 11.1–17% of CPA cases [27, 30, 31], and, where a primary underlying disease is identified, previous pneumothorax (±bullae) is also common [30].

7.8.7 Lung Cancer and Thoracic Surgery

In a recent study, prior treated lung cancer was identified in 10.3% of CPA cases, and thoracic surgery was identified in 14.3% [30]. The relationship of cancer to CPA is complex as chemotherapy, chest radiotherapy and/or thoracic surgery are normal treatments for lung cancer and may themselves predispose for the disease [27, 31, 42].

7.8.8 Rheumatoid Arthritis

Rheumatoid arthritis (RA) (with little or no immunosuppressive treatment) was identified as an underlying condition in 4% of CPA patients in a recent study [30], and upper lobe fibrosis and/or cavitation associated with RA has also been identified as an underlying disease in 2.4% of aspergilloma cases [41].

7.8.9 General Comments on Pathogenesis of CPA

The studies discussed here demonstrate the importance of underlying conditions in the development of CPA. Many of these underlying conditions have effects on the physical structure of the lung. Pneumothoraces, lung cancer and thoracic surgery, by their nature and by their treatment, result in lung damage, while tuberculosis can leave cavities in the lung [33–35]. RA can lead to the development of pulmonary fibrosis, pneumonia can cause extensive damage and scarring, and sarcoidosis, particularly the late stage fibrotic form, results in lung fibrosis and cavities [41, 48]. Lung fibrosis can also occur in ABPA [49]. These sequelae result in areas of damaged lung, which *Aspergillus* can colonise. Once inhaled, the fungus can grow and either forms a simple fungal ball or go on to invade the lung parenchyma and cause/expand cavities. Other conditions, such as ABPA or SAFS, have a strong fungal component themselves, and the presence of the fungus in these patients may precipitate colonisation and development of CPA. Additionally, genetic factors may be important in the development of CPA, and some have been identified, but this work is in its infancy, as it is for most respiratory conditions [50–53].

7.8.9.1 Diagnosis

The key diagnostic tests are serum *Aspergillus* IgG testing, also known as *Aspergillus* precipitins, and radiology showing one or more cavities or nodules.

A. fumigatus IgG antibodies are detectable in ~90% of patients. Alternative approaches to diagnosis include detectable *A. flavus* or *A. niger* IgG antibodies, *A. fumigatus* IgE antibodies and biopsy/excision of lesions showing hyphae consistent with *Aspergillus* within a cavity. Sputum culture positive rates are ~25%, and *Aspergillus* PCR is more sensitive, but many patients are still negative.

7.8.9.2 Outlook and Prognosis

CPA progresses at a variable rate and is often diagnosed late. Severe disease carries a 15–30% mortality in the first 6 months after diagnosis. Death is mainly due to pneumonia and lung bleeding. Those with minor involvement will do well for many years, if progressive lung destruction can be halted. Azole resistance in *A. fumigatus* is becoming an increasing problem, especially in patients with aspergillomas and those with low levels of itraconazole.

7.9 Routes of Infection in Chronic and Allergic Fungal Disease

It is presumed that fungi are able to grow and persist in the airways of individuals with the discussed underlying diseases, giving rise to a dynamic, responsive and potent source of allergens as well as secreted fungal proteins such as proteases that may damage the airway epithelium. The combination of tissue damage and a dynamic source of allergens is thought to be important in triggering allergic fungal disease. Other evidence suggests that submicroscopic fragments of dead fungi are present in air and that these allergen-bearing particles may also trigger allergic responses in the lung. The dynamics of particle deposition in the lung means that the smallest particles or spores penetrate furthest. Thus, fungi with small spores can penetrate into the alveolae, whereas other fungi with larger spores are restricted to the nose and upper airway (Fig. 7.2). Lung epithelium also differs in structure and complexity depending on its position in the lung. For example, alveolar epithelium is a relatively simple cell monolayer, whereas bronchial epithelium cells are more substantial and differentiated into several cell types. The combination of this difference in epithelium composition with the different penetration of fungal spores means that different fungi are likely to encounter different epithelium structures and that the differences in the interaction may mean that immune responses could differ dramatically depending on fungal species.

It seems clear that neither live fungus nor hyphal fragments penetrate the epithelium to invade lung tissue to any great extent. Exacerbated symptoms of asthma arise from formation of mucus plugs in the airways that restrict air flow and from potentially continuous allergen exposure with heightened immune responses (Table 7.1 and Fig. 7.1).

Deposition of fungal spores in the lung is dependent on spore size, branching and tubule diameter. Different spore sizes are predicted to penetrate the lung to varying

Table 7.1 Prevalence and annual burden of fungal disease in the EU

	Predominant risk groups	At-risk population	Prevalence	Annual burden
ABPA	Asthma	34,700,000	2.1%	729,000 (243–1215)
ABPA	Cystic fibrosis	29,000	15%	4300
SAFS	Severe asthma	3,470,000	33%	1,145,000
CPA	COPD, sarcoidosis, TB, ABPA	>13,600,000	1–10%	204,000
IPA	HSCT, neutropenia, corticosteroids	~5–50,000,000	1–10%	~50,000

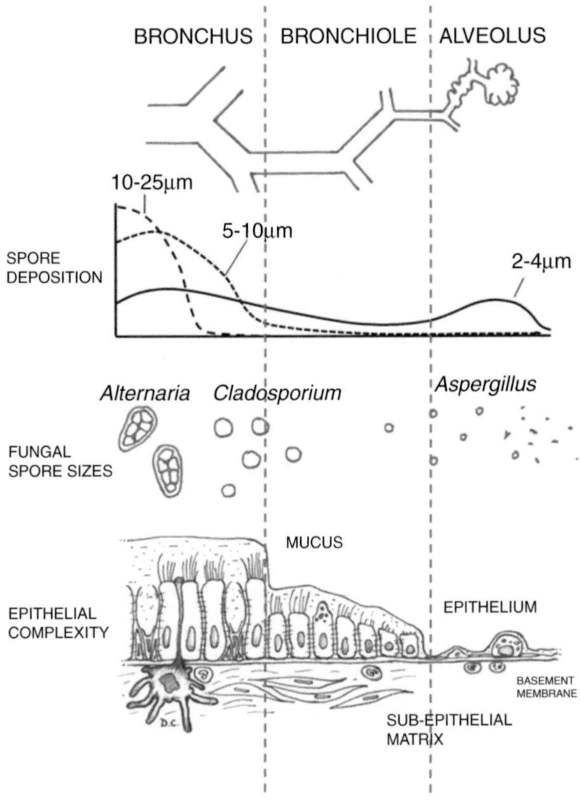

Fig. 7.1 Deposition of fungal spores in the lung

degrees with only the smallest spores penetrating to the alveolus. The structure of the airway lining differs considerably from the upper airway through to the alveolae with the higher airways having the most complex epithelial structure. Thus, spores of *Alternaria* will not penetrate further than the bronchus and will only encounter the highly differentiated epithelium consisting of epithelial cells, goblet cells and Clara cells, whereas *Aspergillus* spores will be deposited throughout the airway but predominantly in the alveolus.

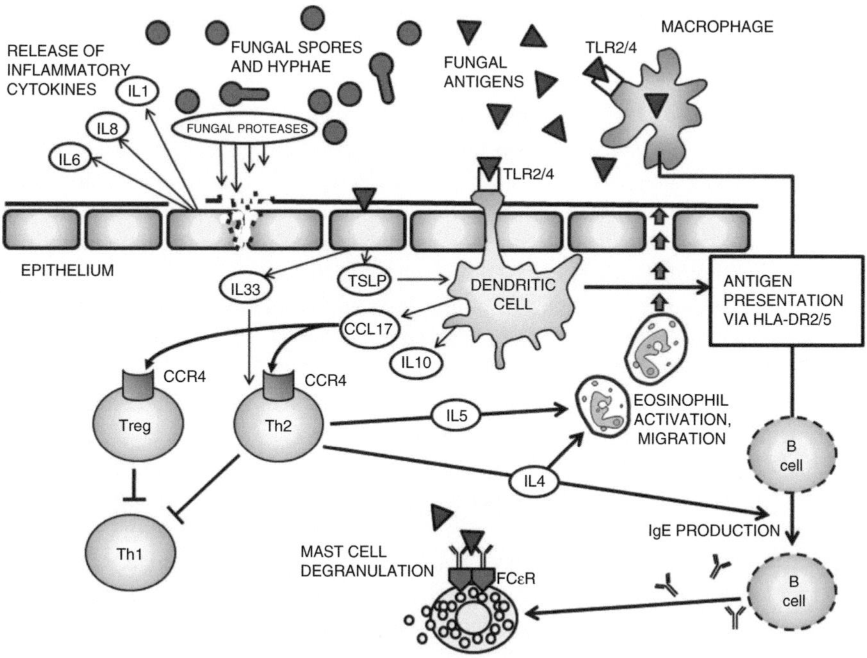

Fig. 7.2 Immunology of the ABPA response. Glucan and other surface components of *Aspergillus fumigatus* germinating spores and hyphae activate resident macrophages, dendritic and respiratory epithelial cells via innate recognition receptors, such as dectin-1 or toll-like receptor (TLR2/4) to produce T-helper cell (Th2) promoting cytokines; chemokines and co-stimulatory molecules that include thymic stromal lymphopoetin (TSLP), interleukin (IL)-25, IL-33 and CCL17. These stimulate differentiation, chemotaxis and activation of CD4+ Th2 cells. CCL17 also attracts regulatory T cells (Treg) capable of suppressing protective Th1. Th2 cells produce IL-4 and IL-5 that attract and activate eosinophils. Fungal antigens are captured and presented to the adaptive immune system by professional antigen-presenting cells such as macrophages and dendritic cells leading to the presence of B cells that produce IgG specific to fungal proteins. On further exposure to these proteins and with co-stimulation by IL4, these B cells differentiate into IgE-producing B cells or plasmacytes. IgE antibodies bind to the FCEr receptor of mast cells: these receptors dimerise in the presence of fungal antigen triggering an immediate hypersensitivity reaction. Further inflammatory responses are caused by fungal protease-mediated degradation of the epithelial cell tight junction typically leading to release of the broad spectrum IL6 and IL8 cytokines. Combination of the Th2 cell response and mast cell degranulation leads to the typical mucosal inflammation and mucus over secretion seen in ABPA

7.10 Immunology of Allergic and Chronic Fungal Disease

7.10.1 Immunopathogenesis of ABPA

The fact that only 2–4% of atopic asthmatics acquire ABPA in an environment providing constant exposure to fungi suggests that susceptibility may be genetic. Two to four percent of the atopic population is allergic to fungi; however, most individuals with fungal allergy do not have ABPA. These observations suggest that susceptibility to ABPA is not simply a matter of atopic asthma complicated by fungal allergy but that it must depend on some more profound susceptibility to fungal colonisation. Atopic asthma is not a strict requirement for ABPA; however, almost all individuals with ABPA have this underlying condition. This poses difficulties in attempting to define genetic susceptibility factors for ABPA as affected individuals already have a genetically and immunologically complex disease. Furthermore, the use of animal models to discover genes involved in the disease is hindered by the lack of refined models for either ABPA or atopic asthma.

In a normal, healthy immune response, lung epithelial cells, dendritic cells and macrophages regulate the Th1/Th17/Th2/Treg balance, which is critical for pathogen clearance [54]. For most fungal exposure, this response is biased towards Th1cell proliferation which is thought to lead to effective killing and clearance of fungi by neutrophils, macrophages and T cells [55].

In ABPA or other allergic fungal diseases, cells respond to fungal exposure with a Th2 response. *A. fumigatus* germinating spores and hyphae activate dendritic and respiratory epithelial cells via components of the innate immune system [9, 56, 57]. Toll-like receptor (TLR) 2/4, dectin 1 and 2 and other pattern-associated molecular pattern receptors located on epithelial cells, dendritic cells and macrophages resident in the lung produce cytokines, chemokines and co-stimulatory molecules such as thymic stromal lymphopoetin (TSLP), interleukin (IL)-25, IL-33, OX40 ligand (OX40L) and CCL17 (thymus-activated and thymus-regulated chemokine), which stimulate differentiation and activation of CD4+ Th2 cells. CCL17 also attracts regulatory T cells (Treg) capable of suppressing protective Th1 responses.

The Th2 cell response releases IL-4 and IL-5 that attract eosinophils and drive differentiation of B cells to IgE-secreting plasmacytes. Since the lungs may contain a substantial amount of fungus, many B cells will carry fungus-specific IgG that is converted to fungus-specific IgE by chain switching. Fungus-specific IgE binds a specific receptor, FCER, on mast cells and basophils, and these cells react to the binding of fungal allergen and antigen proteins by degranulation and release of histamines and other factors that trigger an immediate hypersensitivity reaction. This results in bronchoconstriction and overproduction of mucus in the airway leading to mucus plugging. The inflammatory response can lead to bronchiectasis that may progress to fibrosis if untreated. Recent work by Becker et al. suggested that the Th2 stimulatory signalling observed in ABPA arises through CR3 receptor-mediated detection of fungi, specifically *A. fumigatus* [24].

7.10.1.1 SAFS

It is not clear why the proportion of individuals sensitised to fungi is so high in severe asthmatics. The tenfold higher rate of fungal allergy in severe asthma compared to normal allergic individuals suggests a role for fungal colonisation in driving asthma to its most extreme form; however, no mechanisms have yet been proven to support this hypothesis.

7.10.2 Immunology of Chronic Pulmonary Aspergillosis

It is thought that the scar or cavity left by the predisposing disease or lung injury forms a weak point in the lung that can be exploited by the infecting fungus. Few immunological features have been associated with the disease; however, many individuals with CPA have high levels of *Aspergillus*-specific IgG, which may arise from the very high fungal burden observed in this condition. The field has also been hampered by lack of an animal model for chronic fungal infection. One recent promising advance has been the use of agarose bead protected fungal hyphae in mouse models of long-term fungal colonisation [58]. In this model system, fungi can persist in mouse airways for up to 28 days. Pro-inflammatory cytokines and chemokines increased early in infection with raised levels of interleukin-4 (IL-4), elevated IgE levels in serum and a mild increase in airway responsiveness. T-cell analysis suggested a Th2-type response, followed by a rise in IL-17 and Foxp3 (+) cells by day 14. A high proportion of patients with chronic pulmonary aspergillosis are poor producers of IFN-γ in response to multiple stimuli, and this is currently being explored as a possible therapeutic tool for CPA [59].

7.10.3 Gene Variants Associated with Chronic and Allergic Fungal Disease

The study of genetic variants associated with chronic and allergic fungal disease has been hampered by the complexity of both the disease and by the associated underlying conditions. For instance, it is not clear whether genetic factors discovered for CPA are somehow related to underlying tuberculosis or COPD.

7.10.3.1 CPA

Little is known about the factors affecting susceptibility, continuing inflammation or disease pathogenesis in CCPA. The most commonly cited susceptibility factor is underlying disease; however, the proportion of patients with any one disease is small, and only a small percentage of individuals with any one underlying disease develop CCPA [30]. Previous genetic association studies involving small numbers of patients have identified associations between CPA and *TNF*, *MBL2*, *TGFB1*, *IL15*, *TLR4* and *IL10* [51–53, 60] but do not explain all cases of CPA and have proved difficult to replicate.

Recent studies [29, 61] using larger CPA populations suggested several SNPs associated with CCPA including three intronic mutations in *IL15* (rs6842735, rs12508866, rs1519551), an intronic insertion-deletion mutation in *IL1B* (rs3917354), a missense non-synonymous coding SNP in *TLR1* (rs4833095),a 3′UTR SNP in *IL1RN* (rs4252041), a *CLEC7A* SNP (rs7309123) previously associated with IA [62] and further SNPs in *DENND1B* (rs2477077), *PLAT* (rs8178890)

Table 7.2 SNPs associated with CCPA

Gene	SNP	Alleles	Model for association	Odds ratio (95% CI)	FDR p-value	Location
IL1RN	**rs4252041**	C/**T**	TT+TC vs. CC	0.23 (0.07, 0.76)	**0.039**	3′ UTR
IL1B	rs3136558	**A**/G	AG+GG vs. AA	0.57 (0.35, 0.92)	0.051	Intronic
	rs3917354	**T**/–	T-+-- vs. TT	0.55 (0.33, 0.91)	**0.046**	Intronic
IL15	**rs1519551**	A/**G**	AA+AG vs. GG	0.48 (0.29, 0.79)	**0.011**	Intronic
	rs6842735	G/**T**	TT+GT vs. GG	1.79 (1.12, 2.88)	**0.038**	Intronic
	rs12508866	T/**C**	CC+TC vs. TT	1.70 (1.09, 2.66)	**0.046**	Intronic
IL17A	rs3748067	G/**A**	AA+GA vs. GG	1.90 (1.10, 3.28)	0.050	3′ UTR
TLR1	rs4833095	**A**/G	AG+GG vs. AA	0.58 (0.36, 0.95)	0.065	Exonic (Asn/Ser)
CLEC7A (dectin-1)	rs7309123	C/**G**	CC+GC vs. GG	0.59 (0.35, 0.99)	0.099	Intronic
PLAT	rs8178890	**G**/A	AA+GA vs.GG	0.38 (0.16, 0.86)	**0.049**	Intronic
	rs879293	G/**A**	AA+GA vs. GG	1.65 (1.01, 2.69)	0.097	Intronic
DENND1B	**rs2477077**	C/**T**	CC+CT vs. TT	0.34 (0.14, 0.83)	**0.041**	Intronic
VEGFA	**rs10434**	**G**/A	GG+AG vs. AA	2.12 (1.16, 3.90)	**0.036**	3′ UTR

From Smith et al. [29, 61]
Risk allele shown in bold. All SNPs are associated with CCPA before correction for multiple testing ($p < 0.05$). SNPs in bold remain significant after Benjamini-Hochberg adjustment for false discovery rate (FDR adjusted p-values shown)
CI confidence interval

and *VEGFA* (rs10434) (Table 7.2) [61]. Additional SNPs in *TLR1, CLEC7A, IL17A* and *IL1B* showed trends towards significance but failed to pass correction for multiple testing (FDR corrected p-values 0.050–0.051) (Table 7.2) [29].

7.10.3.2 ABPA

Why some asthmatic individuals develop ABPA upon exposure to *A. fumigatus* while others are unaffected remains unclear, despite studies. Chronic intranasal administration of mould spores or extracts to unsensitised mice can lead to allergic lung inflammation, hyperreactivity and lung remodelling [63], but the effect in humans is unclear. There are reports of ABPA within families, suggesting a common genetic basis with low penetrance [64, 65], and familiar occurrence of ABPA has been reported in 4.9% of ABPA patients in India, where the disease is common [66]. Although our knowledge of genetic risk factors that might be involved in ABPA is limited, polymorphisms in genes that might play a crucial role for the ABPA immune response (IL4R, IL10, TLR9, SFTPA2 and HLA-DR) have been described in various small genetic association studies (involving ≤38 patients) [51, 60, 67–69]. In addition, the structural gene CFTR has been previously associated with ABPA [70], and a more recent, larger genetic association study has found associations with other genes [71]. This study identified 17 ABPA-associated polymorphisms, three of which remained significantly associated after correction for multiple testing. These were in the immune genes IL13, IL4R and TLR3 [71] (Table 7.3).

Table 7.3 SNPs associated with ABPA

Gene	SNP	Alleles	Model for association	Odds ratio (95% CI)	BH FDR p-value	Location
ADORA2A	rs2236624	C/**T**	CC+CT vs. TT	0.37(0.14–0.99)	0.130	Intronic
DECTIN1	rs11053624	T/**C**	CC+TC vs. TT	2.11 (1.08–4.10)	0.086	5′ near gene
	rs7959451	C/**T**	TT+CT vs. CC	2.00 (1.12–3.55)	0.061	3′ UTR
IL13	**rs20541**	G/**A**	AA+GA vs. GG	2.08 (1.23–3.53)	**0.025**	Exonic (R>Q)
	rs1800925	C/**T**	TT+TC vs. CC	1.86(1.10–3.14)	0.067	5′ near gene
IL17A	rs3819024	A/**G**	GG+GA vs. AA	1.78(1.05–3.02)	0.097	5′ near gene
IL4R	**rs3024656**	**G**/A	GG+GA vs. AA	4.78 (1.39–16.4)	**0.045**	Intronic
	rs1029489	G/**A**	AA+GA vs. GG	2.00 (1.14–3.52)	0.054	3′ near gene
	rs6498012	G/C	GG+GC vs. CC	0.49 (0.25–0.98)	0.122	Intronic
MBL2	rs2099903	C/**A**	CC+CA vs. AA	0.31(0.11–0.88)	0.086	3′ UTR
PLAT	rs8178880	**A**/G	GG+AG vs. AA	0.26(0.07–0.92)	0.108	Intronic
PLG	rs4252053	A/**G**	GG+AG vs. AA	1.97(1.10–3.54)	0.075	5′ near gene
TLR3	**rs1879026**	**G**/T	TT+GT vs. GG	0.44(0.24–0.80)	**0.026**	Intronic
	rs10025405	A/**G**	GG+GA vs. AA	1.83 (1.05–3.18)	0.100	Intergenic
	rs5743303	A/**T**	TT+AT vs. AA	1.95(1.13–3.36)	0.56	5′ near gene
	rs5743305	**T**/A	AA+TA vs. TT	0.54(0.32–0.91)	0.67	5′ near gene
	rs7668666	C/**A**	AA+CA vs. CC	1.75(1.04–2.96)	0.105	Intronic

From Overton et al. [71]
Risk allele shown in bold. All SNPs are associated with ABPA before correction for multiple testing ($p < 0.05$). SNPs in bold remain significant after Benjamini-Hochberg adjustment for false discovery rate (FDR adjusted p-values shown)
CI Confidence interval

7.10.3.3 SAFS

Recent work in our laboratory suggests that there are some genetic susceptibility factors for SAFS. Additional and broader genetic association studies in SAFS, combined with experimental work, are likely to contribute to our understanding of different phenotypes of problematic asthma.

7.11 Discussion

Chronic and allergic fungal diseases are both common and complex. They are almost exclusively secondary infections that complicate an existing condition or display a specialised opportunistic mode of infection utilising lung damage caused by a previous disease. The manner in which allergic disease can progress to chronic disease suggests that there may be shared susceptibility for both allergic and chronic fungal disease, but the symptoms and features of the two types of disease are quite distinct.

Study of genetic factors underlying chronic and allergic fungal disease has been hampered by a number of factors: until recently clinical guidelines and descriptions for either disease were not available, so few cases were diagnosed, symptoms for either disease are diffuse and easily misdiagnosed so strict phenotyping of patients for genetic typing has proved problematic, and, finally, the nature of the underlying disease needs to be considered, and this has posed problems in choosing the right control group for genetic comparisons.

The gene variants associated with either disease can be grouped into those affecting antigen presentation for the adaptive immune response (HLA genes), genes involved in the innate immune response particularly pattern recognition receptors (e.g. dectin-1, TLR genes, CLEC7A, MBL and SP-A) and genes involved in immune cell attraction, maturation and migration (e.g. PLAT, CCL2). The genes selected for analysis were chosen from our existing knowledge of the innate immune response to fungi, and so these results are not unexpected. Although these known variants are significant, they are all present at low frequency in the affected population. No variant yet studied is capable of explaining the full range or frequency of genetic susceptibility to fungal infection.

Future research in this area is likely to include more wide-ranging genetic techniques such as whole genome and exome sequencing that will shed light on the true range of factors that underlie these diseases.

References

1. Schleich F, Brusselle G, Louis R, et al. Heterogeneity of phenotypes in severe asthmatics. The Belgian Severe Asthma Registry (BSAR). Respir Med. 2014;108(12):1723–32.
2. Shah A, Panjabi C. Allergic bronchopulmonaryAspergillosis: a perplexing clinical entity. Allergy Asthma Immunol Res. 2016;8(4):282–97.
3. Tay TR, Bosco J, Gillman A, et al. Coexisting atopic conditions influence the likelihood of allergic bronchopulmonary aspergillosis in asthma. Ann Allergy Asthma Immunol Off Publ Am Coll Allergy Asthma Immunol. 2016;117(1):29–32. e1
4. Denning DW, Pashley C, Hartl D, et al. Fungal allergy in asthma-state of the art and research needs. Clin Transl Allergy. 2014;4:14.
5. Singh M, Das S, Chauhan A, et al. The diagnostic criteria for allergic bronchopulmonary aspergillosis in children with poorly controlled asthma need to be re-evaluated. Acta Paediatr. 2015;104(5):e206–9.
6. Maurya V, Gugnani HC, Sarma PU, Madan T, Shah A. Sensitization to *Aspergillus* antigens and occurrence of allergic bronchopulmonary aspergillosis in patients with asthma. Chest. 2005;127(4):1252–9.
7. Denning DW, Pleuvry A, Cole DC. Global burden of allergic bronchopulmonary aspergillosis with asthma and its complication chronic pulmonary aspergillosis in adults. Med Mycol. 2012;51:361–70.
8. Greenberger PA, Bush RK, Demain JG, et al. Allergic bronchopulmonary Aspergillosis. J Allergy Clin Immunol Pract. 2014;2(6):703–8.

9. Knutsen AP, Slavin RG. Allergic bronchopulmonary aspergillosis in asthma and cystic fibrosis. Clin Dev Immunol. 2011;2011:843763.
10. Agarwal R, Aggarwal AN, Gupta D, Jindal SK. *Aspergillus* hypersensitivity and allergic bronchopulmonary aspergillosis in patients with bronchial asthma: systematic review and meta-analysis. Int J Tuberc Lung Dis. 2009;13(8):936–44.
11. Maturu VN, Agarwal R. Prevalence of *Aspergillus* sensitization and allergic bronchopulmonary aspergillosis in cystic fibrosis: systematic review and meta-analysis. Clin Exp Allergy. 2015;45(12):1765–78.
12. Pana ZD, Farmaki E, Roilides E. Host genetics and opportunistic fungal infections. Clin Microbiol Infect. 2014;20(12):1254–64.
13. Agarwal R. Allergic bronchopulmonary aspergillosis. Chest. 2009;135(3):805–26.
14. Stevens DA, Moss RB, Kurup VP, et al. Allergic bronchopulmonary aspergillosis in cystic fibrosis – state of the art: cystic fibrosis foundation consensus conference. Clin Infect Dis. 2003;37(Suppl 3):S225–64.
15. Latge JP. *Aspergillus fumigatus* and aspergillosis. Clin Microbiol Rev. 1999;12(2):310–50.
16. Beauvais A, Fontaine T, Aimanianda V, Latge JP. *Aspergillus* cell wall and biofilm. Mycopathologia. 2014;178(5–6):371–7.
17. Chai LY, van de Veerdonk F, Marijnissen RJ, et al. Anti-Aspergillus human host defence relies on type 1T helper (Th1), rather than type 17T helper (Th17), cellular immunity. Immunology. 2010;130(1):46–54.
18. Eickmeier O, Rieber N, Eckrich J, et al. Immune response, diagnosis and treatment of allergic bronchopulmonary aspergillosis in cystic fibrosis lung disease. Curr Pharm Des. 2013;19(20):3669–78.
19. Gresnigt MS, Netea MG, van de Veerdonk FL. Pattern recognition receptors and their role in invasive aspergillosis. Ann N Y Acad Sci. 2012;1273:60–7.
20. Kita H. ILC2s and fungal allergy. Allergol Int. 2015;64(3):219–26.
21. Thakur R, Anand R, Tiwari S, et al. Cytokines induce effector T-helper cells during invasive aspergillosis; what we have learned about T-helper cells? Front Microbiol. 2015;6:429.
22. Agarwal R, Chakrabarti A, Shah A, et al. Allergic bronchopulmonary aspergillosis: review of literature and proposal of new diagnostic and classification criteria. Clin Exp Allergy. 2013;43(8):850–73.
23. Chaudhary N, Datta K, Askin FB, Staab JF, Marr KA. Cystic fibrosis transmembrane conductance regulator regulates epithelial cell response to *Aspergillus* and resultant pulmonary inflammation. Am J Respir Crit Care Med. 2012;185(3):301–10.
24. Becker KL, Gresnigt MS, Smeekens SP, et al. Pattern recognition pathways leading to a Th2 cytokine bias in allergic bronchopulmonary aspergillosis patients. Clin Exp Allergy. 2015;45(2):423–37.
25. Soubani AO, Chandrasekar PH. The clinical spectrum of pulmonary aspergillosis. Chest. 2002;121(6):1988–99.
26. Kosmidis C, Denning DW. The clinical spectrum of pulmonary aspergillosis. Thorax. 2015;70(3):270–7.
27. Denning DW, Riniotis K, Dobrashian R, Sambatakou H. Chronic cavitary and fibrosing pulmonary and pleural aspergillosis: case series, proposed nomenclature change, and review. Clin Infect Dis. 2003;37(Suppl 3):S265–80.
28. Roberts CM, Citron KM, Strickland B. Intrathoracic aspergilloma: role of CT in diagnosis and treatment. Radiology. 1987;165(1):123–8.
29. Smith NL, Hankinson J, Simpson A, Bowyer P, Denning DW. A prominent role for the IL1 pathway and IL15 in susceptibility to chronic cavitary pulmonary aspergillosis. Clin Microbiol Infect. 2013;20(8):O480–8.
30. Smith NL, Denning DW. Underlying conditions in chronic pulmonary aspergillosis including simple aspergilloma. Eur Respir J. 2011;37(4):865–72.
31. Camuset J, Nunes H, Dombret MC, et al. Treatment of chronic pulmonary aspergillosis by voriconazole in nonimmunocompromised patients. Chest. 2007;131(5):1435–41.

32. Addrizzo-Harris DJ, Harkin TJ, McGuinness G, Naidich DP, Rom WN. Pulmonary aspergilloma and AIDS. A comparison of HIV-infected and HIV-negative individuals. Chest. 1997;111(3):612–8.
33. *Aspergillus* in persistent lung cavities after tuberculosis. A report from the Research Committee of the British Tuberculosis Association. Tubercle. 1968;49(1):1–11.
34. Anonymous. Aspergilloma and residual tuberculous cavities – the results of a resurvey. Tubercle. 1970;51(3):227–45.
35. Sonnenberg P, Murray J, Glynn JR, et al. HIV-1 and recurrence, relapse, and reinfection of tuberculosis after cure: a cohort study in South African mineworkers. Lancet. 2001;358(9294):1687–93.
36. Lee JJ, Chong PY, Lin CB, Hsu AH, Lee CC. High resolution chest CT in patients with pulmonary tuberculosis: characteristic findings before and after antituberculous therapy. Eur J Radiol. 2008;67(1):100–4.
37. Andrejak C, Lescure FX, Pukenyte E, et al. *Mycobacterium xenopi* pulmonary infections: a multicentric retrospective study of 136 cases in north-east France. Thorax. 2009;64(4):291–6.
38. Maliwan N, Zvetina JR. Clinical features and follow up of 302 patients with *Mycobacterium kansasi*i pulmonary infection: a 50 year experience. Postgrad Med J. 2005;81(958):530–3.
39. Shah A, Khan ZU, Chaturvedi S, et al. Allergic bronchopulmonary aspergillosis with coexistent aspergilloma: a long-term followup. J Asthma. 1989;26(2):109–15.
40. Israel RH, Poe RH, Bomba PA, Gross RA. The rapid development of an aspergilloma secondary to allergic bronchopulmonary aspergillosis. Am J Med Sci. 1980;280(1):41–4.
41. Jewkes J, Kay PH, Paneth M, Citron KM. Pulmonary aspergilloma: analysis of prognosis in relation to haemoptysis and survey of treatment. Thorax. 1983;38(8):572–8.
42. Saraceno JL, Phelps DT, Ferro TJ, Futerfas R, Schwartz DB. Chronic necrotizing pulmonary aspergillosis: approach to management. Chest. 1997;112(2):541–8.
43. Denning DW, O′Driscoll BR, Hogaboam CM, Bowyer P, Niven RM. The link between fungi and severe asthma: a summary of the evidence. Eur Respir J. 2006;27(3):615–26.
44. Bulpa P, Dive A, Sibille Y. Invasive pulmonary aspergillosis in patients with chronic obstructive pulmonary disease. Eur Respir J. 2007;30(4):782–800.
45. Guinea J, Torres-Narbona M, Gijón P, et al. Pulmonary aspergillosis in patients with chronic obstructive pulmonary disease: incidence, risk factors, and outcome. Clin Microbiol Infect. 2009;16(7):870–7.
46. Israel HL, Ostrow A. Sarcoidosis and aspergilloma. Am J Med. 1969;47(2):243–50.
47. Panjabi C, Sahay S, Shah A. Aspergilloma formation in cavitary sarcoidosis. J Bras Pneumol. 2009;35(5):480–3.
48. Wollschlager C, Khan F. Aspergillomas complicating sarcoidosis. A prospective study in 100 patients. Chest. 1984;86(4):585–8.
49. Lee TM, Greenberger PA, Patterson R, Roberts M, Liotta JL. Stage V (fibrotic) allergic bronchopulmonary aspergillosis. A review of 17 cases followed from diagnosis. Arch Intern Med. 1987;147(2):319–23.
50. Carvalho A, Pasqualotto AC, Pitzurra L, et al. Polymorphisms in toll-like receptor genes and susceptibility to pulmonary aspergillosis. J Infect Dis. 2008;197(4):618–21.
51. Vaid M, Kaur S, Sambatakou H, et al. Distinct alleles of mannose-binding lectin (MBL) and surfactant proteins A (SP-A) in patients with chronic cavitary pulmonary aspergillosis and allergic bronchopulmonary aspergillosis. Clin Chem Lab Med. 2007;45(2):183–6.
52. Sambatakou H, Pravica V, Hutchinson IV, Denning DW. Cytokine profiling of pulmonary aspergillosis. Int J Immunogenet. 2006;33(4):297–302.
53. Crosdale DJ, Poulton KV, Ollier WE, Thomson W, Denning DW. Mannose-binding lectin gene polymorphisms as a susceptibility factor for chronic necrotizing pulmonary aspergillosis. J Infect Dis. 2001;184(5):653–6.
54. Romani L. Immunity to fungal infections. Nat Rev Immunol. 2011;11(4):275–88.

55. Croft CA, Culibrk L, Moore MM, Tebbutt SJ. Interactions of *Aspergillus fumigatus* conidia with airway epithelial cells: a critical review. Front Microbiol. 2016;7:472.
56. Hartl D, Buckland KF, Hogaboam CM. Chemokines in allergic aspergillosis – from animal models to human lung diseases. Inflamm Allergy Drug Targets. 2006;5(4):219–28.
57. Kreindler JL, Steele C, Nguyen N, et al. Vitamin D3 attenuates Th2 responses to *Aspergillus fumigatus* mounted by CD4+ T cells from cystic fibrosis patients with allergic bronchopulmonary aspergillosis. J Clin Invest. 2010;120(9):3242–54.
58. Urb M, Snarr BD, Wojewodka G, et al. Evolution of the immune response to chronic airway colonization with *Aspergillus fumigatus* hyphae. Infect Immun. 2015;83(9):3590–600.
59. Smith NL, Denning DW. Clinical implications of interferon-gamma genetic and epigenetic variants. Immunology. 2014;143(4):499–511.
60. Carvalho A, Pasqualotto AC, Pitzurra L, et al. Polymorphisms in toll-like receptor genes and susceptibility to pulmonary aspergillosis. J Infect Dis. 2008;197(4):618–21.
61. Smith NL, Hankinson J, Simpson A, Denning DW, Bowyer P. Reduced expression of TLR3, TLR10 and TREM1 by human macrophages in CCPA, and novel associations of VEGFA, DENND1B and PLAT. Clin Microbiol Infect. 2014;20:O960–8.
62. Sainz J, Lupianez CB, Segura-Catena J, et al. Dectin-1 and DC-SIGN polymorphisms associated with invasive pulmonary *Aspergillosis* infection. PLoS ONE. 2012;7(2):e32273.
63. Denis O, van den Brule S, Heymans J, et al. Chronic intranasal administration of mould spores or extracts to unsensitized mice leads to lung allergic inflammation, hyper-reactivity and remodelling. Immunology. 2007;122(2):268–78.
64. Halwig JM, Kurup VP, Greenberger PA, Patterson R. A familial occurrence of allergic bronchopulmonary aspergillosis: a probable environmental source. J Allergy Clin Immunol. 1985;76(1):55–9.
65. Graves TS, Fink JN, Patterson R, Kurup VP, Scanlon GT. A familial occurrence of allergic bronchopulmonary aspergillosis. Ann Intern Med. 1979;91(3):378–82.
66. Shah A, Kala J, Sahay S, Panjabi C. Frequency of familial occurrence in 164 patients with allergic bronchopulmonary aspergillosis. Ann Allergy Asthma Immunol Off Publ Am Coll Allergy Asthma Immunol. 2008; 101(4): 363–369.
67. Knutsen AP, Kariuki B, Consolino JD, Warrier MR. IL-4 alpha chain receptor (IL-4Ralpha) polymorphisms in allergic bronchopulmonary aspergillosis. Clin Mol Allergy. 2006;4(1):3–9.
68. Brouard J, Knauer N, Boelle PY, et al. Influence of interleukin-10 on Aspergillus fumigatus infection in patients with cystic fibrosis. J Infect Dis. 2005;191(11):1988–91.
69. Chauhan B, Hutcheson PS, Slavin RG, Bellone CJ. MHC restriction in allergic bronchopulmonary aspergillosis. Front Biosci. 2003;8:s140–8.
70. Agarwal R, Khan A, Aggarwal AN, Gupta D. Link between CFTR mutations and ABPA: a systematic review and meta-analysis. Mycoses. 2012;55(4):357–65.
71. Overton NLD, Denning DW, Bowyer P, Simpson A. Genetic susceptibility to allergic bronchopulmonary aspergillosis in asthma: a genetic association study. Allergy Asthma Clin Immunol. 2016;12:47. ecollection

Biomarker Applications in Diagnostics of Fungal Infections

8

Johan Maertens and Katrien Lagrou

Abstract

Diagnosing invasive mold disease has long been problematic owing to the inability to culture the causal fungal agent from blood or other body fluids. This has fueled an interest in nonculture-based techniques such as the detection of galactomannan in blood and bronchoalveolar fluid, the detection of beta-D-glucan in blood, and the detection of fungal DNA by PCR-based platforms. The past decades have witnessed important improvements in our understanding of the strengths and limitations of the antigen assays and in the standardization of PCR-based DNA techniques. These assays are now being incorporated into care pathways and diagnostic algorithms; they help us to steward and monitor antifungal therapies and to predict treatment outcomes.

8.1 Introduction

Invasive fungal infections are usually caused by yeast or mold pathogens. Diagnosis of invasive yeast infections is often based on a positive culture from a sterile body site (e.g., blood culture positive for *Candida* spp.) or on a specific serological test (e.g., cryptococcal antigen test). Diagnosis of invasive mold infections is less

J. Maertens (✉)
Department of Hematology, University Hospitals Leuven,
Herestraat 49, 3000 Leuven, Belgium
e-mail: johan.maertens@uzleuven.be

K. Lagrou
Department of Microbiology and Immunology, KU Leuven – University of Leuven,
Leuven, Belgium

Department of Laboratory Medicine and National Reference Center for Medical Mycology,
University Hospitals Leuven, Leuven, Belgium

A. Carvalho (ed.), *Immunogenetics of Fungal Diseases*,
DOI 10.1007/978-3-319-50842-9_8

straightforward; culture is frequently negative, and non-culture-based mycological tests exhibit major shortcomings, although advances have been made over the past two decades. Herein, we will focus on the availability and the use of biomarkers for diagnosing invasive mold disease with a particular emphasis on invasive aspergillosis.

Invasive mold infections, usually affecting the respiratory tract, occur almost exclusively in patients with varied degrees of immunodeficiency and produce a wide range of clinical manifestations. The risk is determined by the nature and the extent of the compromised immunity as well as the prophylactic use of antifungals and the accommodation in protective environments [1]. Patients considered at high-risk include allogeneic stem cell transplant recipients, those being treated for acute myeloid leukemia, myelodysplastic syndromes or aplastic anemia, and subgroups of solid organ transplant recipients [1]. However, over the past decade, several novel risk groups have been identified, including (but not restricted to) patients with chronic obstructive lung disease, liver cirrhosis, autoimmune disorders, and influenza pneumonia. Many of these latter patients do not reside in hemato-oncology or transplantation units but are being hospitalized in intensive care facilities [2, 3]. However, many cases of invasive mold disease still remain undiagnosed or are only identified at autopsy because of difficulties in making an early diagnosis [4]. This shortcoming has resulted in a widespread and well-accepted practice of starting antifungals prophylactically or empirically, in the absence of any confirmation of fungal infection or disease. Although this approach is considered "standard of care" by many treating physicians, this also results in unnecessary antifungal drug treatment, adverse drug reactions, and increased healthcare expenditure [5]. Diagnostic tools targeting fungal biomarkers (galactomannan, β-D-glucan, fungal DNA) have been developed over the past decades. These assays display improved performance characteristics compared with culture and microscopic examination, the more conventional diagnostic tools. In recent clinical practice, these novel tests are being increasingly used to determine a treatment strategy and to influence patient management [6]. However, understanding test performance in different at-risk populations with different prevalence of disease and in different clinical specimens is required. Assessing the clinical utility of these tests and feeding back the interpretation of test results to treating physicians has become a key element of antifungal stewardship, especially in centers with a large population of immunocompromised patients.

8.2 Available Biomarkers

8.2.1 Conventional Tools

Culture and microscopic examination have always been the cornerstones for making a microbiological diagnosis of IFD. However, culture is time-consuming and requires considerable expertise. In addition, blood cultures are notoriously negative (with the exception of *Fusarium* spp.), even in disseminated disease, and culture from any respiratory specimen has only low to moderate sensitivity and predictive value [7–9]. In an attempt to minimize the overinterpretation of the clinical significance of a positive culture for *Aspergillus* species, Bouza and colleagues developed a helpful score based on easily obtainable clinical and microbiological information, including (a) a sample obtained by invasive procedures (1 point), (b) two or more positive samples from the same patient (1 point), (c) underlying leukemia (2 points), (d) presence of neutropenia (5 points), and (e) corticosteroid treatment (2 points) [10]. Patients with a score of 0 had only a 2.5% probability of invasive aspergillosis. Those with a score of 1 or 2 had an increased probability of 10.3%. The probabilities rose to 40% and 70%, respectively, for patients with a score of 3 or 4 or a score of ≥5. This score helps to rule out the probability of proven or probable aspergillosis in an unselected population and better defines the subpopulation which needs more aggressive diagnostic work-up for the confirmation of disease. Similar scores have not yet been developed for other mold pathogens.

However, the lack of efficient diagnostic tools has led to the development of surrogate markers, based on the detection of fungal cell wall components or fungal DNA in clinical specimens.

8.2.2 Galactomannan

The fungal cell wall is almost exclusively composed of polysaccharides, including galactomannan (GM), a molecule composed of mannose residues with side chains of β-(1-5)-linked galactofuranosyl units. During the initial phase of logarithmic fungal growth, GM is incorporated into the cell wall, but as apical growth continues, the hyphal tip becomes weaker and releases GM [11]. Using an in vitro model of the human alveolus, Hope et al. demonstrated that the kinetics of GM release and subsequent levels are closely related to the dynamics of angioinvasion, concluding that that GM is only released into the circulation after the fungus has invaded the endothelial compartment [12].

GM can be detected in various body fluids by a commercially available sandwich enzyme-linked immunosorbent assay (ELISA; Platelia *Aspergillus*®, Bio-Rad, Marnes-la-Coquette, France). This test uses EB-A2, a rat monoclonal antibody which specifically binds to four galactofuranosyl residues, both as capture and detecting antibody [13]. In the presence of antigen in a clinical specimen, a monoclonal antibody-antigen-monoclonal antibody complex is formed. A chromogenic substrate is added to reveal the presence of such complexes by turning blue. Microplates are read using an optical reader that calculates the ratio of the optical density relative to a control provided by the manufacturer (the so-called optical density index) [14]. The test is included as a mycological criterion within the EORTC/MSG consensus definitions and has become the mainstay for diagnosing probable invasive aspergillosis [15]. This simple ELISA can be performed at the local laboratory level; however, no external quality control exists yet. The assay has been extensively evaluated and is the subject of meta-analyses and systematic reviews [16–18]. Sensitivities between 17% and 100% have been reported depending on the index cutoff used to determine positivity and on the nature of the population at risk. Indeed, the test performs best in adult and pediatric neutropenic patients (frequently undergoing intensive chemotherapy for acute leukemia) and less well in non-neutropenic patients, including organ transplant recipients and stem cell transplant recipients with graft-versus-host disease [16–18]. This probably reflects differences in immunopathogenesis of disease and fungal burden and represents a serious limitation of the assay when used as a screening tool in unselected immunosuppressed patients [19, 20]. Earlier studies used an index of ≥1.5 to define positivity, as initially recommended by the manufacturer. More recently, the United States Food and Drug Administration (US FDA) has approved a cutoff index value of ≥0.5 based on testing of two separate blood samples or a single sample with a value of ≥1.0 (restricted to patients with hematological malignancies or recipients of hematopoietic stem cell transplant) [21]. The European Conference on Infections in Leukemia (ECIL) guidelines recommend a single value of ≥0.7 or multiple (consecutive) values of ≥0.5 for blood specimens [22]. Of note, the 2008 EORTC-MSG revised consensus document has no specified cutoffs for positivity, but refers to the manufacturer's instructions [15]. However, improved sensitivity with the use of lower cutoffs comes with a loss of specificity.

Although fairly specific for *Aspergillus* species, cross-reactivity with non-*Aspergillus* molds (including but not limited to *Fusarium* spp., *Penicillium* spp., *Acremonium* spp., *Alternaria* spp, and *Histoplasma capsulatum*) may occur. In addition, galactofuranosyl residues are also present in other macromolecules, resulting in false-positive test results. Table 8.1 summarizes established causes of false positivity and false negativity.

GM testing can also be applied to other types of specimens, including bronchoalveolar lavage (BAL) fluid [23, 24]. Diagnostic bronchoscopy with lavage is performed when radiographic abnormalities of the lung have been detected, usually by pulmonary CT-scanning. In this setting, the pretest probability of (fungal) disease is much higher than when screening a blood sample from an asymptomatic patient; hence specificity becomes crucial such that a higher threshold of positivity is needed. Cutoff values of 1.0 have been recommended (and approved by the US FDA [21]), although it is likely that even higher thresholds are needed [25]. Recently, an index cutoff of 1.0 has also been suggested for analyzing cerebrospinal fluid (CSF) samples from patients with (suspected) cerebral aspergillosis [26]. Stringent criteria still need to be developed for use with other body fluids (urine, abscesses, pleural fluid, ascites, etc.)

8.2.3 Beta-1,3-D-glucan

Unlike GM, β-D-glucan (BDG) is a polysaccharide component of the cell wall of many pathogenic fungi including *Candida* spp., *Fusarium* spp., and *Pneumocystis*. The main exceptions are *Mucorales* and some *Cryptococcus* species [27]. Four assays are now commercially available, of which the Fungitell® assay (Associates of Cape Cod, Inc., East Falmouth, MA, USA) has been approved by the US FDA

Table 8.1 Limitations of antigen assays in diagnosing fungal disease

	Galactomannan (GM)	Beta-D-glucan (BDG)
Reactivity with fungal species	*Aspergillus* sp., *Fusarium* sp., *Paecilomyces* sp., *Acremonium* sp., *Penicillium* sp., *Alternaria* sp., *Histoplasma capsulatum*, *Blastomyces dermatitidis*, *Cryptococcus neoformans*, *Emmonsia* sp., *Wangiella dermatitidis*, *Prototheca*, *Myceliophthora*, *Geotrichum capitatum*, *Chaetomium globosum*	*Pneumocystis jiroveci*, *Aspergillus* sp., *Fusarium* sp., *Histoplasma capsulatum*, *Candida* sp., *Acremonium* sp., *Trichosporon* sp., *Sporothrix schenckii*, *Saccharomyces cerevisiae*, *Coccidioides immitis*, *Prototheca*
False-positive test results	Semisynthetic β-lactam antibiotics[a]	Semisynthetic β-lactam antibiotics
	Multiple myeloma	Human blood products, including immunoglobulins, albumin, plasma, coagulation factor infusions, filtered through cellulose membranes
	Blood products collected using Fresenius Kabi bags	Cellulose hemodialysis/hemofiltration membranes
	Gluconate-containing plasma expanders (e.g., Plasmalyte)	Exposure to (surgical) gauze
	Flavored ice pops/frozen dessert containing sodium gluconate	Bacterial bloodstream infections (e.g., *Pseudomonas aeruginosa*)
	Bifidobacterium sp. (gut)	
	Severe mucositis or gastrointestinal graft-versus-host disease	
	Enteral nutritional supplements	
False-negative test results	Concomitant use of mold-active antifungal agents	Concomitant use of antifungal agents
	Mucolytic agents (BAL) such as Sputasol or SLsolution	

[a]Include ampicillin, amoxicillin-clavulanate, and piperacillin-tazobactam (currently this problem seems largely abated compared to previous reports)

and carries the European CE label for the presumptive diagnosis of invasive fungal infection [28]. The remainder are only marketed in Japan. Fungitell detects BDG through a pathway in the *Limulus* amebocytes lysate (LAL), an aqueous extract of blood cells from the horseshoe crab, *Limulus polyphemus*. Bacterial endotoxins and BDG can activate different coagulation cascades in the LAL; bacterial endotoxins specifically activate factor B and C, whereas BDG activates factor G. The Fungitell assay uses a modified pathway in the LAL by removing factor C. Thus, in the absence of factor C, the coagulation cascade is activated only in the presence of BDG [14]. Also this test has been included in the EORTC/MSG definitions of invasive fungal disease [15]. Of note, cutoff values for determining positivity differ markedly between these assays [14].

Any systematic review of this test is hampered by significant heterogeneity among the patient populations, testing strategies, and the inclusion of retrospective and case-controlled studies alongside prospective cohort studies with low numbers of documented fungal diseases [29–32]. Most studies report good sensitivity, but specificity and positive predictive value for diagnosing mold infections is poor due to a high rate of false-positive results (Table 8.1), regardless of the specimen [33]. However, the negative predictive value is around 80–90%. Unfortunately, the BDG assay is not pathogen specific and therefore cannot differentiate fungal species. In addition, pretest preparations may limit its routine applicability.

8.2.4 Polymerase Chain Reaction

Polymerase chain reaction (PCR)-based methods have been developed for the diagnosis of fungal diseases. The main advantage is the very high sensitivity for the real-time detection of fungal DNA. In addition, PCR-based methods can be applied to any specimen type, including whole blood, serum, plasma, BAL fluid, CSF, and tissue samples. However, lack of standardization due to the use of in-house assays using varied protocols involving different specimens, extraction techniques, molecular targets, amplification platforms, and detection techniques has hampered the acceptance of these diagnostic assays. For this very reason, PCR has not yet been included in the EORTC/MSG consensus definitions as a reliable microbiological marker [15]. Fortunately, over the past decade, the European Aspergillus PCR Initiative (EAPCRI), established to remedy this situation for diagnosing invasive aspergillosis, has made tremendous progress in standardizing protocols for efficient DNA extraction and amplification [34–40]. Clinical validation in multicentre prospective studies is ongoing.

Commercially available as well as in-house platforms using genus-/species-specific genes and panfungal targets have been developed, and the usefulness of PCR for diagnosing invasive fungal disease has been recently reviewed [41, 42]. Superior performance compared to the serological biomarkers has been suggested and high negative predictive values have been consistently documented, despite all methodological variabilities [43–45]. Whereas two positive results seem to be required to rule in disease, it has been suggested that a single negative PCR result is sufficient to exclude *Aspergillus* disease at that time point.

8.2.5 Lateral-Flow Device for Invasive Aspergillosis

A lateral-flow device (LFD) was developed for a point-of-care diagnosis of invasive aspergillosis. This assay uses a monoclonal antibody that is highly specific to growing *Aspergillus* species (but different from the one used in the Platelia assay) [46, 47]. Compared to GM and BDG assays, the LFD test is quick (15 min to perform) and does not require expensive equipment or specific laboratory facilities to be run. Furthermore, cross-reactions with drugs or contaminants that have been shown to cause false-positive reaction in the GM and BDG tests have not (yet) been seen. A recent meta-analysis of seven studies (with mainly solid organ transplant recipients) yielded a pooled sensitivity, specificity, and DOR for proven/probable versus no aspergillosis cases of 86%, 93%, and 65.9%, respectively when using BAL fluid and 68%, 87%, and 11.9% when using serum samples (in which case a heating step is required) [48]. More data on the impact of antifungal prophylaxis or therapy on the performance are needed [49]. Of note, similar lateral-flow devices have proven to be very successful for the diagnosis of cryptococcal disease and are currently being developed for diagnosing non-*Aspergillus* mold infections (including *Fusarium* and *Scedosporium* species).

8.2.6 Biomarkers in Development

Despite significant recent advances, the available tools for diagnosing invasive fungal disease are far from perfect and clinicians still struggle to make a timely diagnosis. Therefore, the search for novel targets and platforms that may further improve our diagnostic capabilities continues. An electronic nose (eNose) can discriminate various lung diseases through an analysis of exhaled volatile organic compounds. An eNose is cheap and noninvasive and yields results within minutes. A proof-of-principle study showing that neutropenic patients with aspergillosis have a distinct exhaled breath profile (or "breath print") that can be discriminated with an eNose has recently been published. This study showed a sensitivity of 100% and a specificity of 83% [50].

Using gas chromatography and mass spectrometry, US researchers were able to measure fungal volatile metabolites in breath samples of patients with invasive aspergillosis [51]. Detection of α-trans-bergamotene, β-trans-bergamotene, a β-vatirenene-like sesquiterpene, or trans-geranylacetone identified these patients with 94% sensitivity and 93% specificity. Although both techniques perform well for diagnosing invasive aspergillosis, more extensive validation is needed.

In recent years, gliotoxin (GT), a virulence factor during hyphal growth, has been proposed as a diagnostic biomarker of invasive aspergillosis. *Aspergillus fumigatus* is the most important GT-producing fungal pathogen, although also non-*fumigatus Aspergillus* species can produce GT, as well as less common opportunistic pathogens such as *Penicillium* spp., *Gliocladium* spp., and *Pseudallescheria* spp. [52]. Unfortunately, GT is hard to detect in body fluids. Bis(methylthio)gliotoxin (bmGT), the inactive derivative of GT, is more stable and appears to be a more reliable indicator of infection than GT [52]. Preliminary work demonstrated that bmGT is produced by a higher percentage of isolates of *A. fumigatus* than GT. A recent prospective study comparing the diagnostic accuracy of bmGT detection (by high-performance thin layer chromatography) with GM detection (Platelia assay) in 79 patients at risk for invasive aspergillosis suggests a higher sensitivity and positive predictive value for bmGT than GM and similar specificity and negative predictive value [53]. Importantly, combining both tests increased the predictive value of the individual biomarkers. Although promising, additional analysis with larger cohorts of patients, as well as the development of an immunochemical method, are needed before this test can be implemented in clinical management.

8.3 Clinical Validity of Available Biomarkers

Assessing the clinical utility of a diagnostic test – i.e., how will the result determine a treatment strategy and potentially influence patient management and outcome – has become a key element of antifungal stewardship programs.

Based on factors related to host, underlying disease and condition, and fungal exposure, patients can generally be stratified into three risk groups for IFD (high, intermediate, and low), and risk-adapted antifungal strategies can be applied accordingly [54]. One generally considers a prevalence of ≥10% as being at high risk and ≤5% as being at low risk with intermediate lying in between. Importantly, risk assessment is a dynamic process and patients may gradually move to higher- or lower-risk categories (e.g., patients with refractory initially low-risk disease in need of intensive chemotherapy may become high-risk patients) [54]. Adequate risk assessment is an important element for the interpretation of test results. In clinical practice, physicians don't usually rely on the clinical sensitivity and specificity but rather on the positive and negative predictive values. These latter are influenced by the prevalence of disease in a population which determines the pretest probability of disease. Hence a diagnostic test for IFD with a sensitivity of 71% and a specificity of 89% will have a positive predictive value of only 12% in a population with a pretest probability of 2% (e.g., a kidney transplant recipient or a patient with first-line lymphoma therapy) [55]. However, the negative predictive value of 99.3% enables the fungal disease to be ruled out with a high degree of confidence. Using the same test in a population with a pretest probability of 15% increases the positive predictive value to almost 60% (or a six out of ten chance that the patient has IFD), while the negative predictive value remains high at 94%. Unlike predictive values, likelihood ratios (LR) are not influenced by prevalence; they inform us on how more likely the patient is to have IFD after the test results have become available, allowing us to calculate posttest probabilities (using Fagan's nomogram). For instance, if the prevalence of disease is 15% and the test has a positive LR of 50, then the chances of a patient with a positive result having IFD are 90%. Conversely, for a test with a negative LR of 0.1, the chances of a patient with a negative result having IFD are only 1.7%. Such a probability increase from 15% to 90% or decrease to 1.7% is clinically meaningful and should be used to guide antifungal management.

The importance of pretest prevalence is further evidenced by the impact of the use of mold-active antifungal drugs, either as prophylaxis or as treatment, on the performance characteristics of diagnostic tests [56, 57]. Biomarker assays remain frequently negative (or falsely positive) in the presence of drugs that reduce the pretest probability of IFD to less than 5% (e.g., posaconazole prophylaxis during remission-induction therapy of acute myeloid leukemia) [58].

Finally, the results of all these assays should not be interpreted in isolation. Nowadays an adequate and rapid diagnosis of IFD relies heavily on a few well-defined radiological features on pulmonary CT scan (nodules with or without a halo, cavities, and/or air crescent signs, as defined by the EORTC/MSG consensus criteria) [59]. Unfortunately these abnormalities are time-dependent, largely restricted to profoundly neutropenic patients, and nonspecific for invasive pulmonary mold disease. Moreover, nonspecific radiological abnormalities may precede these classical signs, especially in less immunocompromised patients and in those with moderate or transient neutropenia [60]. Biomarkers have the capacity to improve the specificity of these radiological features.

8.4 Clinical Application of Biomarkers

8.4.1 Low-Risk Patients

Mold-active prophylaxis is not justified for low-risk patients (incidence ≤5%) as the number need to harm will exceed the number need to treat to prevent a fungal infection [61]. Also screening for biomarkers is unlikely to be clinically useful and certainly not cost-effective [58]. Only testing for biomarkers in patients with a clinical picture suggestive of an invasive mold infection, usually a new lung infiltrate, appears to be appropriate.

8.4.2 High-Risk Patient on Mold-Active Drugs

As evidenced by a recent Spanish study, the clinical utility of twice weekly biomarker (GM) screening on blood samples of high-risk patients is severely compromised when mold-active prophylaxis is given or empirical therapy has been started [58]. Because of a relative high number of false-positive GM assays and the low incidence of IFD in effectively prophylaxed asymptomatic patients, the positive predictive value was only 11.8%. However, biomarkers may still be useful to confirm a diagnosis in the event of failure of prophylaxis or breakthrough cases of invasive aspergillosis. Indeed, when used to diagnose invasive aspergillosis in case of clinical suspicion, the positive predictive value increased to 89.6%. For these patients, an efficient co-positioning of effective prophylaxis and diagnostic strategies seems feasible. For instance, empirical antifungal therapy could be replaced with a diagnostic strategy that employs early pulmonary CT scan and serum/plasma and BAL GM detection [62]. Given its high sensitivity and specificity, PCR detection of fungal DNA might be used as well.

8.4.3 High-Risk Patient Not Receiving Mold-Active Drugs

In a high-risk population not receiving mold-active prophylaxis (fluconazole is permitted), a biomarker screening strategy using assays with high sensitivity and high negative predictive value can identify patients who do not have fungal infection and do not need antifungal therapy. All currently available noninvasive diagnostic tests (GM, BDG, PCR) can be used for this [63]. Of course, the rather low prevalence of fungal disease (even in high-risk patients not receiving prophylaxis) and the ubiquitous nature of contaminating fungal pathogens mean that false-positive assays will be seen. This will overestimate the need for antifungal therapy, albeit at a much lower rate than when empirical therapy would be initiated. Moreover, this drawback can be largely overcome by more frequent testing (twice or thrice weekly) or by combining different biomarkers [41, 64, 65]. Of note, antifungal therapy should not be initiated for patients with a single positive biomarker who have no clinical signs of invasive fungal disease; however, this should trigger repeat sampling and further intensive diagnostic work-up that includes imaging and, if needed, bronchoscopy with lavage. This approach can be used without excess morbidity or mortality [66]. Of course, such an approach will inevitably result in more documented cases of probable invasive fungal disease.

8.5 Can Biomarkers Be Used for Early Response Assessment?

Serum GM kinetics has been proposed as a good marker for predicting the outcome of patients with invasive aspergillosis, due to the excellent correlation observed in recent studies [67, 68]. In general, GM normalization after the initial 2 weeks of antifungal therapy is more prevalent in responders than in nonresponders (although the kinetics may depend upon the antifungal treatment), whereas persistently positive GM is associated with higher mortality [69, 70]. Given the performance characteristics of the assay, the correlation between GM values and patient outcome has predominantly been observed in studies composed of hematological patients only [71]. However, at present, no data suggest that the duration of antifungal therapy should be adjusted to the kinetics of biomarkers, including GM. Finally, whether a high baseline serum GM value or persistently positive assays supports the use of combination antifungal therapy, as carefully suggested in a recent study, remains to be determined [72]. The kinetics of BDG have been less vigorously studied, but preliminary data shows that prolonged persistence of BDG can occur despite resolution of the fungal infection.

8.6 Conclusion

Patients at risk for IFD constitute a heterogenous group and are frequently subjected to preventative strategies. Hence, different approaches may need to be used in different patient groups to maximize diagnostic accuracy. Understanding test performance in specific patient populations as well as in different clinical specimens and acknowledging the strengths as well as the limitations of testing strategies is imperative to maximize clinical benefit in an economically useful way.

References

1. Herbrecht R, Bories P, Moulin JC, et al. Risk stratification for invasive aspergillosis in immunocompromisedpatients.AnnNYAcadSci.2012;1272:23–30.doi:10.1111/j.1749-6632.2012.06829.x.
2. Meersseman W, Van Wijngaerden E. Invasive aspergillosis in the ICU: an emerging disease. Intensive Care Med. 2007;33(10):1679–81.
3. Taccone FS, Van den Abeele AM, Bulpa P, et al. Epidemiology of invasive aspergillosis in critically ill patients: clinical presentation, underlying conditions, and outcomes. Crit Care. 2015;19:7. doi:10.1186/s13054-014-0722-7.
4. Sinkó J, Csomor J, Nikolova R, et al. Invasive fungal disease in allogeneic hematopoietic stem cell transplant recipients: an autopsy-driven survey. Transpl Infect Dis. 2008;10(2): 106–9.
5. Maertens J, Buvé K, Anaissie E. Broad-spectrum antifungal prophylaxis in patients with cancer at high risk for invasive mold infections: counterpoint. J Natl Compr Cancer Netw. 2008;6(2):183–9.
6. Maertens J, Huysmans G, Theunissen K. Early diagnosis and preemptive therapy of pulmonary mold infections in high-risk patients. Curr Infect Dis Rep. 2008;10(6):459–65.
7. Arendrup MC, Bille J, Dannaoui E, et al. ECIL-3 classical diagnostic procedures for the diagnosis of invasive fungal diseases in patients with leukaemia. Bone Marrow Transplant. 2012;47(8):1030–45. doi:10.1038/bmt.2011.246.
8. Rickerts V, Mousset S, Lambrecht E, et al. Comparison of histopathological analysis, culture, and polymerase chain reaction assays to detect invasive mold infections from biopsy specimens. Clin Infect Dis. 2007;44(8):1078–83.
9. Guinea J, Torres-Narbona M, Gijón P, et al. Pulmonary aspergillosis in patients with chronic obstructive pulmonary disease: incidence, risk factors, and outcome. Clin Microbiol Infect. 2010;16(7):870–7. doi:10.1111/j.1469-0691.2009.03015.x.
10. Bouza E, Guinea J, Peláez T, et al. Workload due to Aspergillus fumigatus and significance of the organism in the microbiology laboratory of a general hospital. J Clin Microbiol. 2005;43(5):2075–9.
11. Morton CO, Loeffler J, De Luca A, et al. Dynamics of extracellular release of Aspergillus fumigatus DNA and galactomannan during growth in blood and serum. J Med Microbiol. 2010;59(4):408–13. doi:10.1099/jmm.0.017418-0.
12. Hope WW, Kruhlak MJ, Lyman CA, et al. Pathogenesis of Aspergillus fumigatus and the kinetics of galactomannan in an in vitro model of early invasive pulmonary aspergillosis: implications for antifungal therapy. J Infect Dis. 2007;195(3):455–66.
13. Barton RC. Laboratory diagnosis of invasive aspergillosis: from diagnosis to prediction of outcome. Sci (Cairo). 2013;2013:459405. doi:10.1155/2013/459405.
14. Miceli MH, Maertens J. Role of non-culture-based tests, with an emphasis on galactomannan testing for the diagnosis of invasive Aspergillosis. Semin Respir Crit Care Med. 2015;36(5):650–61. doi:10.1055/s-0035-1562892.
15. De Pauw B, Walsh TJ, Donnelly JP, et al. Revised definitions of invasive fungal disease from the European Organization for Research and Treatment of Cancer/Invasive Fungal Infections Cooperative Group and the National Institute of Allergy and Infectious Diseases Mycoses Study Group (EORTC/MSG) Consensus Group. Clin Infect Dis. 2008;46(12):1813–21. doi:10.1086/588660.
16. Mennink-Kersten MA, Donnelly JP, Verweij PE. Detection of circulating galactomannan for the diagnosis and management of invasive aspergillosis. Lancet Infect Dis. 2004;4(6):349–57.
17. Pfeiffer CD, Fine JP, Safdar N. Diagnosis of invasive aspergillosis using a galactomannan assay: a meta-analysis. Clin Infect Dis. 2006;42(10):1417–27.
18. Leeflang MM, Debets-Ossenkopp YJ, Wang J, et al. Galactomannan detection for invasive aspergillosis in immunocompromised patients. Cochrane Database Syst Rev. 2015;12:CD007394. doi:10.1002/14651858.CD007394.

19. Chamilos G, Luna M, Lewis RE, et al. Invasive fungal infections in patients with hematologic malignancies in a tertiary care cancer center: an autopsy study over a 15-year period (1989–2003). Haematologica. 2006;91(7):986–9.
20. Lewis RE, Kontoyiannis DP. Invasive aspergillosis in glucocorticoid-treated patients. Med Mycol. 2009;47(Suppl 1):S271–81. doi:10.1080/13693780802227159.
21. Galactomannan – Food and Drug Administration – www.fda.gov/downloads/drugs/guidance-complianceregulatoryinformation/guidances/ucm472606.pdf
22. Marchetti O, Lamoth F, Mikulska M, et al. ECIL recommendations for the use of biological markers for the diagnosis of invasive fungal diseases in leukemic patients and hematopoietic SCT recipients. Bone Marrow Transplant. 2012;47(6):846–54. doi:10.1038/bmt.2011.178.
23. Zou M, Tang L, Zhao S, et al. Systematic review and meta-analysis of detecting galactomannan in bronchoalveolar lavage fluid for diagnosing invasive aspergillosis. PLoS ONE. 2012;7(8):e43347. doi:10.1371/journal.pone.0043347.
24. Guo YL, Chen YQ, Wang K, et al. Accuracy of BAL galactomannan in diagnosing invasive aspergillosis: a bivariate meta-analysis and systematic review. Chest. 2010;138(4):817–24. doi:10.1378/chest.10-0488.
25. D'Haese J, Theunissen K, Vermeulen E, et al. Detection of galactomannan in bronchoalveolar lavage fluid samples of patients at risk for invasive pulmonary aspergillosis: analytical and clinical validity. J Clin Microbiol. 2012;50(4):1258–63. doi:10.1128/JCM.06423-11.
26. Chong GM, Maertens JA, Lagrou K, et al. Diagnostic performance of galactomannan antigen testing in cerebrospinal fluid. J Clin Microbiol. 2016;54(2):428–4231. doi:10.1128/JCM.02913-15.
27. Lamoth F, Cruciani M, Mengoli C, et al. β-Glucan antigenemia assay for the diagnosis of invasive fungal infections in patients with hematological malignancies: a systematic review and meta-analysis of cohort studies from the Third European Conference on Infections in Leukemia (ECIL-3). Clin Infect Dis. 2012;54(5):633–43. doi:10.1093/cid/cir897.
28. White PL, Wingard JR, Bretagne S, et al. Aspergillus polymerase chain reaction: systematic review of evidence for clinical use in comparison with antigen testing. Clin Infect Dis. 2015;61(8):1293–303. doi:10.1093/cid/civ507.
29. Hou TY, Wang SH, Liang SX, et al. The screening performance of serum 1,3-beta-D-glucan in patients with invasive fungal diseases: a meta-analysis of prospective cohort studies. PLoS ONE. 2015;10(7):e0131602. doi:10.1371/journal.pone.0131602.
30. He S, Hang JP, Zhang L, et al. A systematic review and meta-analysis of diagnostic accuracy of serum 1,3-β-D-glucan for invasive fungal infection: focus on cutoff levels. J Microbiol Immunol Infect. 2015;48(4):351–61. doi:10.1016/j.jmii.2014.06.009.
31. Lu Y, Chen YQ, Guo YL, et al. Diagnosis of invasive fungal disease using serum (1→3)-β-D-glucan: a bivariate meta-analysis. Intern Med. 2011;50(22):2783–91.
32. Karageorgopoulos DE, Vouloumanou EK, Ntziora F, et al. β-D-glucan assay for the diagnosis of invasive fungal infections: a meta-analysis. Clin Infect Dis. 2011;52(6):750–70. doi:10.1093/cid/ciq206.
33. Theel ES, Jespersen DJ, Iqbal S, et al. Detection of (1, 3)-β-D-glucan in bronchoalveolar lavage and serum samples collected from immunocompromised hosts. Mycopathologia. 2013;175(1–2):33–41. doi:10.1007/s11046-012-9579-y.
34. White PL, Wiederhold NP, Loeffler J, et al. Comparison of nonculture blood-based tests for diagnosing invasive Aspergillosis in an animal model. J Clin Microbiol. 2016;54(4):960–6. doi:10.1128/JCM.03233-15.
35. Loeffler J, Mengoli C, Springer J, et al. Analytical comparison of in vitro-spiked human serum and plasma for PCR-based detection of Aspergillus fumigatus DNA: a study by the European Aspergillus PCR Initiative. J Clin Microbiol. 2015;53(9):2838–45. doi:10.1128/JCM.00906-15.
36. White PL, Barnes RA, Springer J, et al. Clinical performance of Aspergillus PCR for testing serum and plasma: a study by the European Aspergillus PCR initiative. J Clin Microbiol. 2015;53(9):2832–7. doi:10.1128/JCM.00905-15.

37. Lyon GM, Abdul-Ali D, Loeffler J, et al. Development and evaluation of a calibrator material for nucleic acid-based assays for diagnosing aspergillosis. J Clin Microbiol. 2013;51(7):2403–5. doi:10.1128/JCM.00744-13.
38. White PL, Mengoli C, Bretagne S, et al. Evaluation of Aspergillus PCR protocols for testing serum specimens. J Clin Microbiol. 2011;49(11):3842–8. doi:10.1128/JCM.05316-11.
39. White PL, Perry MD, Loeffler J, et al. Critical stages of extracting DNA from Aspergillus fumigatus in whole-blood specimens. J Clin Microbiol. 2010;48(10):3753–5. doi:10.1128/JCM.01466-10.
40. White PL, Bretagne S, Klingspor L, et al. Aspergillus PCR: one step closer to standardization. J Clin Microbiol. 2010;48(4):1231–40. doi:10.1128/JCM.01767-09.
41. Arvanitis M, Ziakas PD, Zacharioudakis IM, et al. PCR in diagnosis of invasive aspergillosis: a meta-analysis of diagnostic performance. J Clin Microbiol. 2014;52(10):3731–42. doi:10.1128/JCM.01365-14.
42. Kourkoumpetis TK, Fuchs BB, Coleman JJ, et al. Polymerase chain reaction-based assays for the diagnosis of invasive fungal infections. Clin Infect Dis. 2012;54(9):1322–31. doi:10.1093/cid/cis132.
43. Mengoli C, Cruciani M, Barnes RA, et al. Use of PCR for diagnosis of invasive aspergillosis: systematic review and meta-analysis. Lancet Infect Dis. 2009;9(2):89–96. doi:10.1016/S1473-3099(09)70019-2.
44. Arvanitis M, Anagnostou T, Mylonakis E. Galactomannan and polymerase chain reaction-based screening for invasive Aspergillosis among high-risk hematology patients: a diagnostic meta-analysis. Clin Infect Dis. 2015;61(8):1263–72. doi:10.1093/cid/civ555.
45. Heng SC, Morrissey O, Chen SC, et al. Utility of bronchoalveolar lavage fluid galactomannan alone or in combination with PCR for the diagnosis of invasive aspergillosis in adult hematology patients: a systematic review and meta-analysis. Crit Rev Microbiol. 2015;41(1):124–34. doi:10.3109/1040841X.2013.804033.
46. Thornton C, Johnson G, Agrawal S. Detection of invasive pulmonary aspergillosis in haematological malignancy patients by using lateral-flow technology. J Vis Exp. 2012;(61). pii: 3721. doi:10.3791/3721.
47. Thornton CR. Development of an immunochromatographic lateral-flow device for rapid serodiagnosis of invasive aspergillosis. Clin Vaccine Immunol. 15(7):1095–105. doi:10.1128/CVI.00068-08.
48. Pan Z, Fu M, Zhang J, et al. Diagnostic accuracy of a novel lateral-flow device in invasive aspergillosis: a meta-analysis. J Med Microbiol. 2015;64(7):702–7. doi:10.1099/jmm.0.000092.
49. Eigl S, Prattes J, Reinwald M, et al. Influence of mould-active antifungal treatment on the performance of the Aspergillus-specific bronchoalveolar lavage fluid lateral-flow device test. Int J Antimicrob Agents. 2015;46(4):401–5. doi:10.1016/j.ijantimicag.2015.05.017.
50. de Heer K, van der Schee MP, Zwinderman K, et al. Electronic nose technology for detection of invasive pulmonary aspergillosis in prolonged chemotherapy-induced neutropenia: a proof-of-principle study. J Clin Microbiol. 2013;51(5):1490–5. doi:10.1128/JCM.02838-12.
51. Koo S, Thomas HR, Daniels SD, et al. A breath fungal secondary metabolite signature to diagnose invasive aspergillosis. Clin Infect Dis. 2014;59(12):1733–4170. doi:10.1093/cid/ciu725.
52. Domingo MP, Colmenarejo C, Martínez-Lostao L, et al. Bis(methyl)gliotoxin proves to be a more stable and reliable marker for invasive aspergillosis than gliotoxin and suitable for use in diagnosis. Diagn Microbiol Infect Dis. 2012;73(1):57–64. doi:10.1016/ j. diagmicrobio.2012.01.012.
53. Vidal-García M, Domingo MP, De Rueda B, et al. Clinical validity of bis(methylthio)gliotoxin for the diagnosis of invasive aspergillosis. Appl Microbiol Biotechnol. 2016;100(5):2327–34. doi:10.1007/s00253-015-7209-6.
54. Nucci M, Anaissie E. How we treat invasive fungal diseases in patients with acute leukemia: the importance of an individualized approach. Blood. 2014;124(26):3858–6389. doi:10.1182/blood-2014-04-516211.

55. Donnelly JP, Leeflang MM. Galactomannan detection and diagnosis of invasive aspergillosis. Clin Infect Dis. 2010;50(7):1070–1. author reply 1071–2 doi:10.1086/651161.
56. Marr KA, Balajee SA, McLaughlin L, et al. Detection of galactomannan antigenemia by enzyme immunoassay for the diagnosis of invasive aspergillosis: variables that affect performance. J Infect Dis. 2004;190(3):641–9.
57. Marr KA, Laverdiere M, Gugel A, et al. Antifungal therapy decreases sensitivity of the Aspergillus galactomannan enzyme immunoassay. Clin Infect Dis. 2005;40(12):1762–9.
58. Duarte RF, Sánchez-Ortega I, Cuesta I, et al. Serum galactomannan-based early detection of invasive aspergillosis in hematology patients receiving effective antimold prophylaxis. Clin Infect Dis. 2014;59(12):1696–702. doi:10.1093/cid/ciu673.
59. Maschmeyer G, Donnelly JP. How to manage lung infiltrates in adults suffering from haematological malignancies outside allogeneic haematopoietic stem cell transplantation. Br J Haematol. 2016;173(2):179–819. doi:10.1111/bjh.13934.
60. Nucci M, Nouér SA, Cappone D, et al. Early diagnosis of invasive pulmonary aspergillosis in hematologic patients: an opportunity to improve the outcome. Haematologica. 2013;98(11):1657–60. doi:10.3324/haematol.2013.094359.
61. De Pauw BE, Donnelly JP. Prophylaxis and aspergillosis – has the principle been proven? N Engl J Med. 2007;356(4):409–11.
62. Aguilar-Guisado M, Martín-Peña A, Espigado I, et al. Universal antifungal therapy is not needed in persistent febrile neutropenia: a tailored diagnostic and therapeutic approach. Haematologica. 2012;97(3):464–71. doi:10.3324/haematol.2011.049999.
63. Barnes RA, White PL, Bygrave C, et al. Clinical impact of enhanced diagnosis of invasive fungal disease in high-risk haematology and stem cell transplant patients. J Clin Pathol. 2009;62(1):64–9. doi:10.1136/jcp.2008.058354.
64. Barnes RA, Stocking K, Bowden S, et al. Prevention and diagnosis of invasive fungal disease in high-risk patients within an integrative care pathway. J Infect. 2013;67(3):206–14. doi:10.1016/j.jinf.2013.04.020.
65. Aguado JM, Vázquez L, Fernández-Ruiz M, et al. Serum galactomannan versus a combination of galactomannan and polymerase chain reaction-based Aspergillus DNA detection for early therapy of invasive aspergillosis in high-risk hematological patients: a randomized controlled trial. Clin Infect Dis. 2015;60(3):405–14. doi:10.1093/cid/ciu833.
66. Morrissey CO, Chen SC, Sorrell TC, et al. Galactomannan and PCR versus culture and histology for directing use of antifungal treatment for invasive aspergillosis in high-risk haematology patients: a randomized controlled trial. Lancet Infect Dis. 2013;13(6):519–28. doi:10.1016/S1473-3099(13)70076-8.
67. Fisher CE, Michal Stevens A, Leisenring W, et al. The serum galactomannan index predicts mortality in hematopoietic stem cell transplant recipients with invasive Aspergillosis. Clin Infect Dis. 2013;57(7):1001–4. doi:10.1093/cid/cit393.
68. Maertens J, Buvé K, Theunissen K, et al. Galactomannan serves as a surrogate endpoint for outcome of pulmonary invasive aspergillosis in neutropenic hematology patients. Cancer. 2009;115(2):355–62. doi:10.1002/cncr.24022.
69. Chai LYA, Kullberg BJ, Johnson EM, et al. Early serum galactomannan trend as a predictor of outcome of invasive Aspergillosis. J Clin Microbiol. 2012;50(7):2330–6. doi:10.1128/JCM.06513-11.
70. Koo S, Bryar JM, Baden LR, et al. Prognostic features of galactomannan antigenemia in galactomannan-positive invasive Aspergillosis. J Clin Microbiol. 2010;48(4):1255–60. doi:10.1128/JCM.02281-09.
71. Neofytos D, Railkar R, Mullane KM, et al. Correlation between circulating fungal biomarkers and clinical outcome in invasive Aspergillosis. PLoS ONE. 2015;10(6):e0129022. doi:10.1371/journal.pone.0129022.
72. Marr KA, Schlamm HT, Herbrecht R, et al. Combination antifungal therapy for invasive aspergillosis: a randomized trial. Ann Intern Med. 2015;162(2):81–9. doi:10.7326/M13-2508.

Immunotherapy of Invasive Fungal Disease

9

Thomas Lehrnbecher and Darius Armstrong-James

Abstract

Despite the availability of new antifungal compounds, morbidity and mortality of invasive fungal disease are still unacceptably high, in particular in immunocompromised patients such as patients with hematological malignancies, allogeneic hematopoietic stem cell, solid organ transplant recipients, or advanced HIV infection. However, our knowledge of the immunopathogenesis of invasive fungal disease has greatly expanded over the last decades, which, in turn, provides critical information to augment host immunity against fungal pathogens. Potential approaches for enhancing the host immune system in the combat against invasive fungal disease include the administration of effector and regulatory cells (e.g., granulocytes, antifungal T cells, natural killer cells, dendritic cells) and the administration of recombinant cytokines, antibodies, interferons, and growth factors (e.g., interferon-γ, granulocyte colony-stimulating factor, and granulocyte-macrophage colony-stimulating factor). Although promising results are reported on in vitro data and animal studies, the real challenge in the future is to perform appropriately designed and powered clinical trials.

T. Lehrnbecher, MD (✉)
Pediatric Hematology and Oncology, Hospital for Children and Adolescents, Johann Wolfgang Goethe University, Theodor-Stern-Kai 7, 60590 Frankfurt, Germany
e-mail: Thomas.Lehrnbecher@kgu.de

D. Armstrong-James, FRCP, PhD
Fungal Pathogens Laboratory, National Heart and Lung Institute, Imperial College London, Exhibition Road, London SW7 2AZ, UK
e-mail: d.armstrong@imperial.ac.uk

A. Carvalho (ed.), *Immunogenetics of Fungal Diseases*,
DOI 10.1007/978-3-319-50842-9_9

9.1 Introduction

Patients with hematological malignancies, patients undergoing allogeneic hematopoietic stem cell transplantation (HSCT) or solid organ transplantation, and those with advanced HIV infection are at a particular high risk for invasive fungal infection [4, 60]. The majority of these infections are caused by *Aspergillus* spp (mostly due to *A. fumigatus*, followed by *A. flavus*, *A. niger*, and *A. versicolor*), *Cryptococcus neoformans*, and *Candida* spp (with an increasing frequency of non-albicans *Candida* spp) [16, 62, 73]. In patients with infections due to non-*Aspergillus* molds, mucormycetes, *Scedosporium* spp, and *Fusarium* spp are predominantly seen [115]. Pneumocystis pneumonia is also a significant problem, especially in advanced HIV infection [4]. Despite the availability of new classes of antifungal compounds, such as broad-spectrum triazoles or echinocandins, the mortality of invasive fungal disease is still unacceptably high [24, 28, 58]. The poor outcome in these patients is due to a number of factors including delayed diagnosis and initiation of appropriate treatment and, more importantly, due to the long-lasting and often profound impaired immune response of affected patients [58,105].

Over the last decades, not only the understanding of the complex web of immunity and the impairment of the different arms of the immune system by the treatment of malignancy has greatly advanced but also at the same time our knowledge on the immunopathogenesis of invasive fungal infections [50, 52, 86, 87]. Since the significance of immune reconstitution in order to achieve a favorable outcome in invasive fungal infections has been increasingly recognized, there is growing interest in the role of immunomodulation as adjunctive treatment in immunocompromised patients suffering from aspergillosis, cryptococcosis, candidiasis, and mucormycosis. This chapter will highlight the recent development in the field of immunotherapy in invasive fungal disease. Although important interactions of the different arms of the immune system are well recognized, each arm will separately be described.

9.2 Adoptive Transfer of Immune Cells

9.2.1 Granulocyte Transfusions

In patients suffering from cancer or undergoing HSCT, severe and prolonged neutropenia is one of the most important risk factors for invasive fungal disease [26, 27, 51]. It has also been demonstrated that the outcome of an infectious complication is better in patients in whom neutropenia resolves shortly after the onset of infection as compared to those patients with persistent neutropenia [14]. In addition, the functional activity of neutrophils in HSCT recipients has recently been described as a prognostic factor in invasive aspergillosis [104]. Therefore, it is not surprising that the transfusion of granulocytes from healthy individuals has been considered since a long time as adjunctive

Table 9.1 Current immunotherapeutic approaches for fungal diseases

Modality	Agent	Target	Disease state	Current usage	References
Adoptive transfer of immune cells	Granulocyte transfusions	*Candida*, *Aspergillus*, and *Mucor* spp	Neutropenia	Clinical	[90, 64, 93, 80, 98, 79]
	T cells	*Candidiasis*, *Aspergillosis*, and *Mucormycosis*	Hematopoietic stem cell transplantation	Clinical/preclinical	[7, 11, 36, 47, 74, 76, 105; 109]
	Dendritic cells	*Aspergillus fumigatus*	Hematopoietic stem cell transplantation	Preclinical	[18]
Hematopoietic growth factors, cytokines, and interferons	G-CSF, GM-CSF	*Aspergillosis*	Neutropenia	Clinical	[34, 49, 53]
	Interferon-γ	*Aspergillosis*, *Candidiasis*, phaeohyphomycosis, cryptococcosis	Hematopoietic stem cell transplantation, organ transplant		[6, 5, 31, 91, 30, 44]
Opsonins and antibodies	PTX3, monoclonal and polyclonal antibodies	Prophylaxis, *Candidiasis*, cryptococcosis, *Aspergillosis*	Liver transplant	Clinical/preclinical	[22, 37, 48, 72, 103]
Immunomodulatory molecules	Thymosin alpha 1	*Aspergillosis*, phaeohyphomycosis	Hematopoietic stem cell transplantation, chromoblastomycosis		[88]

immunotherapeutic option in neutropenic patients who are at high risk for or suffer from invasive fungal disease. This interest has been further increased when recombinant hematopoietic growth factors such as granulocyte colony-stimulating factor (G-CSF) and granulocyte-macrophage colony-stimulating factor (GM-CSF) became available which markedly enhance the yield of leucocytes from healthy donors [2].

Common adverse events reported in up to 20% of granulocyte transfusions include fever chills and pulmonary reactions presenting as acute respiratory distress syndrome [64, 70, 77, 93, 98]. Unfortunately, current data on the efficacy of granulocyte transfusions are conflicting. Three retrospective studies reported on a potential benefit of granulocyte transfusions in neutropenic patients with severe infectious complications including invasive fungal disease [64, 90, 93]. In addition, a systematic review which analyzed the role of granulocyte transfusions in 34 patients with invasive fusariosis reported that granulocyte transfusions might have contributed to high response rates by effectively bridging periods of neutropenia or marrow suppression, whereas the utility in the absence of neutrophil recovery was questionable [45]. In contrast, a recent retrospective study reported on a significant worse outcome of neutropenic patients when they received granulocyte transfusions for proven/probable invasive aspergillosis, in particular of those patients with pulmonary infection, as compared to patients who did not receive granulocyte transfusions ($P = 0.011$) [80].

To date, two randomized phase III studies have evaluated granulocyte transfusions in neutropenic cancer patients with febrile neutropenia and infection. One study enrolling a total of 74 patients reported that the probability of 28-day survival after randomization did not significantly differ between both groups with 84% and 82%, respectively, and no effect of granulocyte transfusions on survival until day 100 could be detected in patients with fungal ($n = 55$), bacterial, or unknown infection ($n = 17$), even when stratified according to various levels of neutropenia (absolute neutrophil count, ANC<500/μl versus ANC>500/μl) [98]. The authors attributed the lack of benefit primarily to procedural obstacles, such as the long delay from randomization to the first transfusion of granulocytes, the low cell content, and the slow sequence of granulocyte transfusion. These problems led to a dramatic decrease in the recruitment rate in this study, resulting in the premature closure.

The Resolving Infection in Neutropenia with Granulocytes (RING) trial was a multicenter randomized controlled trial in which patients were randomized to receive standard antimicrobial therapy with ($n = 56$) or without ($n = 58$) daily granulocyte transfusions from donors stimulated with G-CSF and dexamethasone [79]. Overall success, defined as survival plus microbial response, was not different between the two groups (42% and 43%, respectively; $P > 0.99$), and success rates did not differ within any infection type. However, in a post hoc analysis, subjects who received an average dose of $\geq 0.6 \times 10^9$ granulocytes/kg per transfusion tended to have a better outcome than those receiving a lower dose. As enrollment was half that of planned, the trial reflects again the problems of evaluating granulocyte transfusions in a randomized manner.

9.2.2 Adoptive Transfer of Antifungal T Cells and Dendritic Cells

In addition to innate immunity, the adaptive immune system plays a major role in the host response to invasive fungal infections [87]. This complex network includes not only different subsets of dendritic cells and T cells but also a multitude of soluble factors, namely, cytokines and interferons (see below). Animal studies demonstrated that exposure to *Aspergillus* antigens which induced T_H1 lung lymphocytes was associated with resistance to invasive *Aspergillus* infection, whereas protection was not observed when mice were exposed to antigens eliciting high-level production of IL-4 which suppresses the T_H1 response [19, 20]. This corroborates the clinical observation which demonstrated that in patients with invasive aspergillosis, a predominant release of interferon (IFN)-γ in culture supernatants on stimulation with *A. fumigatus* antigens, indicating a T_H1 response, was associated with a favorable outcome, whereas a progressive disease was observed in most patients with a predominant T_H2 response characterized by low IFN-γ and increased IL-10 levels [42]. Further studies in solid organ transplant recipients further demonstrate defects in interferon-gamma responses during invasive fungal infection [5, 6].The critical function of T cells in the host response to fungal infection is also supported by the clinical observation that the median time of invasive aspergillosis after HSCT is 82 days (range, 3–6,542 days), a time when neutropenia has resolved but adaptive immune responses are still hampered [41, 67]. Recent analyses also demonstrated that up to 1 year after HSCT, transplant recipients have a significantly lower number of functionally active anti-*Aspergillus* T cells as compared to healthy controls and that lymphopenia is associated with a higher risk of death of transplant recipients suffering from invasive fungal infections [10, 57].

Based on this knowledge, the selective restoration of antifungal cellular immunity seems to be an attractive strategy in the allogeneic HSCT setting, which has already been successfully applied for HSCT recipients suffering from severe viral disease [12, 33]. Unfortunately, in contrast to viral disease, only one clinical trial of adoptive immunotherapy in patients with invasive aspergillosis has been reported to date [76]. Although the study has clear limitations in disease definition and outcome description and also has an unusual low incidence of graft-versus-host disease (GvHD), it is important to note (1) that no toxicity was induced by the infusion of anti-*Aspergillus* T cells and (2) that galactomannan antigenemia fell within 6 weeks of infusion of anti-*Aspergillus* T cells to normal range in all ten patients, whereas it persisted in the 13 controls not receiving anti-*Aspergillus* immunotherapy for as long as monitored. In addition, only one patient received immunotherapy, and 6 out of the 13 controls died of *Aspergillus* pneumonia within 2 weeks of diagnosis.

Based on these promising results, there was an increasing interest in generating and characterizing anti-*Aspergillus* T cells [7, 11, 36, 105, 109]. Due to the relatively low frequency of anti-*Aspergillus* T cells in the peripheral blood of healthy individuals, several approaches to expand sufficient numbers of these cells within a reasonable time frame have been investigated [74]. Although the generated T cells proliferate upon restimulation, the optimal dose of anti-*Aspergillus* T cells that is required for efficacy has not been established to date. In addition, unresolved questions include the optimal $CD4^+/CD8^+$ ratio for the adoptive immunotherapeutic product, whether or not T_H17 cells should be included, and the optimal antigen target. Notably, the *A. fumigatus* proteome is rather complex, and it has been shown that different proteins elicit different, even opposite, T cell responses [8, 68]. In this regard, it has been shown that some cell wall components may potentially inhibit the protective T cell response, for example, by inducing a T_H2 activation [17, 105]. The use of a cellular extract which includes multiple antigens might therefore be problematic, but, on the other hand, might decrease the risk of fungal escape from a generated T cell clone. In addition, T cells generated with cellular fungal extracts might cross-react with other molds and yeast, although this has also been demonstrated for specific peptides [7, 11, 36, 105, 109]. As protocols for generating human antifungal T cells have not only been established for human anti-*Aspergillus* T cells but also for human anti-*Candida* T cells and human anti-mucormycete T cells, one study used cellular extract of different fungi simultaneously to generate multi-specific T cell clones covering a wide variety of medically important fungi [97, 108, 110]. Another elegant approach of generating anti-*Aspergillus* T cells was recently reported by Kumaresan et al. [47]. The group redirected T cells by genetically modifying T cells to express a chimeric antigen receptor (CAR) that recognizes the carbohydrate antigens in beta-glucans, by incorporating the pattern-recognition properties of dectin-1. This approach might offer several important advantages compared to third-party T cells such HLA independency, but the production of these cells is costly, complex, and time-consuming.

Many in vitro studies demonstrate that the generated antifungal T cells are functionally active, have a strong T_H1 cytokine response upon reactivation, and increase the antifungal activity of other cells such as of phagocytes [7, 11, 36, 105, 109]. Importantly, the concomitant use of antifungals does not seem to impair the functional activity of the generated cells, whereas commonly used immunosuppressants impair T cell proliferation and /or the production of important molecules such as IFN-γ, which has to be considered for the clinical application [111, 112].

A potential, but important risk of the immunotherapeutic approach using T cells is the induction of GvHD, which may be caused by the transfer of even a small number of alloreactive T cells. However, in vitro data suggest that the alloreactive potential of the generated antifungal T cells is lower compared to nonselected and unspecific T cells [11, 109], and these data are further supported by clinical data on both virus-specific and antifungal T cells [25, 76].

It has been demonstrated in a murine allogeneic transplant model that dendritic cells stimulated ex vivo with conidia of *Aspergillus* or transfected with conidial RNA-activated, antigen-specific, IFN-γ-producing T lymphocytes in vitro and in vivo [18]. Importantly, the efficacy of the infusion of dendritic cells in protecting the transplanted mice from invasive aspergillosis was superior to that obtained by the adoptive transfer of *Aspergillus*-specific T cells. Despite these promising data and the fact that clinical trials have evaluated dendritic cells to induce antitumor immune responses in cancer patients for a number of years [66], there are no clinical data on the immunotherapeutic use of these cells in patients at high risk or suffering from invasive fungal disease.

9.2.3 Natural Killer (NK) Cells

NK cells represent between 5% and 10% of lymphocytes in the peripheral blood and have the ability to kill tumor cells in vitro, including acute lymphoblastic and myeloid leukemia [39]. Based on these observations, clinical trials are currently being performed which demonstrate that NK cells can safely be transferred to transplant recipients [101, 106]. Importantly, adoptive immunotherapy with NK cells is not associated with an increased risk of GvHD, which is in contrast to the infusion of antifungal T cells. In addition to the ability to kill tumor cells, NK eliminate virus-infected cells, have antibacterial effects, and are active against a wide variety of fungi including *Aspergillus* spp, *Candida* spp, and mucormycetes [94, 95, 100, 113]. Whereas hyphae and germlings of *A. fumigatus* and *R. oryzae* are damaged by both freshly isolated and IL-2 prestimulated human NK cells, conidia are not affected by NK cell populations [15, 95, 96]. This might be due, at least in part, to the fact that conidia of fungi are often protected by cell wall components, melanin pigments, and hydrophobic layers, which are also known to prevent recognition by immune cells [1, 21]. In vitro data clearly indicate that perforin plays an important role in the killing of fungi. In addition, as NK cells produce IFN-γ, NK cells exhibit antifungal activity indirectly via other cells (e.g., via granulocytes).

Animal studies support the important role of NK cells in the host defense against *Aspergillus* spp [63, 75]. For example, in neutropenic mice suffering from pulmonary aspergillosis, the depletion of NK cells by antibodies or reducing the recruitment of NK cells to the lungs resulted in a markedly reduced clearance of the pathogen from the lungs and an increase in mortality. Unfortunately, data on the antifungal activity of NK cells in the clinical setting are lacking. Nevertheless, recipients of unrelated donor HSCT from donors with an activating KIR genotype have a decreased infection rate [107]. In addition, NK cell counts were significantly lower in HSCT recipients with proven/probable aspergillosis than in HSCT recipients not suffering from fungal disease [104]. These data make NK cells an interesting tool in the antifungal immunotherapy in HSCT patients at high risk or suffering from invasive fungal disease.

9.3 Hematopoietic Growth Factors, Cytokines, and Interferons

Both cytotoxic chemotherapy and HSCT may impair the production of as well as the cellular response to cytokines and interferons [50, 52]. These soluble molecules form a complex web of communication molecules in innate and adaptive immune responses, inducing the proliferation, differentiation, and activation or suppression of different target cells. It is important to note that specific cytokines can produce apparently opposing effects, depending on dose and timing of their participation in the immune response. For example, the use of interleukin (IL)-4 during the early stage of infection aggravates the clinical course of candidiasis, whereas neutralization of endogenous IL-4 in the late stage of infection exacerbates an otherwise self-limited infection [86]. This chapter will focus only on the hematopoietic growth factors G-CSF and GM-CSF and on IFN-γ which have been evaluated in the clinical setting of invasive fungal disease, although other cytokines such tumor-necrosis-factor (TNF)-α, IL-12 or IL-18 are potential candidates for antifungal immunotherapy.

9.3.1 Hematopoietic Growth Factors

G-CSF and GM-CSF stimulate the production and activation of professional phagocytes, which play a central role in the antifungal host response. In contrast to G-CSF, the activity of GM-CSF in stimulating the production and enhancing phagocytosis, superoxide generation, and fungicidal activity against *A. fumigatus* is not restricted to neutrophils, since it also involves monocytes and eosinophils [49, 82–84]. It is important to note that GM-CSF also restores the steroid-induced loss of antifungal activity in bronchoalveolar macrophages, which form the second line of defense against inhaled *Aspergillus* conidia [23]. In immunocompromised mice, prophylactic G-CSF provides significant protection against aspergillosis, and the use of G-CSF improves survival in systemic or pulmonary aspergillosis [40, 78, 99].

Multiple trials evaluated G-CSF and GM-CSF in patients receiving therapy for cancer or undergoing HSCT, but it has to be noted that most of the studies were designed to analyze outcomes other than the incidence and the outcome of invasive fungal infection, such as indirect measurements of infectious complications (e.g., days of neutropenia, days of fever, hospital days, duration of antibiotic therapy, and overall financial cost of hospitalization) [49, 53]. However, the limited clinical data support the use of G-CSF in neutropenic patients with invasive aspergillosis, and therefore, a level B III recommendation has been given in the 2008 practical guidelines of the Infectious Diseases Society of America (IDSA) for the treatment of invasive aspergillosis in neutropenic patients who are not already receiving a colony-stimulating factor [32, 114]. In a prospective study, the addition of G-CSF to amphotericin B has been shown to be cost effective compared with amphotericin B monotherapy in managing a presumed deep-seated fungal infection in neutropenic patients [34].

The concern of severe side effects such as capillary leak syndrome might explain the restricted use of GM-CSF by many physicians in patients with invasive fungal disease [9, 13, 89, 92]. However, a recent randomized trial in 208 allogeneic HSCT recipients reported that, compared with G-CSF, prophylactic GM-CSF was associated with lower 100-day transplantation-related mortality, lower 100-day cumulative mortality, and lower 600-day fungal disease-related mortality [116]. Although the antifungal treatment responses were similar among the groups, responses were better in the GM-CSF group than in the G-CSF from day 22 to day 100 ($P = 0.009$).

9.3.2 Interferon-γ

IFN-γ is one of the signature cytokines of a protective T_H1 cell response, but it also plays an important role in NK cell activity and enhances the antifungal activity of neutrophils and macrophages, alone and in combination with G-CSF or GM-CSF [38, 82, 85]. In an animal model, the administration of IFN-γ to mice with invasive aspergillosis resulted in reduced fungal burden and increased survival [65, 102].

On the basis of a randomized trial which demonstrated a benefit of IFN-γ in patients with chronic granulomatous disease, recombinant IFN-γ was approved for this patient population for prophylaxis of invasive fungal disease by the US Food and Drug Administration [43]. Significantly less data of IFN-γ are available in cancer and transplant patients. In a single-center report, refractory fungal infections in four neutropenic patients responded to IFN-γ [31]. Similarly, a benefit of IFN-γ was reported in a limited number of patients suffering from *Candida* infection, aspergillosis or fusariosis [30, 54]. Further case series in organ transplant recipients also suggested the benefit of immunodiagnostic-driven adjunctive IFN-γ therapy [5, 6]. A retrospective analysis of 32 patients, most of them HSCT recipients, demonstrated that the adjunctive administration of IFN-γ is safe [91]. Fever was the most common side effect, and importantly, IFN-γ did not precipitate or exacerbate acute or chronic GVHD [91]. Based on these data, a level B III recommendation has been given in the 2008 IDSA guidelines which suggests a role for IFN-γ as adjunctive immunotherapy for invasive aspergillosis in immunocompromised patients [114]. Recombinant IFN-γ has also been explored in the context of HIV-associated cryptococcal meningitis. A randomized controlled phase II study was performed on the basis of initial encouraging studies in the 1990s [44]. The study demonstrated a significant increase in cerebrospinal fluid (CSF) clearance of *Cryptococcus neoformans* with just two doses. An open-label prospective case series further demonstrated beneficial immunological restoration in the context of candidemia [30].

9.4 Antibodies

Therapy of a malignancy may result in B cell depletion and hypogammaglobulinemia, which are associated with an increased risk for infection [44, 50, 52, 71]. Whereas passive administration of antibodies to B cell-deficient mice infected with *C. albicans* or with *A. fumigatus* increased the fungal clearance [59], clinical data on immunoglobulin therapy are conflicting. An early trial demonstrated that administration of immunoglobulins significantly reduced the incidence of invasive fungal infections in liver transplant patients [103], whereas in 45 HSCT recipients, high-dose immunoglobulin therapy during the first 3 months after transplantation did not significantly decrease fungal infections as compared to 53 controls (9% versus 6%) [46].

Advances in the technology used to produce therapeutic antibodies resulted in a number of protective monoclonal antibodies (mAbs) for various fungi such as *A. fumigatus*, *C. albicans*, *C. neoformans*, and *Histoplasma capsulatum* [22, 55, 61, 69].

In *Candida* infection, there was a great interest in the human recombinant anti-hsp90 monoclonal antibody (Efungumab, Mycograb®, NeuTec Pharma/Novartis). This antibody significantly reduced the mean organ colony count in mice infected with fluconazole-resistant *C. albicans.* [56]. A double-blind, randomized study evaluated the use of this antibody in patients with *Candida* infection and found that significantly less patients receiving lipid-associated amphotericin B plus a 5-day course of the antibody died due to the infection as compared to controls receiving amphotericin B plus placebo (18% versus 4%; $P = 0.025$) [72]. However, due to safety concerns such as the potential induction of a cytokine release syndrome associated with fever and hypotension and the fact that it turned out that the potentiating effect of amphotericin B by the antibody was a nonspecific protein effect [81], the antibody did not receive regulatory approval, and further clinical investigation was stopped.

The administration of antibodies that bind to cryptococcal polysaccharide which has multiple immunosuppressive effects has also been studied extensively in vitro and in animal models [3]. The immunomodulatory effects of mAbs appear to be exerted in a complex and pleiotropic manner through enhancement of opsonization and phagocytosis, direct inhibition of fungal cell growth, and, importantly, modulation of cytokine production and inflammation. Animal studies have demonstrated that the administration of antibodies directed against *C. neoformans* capsular polysaccharide to infected mice not only reduced the tissue fungal burden but also prolonged survival [3]. However, to date, only a phase I dose-escalation study of the murine-derived anti-cryptococcal antibody 18B7 has been performed in HIV-infected individuals, and data on the efficacy are still lacking [48].

As compared to pathogens such as *C. neoformans* or *C. albicans*, significantly less data are available for *Aspergillus* spp. Promising results were reported from in vitro and animal studies on the monoclonal anti-*Aspergillus* antibody MAb A9 [22]. The antibody exerted in vitro cidal effect against *A. fumigatus* reduced the fungal burden in kidney tissues of mice suffering from invasive aspergillosis and enhanced mean survival times. Interestingly, a recent study demonstrated that antibodies generated against streptococci exhibit protection in mice infected with *A. fumigatus* [117]. However, to date, there are no clinical data of the use of mAbs in patients with aspergillosis.

The protein pentraxin 3 (PTX3) is released by a variety of cell types in response to inflammatory cytokines and binds to selected microbial agents, such as conidia of *A. fumigatus*. This soluble pattern-recognition receptor has a nonredundant role in antifungal immunity by activating several effector pathways [35]. As susceptibility of PTX3-deficient mice to *A. fumigatus* was associated with failure to mount an adaptive type 1 immune response that could be restored by the exogenous supply of PTX3 [35], the protein was investigated in an animal model as adjunctive treatment in experimental aspergillosis [37]. The study demonstrated that mice treated with PTX3 after HSCT were completely resistant to infection with *A. fumigatus*, and the protective effect of PTX3 was similar or superior to that observed with amphotericin B. Although it has recently been shown that genetic deficiency of PTX3 may contribute to the risk of invasive aspergillosis in patients undergoing HSCT, clinical studies using PTX3 have not been performed to date [26].

9.5 Other Molecular Approaches

Further studies addressed the therapeutic utility of thymosin alpha 1, which enhances the maturation of dendritic cells exposed to *A. fumigatus* [88]. This approach led to enhanced T_H1 responses in animal models and induction of tolerogenic T_{reg} cells. However, this approach has not been studied in the clinical setting. On the basis of defective toll-like receptor recognition in phaeohyphomycosis due to *Fonsecaea pedrosoi* in animal models, recent encouraging clinical studies demonstrated the utility of adjunctive therapy with the TLR7 agonist imiquimod for chromoblastomycosis [29].

9.6 Conclusions

As in vitro data and animal studies have provided us with critical information to augment host immunity, there is a growing interest in immunotherapeutic approaches in patients at high risk for or suffering from invasive fungal disease. Still, current data are too limited to allow solid conclusions on the risk and the benefit of these strategies. Many questions such as safety, efficacy, timing of immunotherapeutic intervention, dosing, and eligible patients have to be addressed, but can only be answered by appropriately designed and powered clinical trials. This will be the real challenge in the future, and international, multicenter collaboration is required, but might be promising in ultimately improving the outcome in immunocompromised patients suffering from invasive fungal disease.

References

1. Aimanianda V, Bayry J, Bozza S, Kniemeyer O, Perruccio K, Elluru SR, Clavaud C, Paris S, Brakhage AA, Kaveri SV, Romani L, Latge JP. Surface hydrophobin prevents immune recognition of airborne fungal spores. Nature. 2009;460(7259):1117–21.
2. Antachopoulos C, Katragkou A, Roilides E. Immunotherapy against invasive mold infections. Immunotherapy. 2012;4(1):107–20.
3. Antachopoulos C, Walsh TJ. Immunotherapy of cryptococcus infections. Clin Microbiol Infect. 2012;18(2):126–33.
4. Armstrong-James D, Meintjes G, Brown GD. A neglected epidemic: fungal infections in HIV/AIDS. Trends Microbiol. 2014;22(3):120–7.
5. Armstrong-James D, Teo I, Herbst S, Petrou M, Shiu KY, McLean A, Taube D, Dorling A, Shaunak S. Renal allograft recipients fail to increase interferon-gamma during invasive fungal diseases. Am J Transplant. 2012;12(12):3437–40.
6. Armstrong-James D, Teo IA, Shrivastava S, Petrou MA, Taube D, Dorling A, Shaunak S. Exogenous interferon-gamma immunotherapy for invasive fungal infections in kidney transplant patients. Am J Transplant. 2010;10(8):1796–803.
7. Bacher P, Jochheim-Richter A, Mockel-Tenbrink N, Kniemeyer O, Wingenfeld E, Alex R, Ortigao A, Karpova D, Lehrnbecher T, Ullmann AJ, Hamprecht A, Cornely O, Brakhage AA, Assenmacher M, Bonig H, Scheffold A. Clinical-scale isolation of the total Aspergillus fumigatus-reactive T-helper cell repertoire for adoptive transfer. Cytotherapy. 2015;17(10):1396–405.

8. Bacher P, Kniemeyer O, Teutschbein J, Thon M, Vodisch M, Wartenberg D, Scharf DH, Koester-Eiserfunke N, Schutte M, Dubel S, Assenmacher M, Brakhage AA, Scheffold A. Identification of immunogenic antigens from Aspergillus fumigatus by direct multiparameter characterization of specific conventional and regulatory CD4+ T cells. J Immunol. 2014;193(7):3332–43.
9. Bandera A, Trabattoni D, Ferrario G, Cesari M, Franzetti F, Clerici M, Gori A. Interferon-gamma and granulocyte-macrophage colony stimulating factor therapy in three patients with pulmonary aspergillosis. Infection. 2008;36(4):368–73.
10. Beck O, Koehl U, Tramsen L, Mousset S, Latge JP, Muller K, Schwabe D, Bader P, Klingebiel T, Lehrnbecher T. Enumeration of functionally active anti-Aspergillus T-cells in human peripheral blood. J Immunol Methods. 2008;335(1–2):41–5.
11. Beck O, Topp MS, Koehl U, Roilides E, Simitsopoulou M, Hanisch M, Sarfati J, Latge JP, Klingebiel T, Einsele H, Lehrnbecher T. Generation of highly purified and functionally active human TH1 cells against Aspergillus fumigatus. Blood. 2006;107(6):2562–9.
12. Blyth E, Clancy L, Simms R, Ma CK, Burgess J, Deo S, Byth K, Dubosq MC, Shaw PJ, Micklethwaite KP, Gottlieb DJ. Donor-derived CMV-specific T cells reduce the requirement for CMV-directed pharmacotherapy after allogeneic stem cell transplantation. Blood. 2013;121(18):3745–58.
13. Bodey GP, Anaissie E, Gutterman J, Vadhan-Raj S. Role of granulocyte-macrophage colony-stimulating factor as adjuvant treatment in neutropenic patients with bacterial and fungal infection. Eur J Clin Microbiol Infect Dis. 1994;13(Suppl 2):S18–22.
14. Bodey GP, Buckley M, Sathe YS, Freireich EJ. Quantitative relationships between circulating leukocytes and infections in patients with acute leukemia. Ann Intern Med. 1966;64:328–40.
15. Bouzani M, Ok M, McCormick A, Ebel F, Kurzai O, Morton CO, Einsele H, Loeffler J. Human NK cells display important antifungal activity against Aspergillus fumigatus, which is directly mediated by IFN-gamma release. J Immunol. 2011;187(3):1369–76.
16. Bow EJ. Invasive fungal infection in haematopoietic stem cell transplant recipients: epidemiology from the transplant physician's viewpoint. Mycopathologia. 2009;168(6):283–97.
17. Bozza S, Clavaud C, Giovannini G, Fontaine T, Beauvais A, Sarfati J, D'Angelo C, Perruccio K, Bonifazi P, Zagarella S, Moretti S, Bistoni F, Latge JP, Romani L. Immune sensing of Aspergillus fumigatus proteins, glycolipids, and polysaccharides and the impact on Th immunity and vaccination. J Immunol. 2009;183(4):2407–14.
18. Bozza S, Perruccio K, Montagnoli C, Gaziano R, Bellocchio S, Burchielli E, Nkwanyuo G, Pitzurra L, Velardi A, Romani L. A dendritic cell vaccine against invasive aspergillosis in allogeneic hematopoietic transplantation. Blood. 2003;102(10):3807–14.
19. Cenci E, Mencacci A, Bacci A, Bistoni F, Kurup VP, Romani L. T cell vaccination in mice with invasive pulmonary aspergillosis. J Immunol. 2000;165(1):381–8.
20. Cenci E, Mencacci A, Del Sero G, Bacci A, Montagnoli C, d'Ostiani CF, Mosci P, Bachmann M, Bistoni F, Kopf M, Romani L. Interleukin-4 causes susceptibility to invasive pulmonary aspergillosis through suppression of protective type I responses. J Infect Dis. 1999;180(6):1957–68.
21. Chai LY, Netea MG, Sugui J, Vonk AG, van de Sande WW, Warris A, Kwon-Chung KJ, Kullberg BJ. Aspergillus fumigatus conidial melanin modulates host cytokine response. Immunobiology. 2010;215(11):915–20.
22. Chaturvedi AK, Kavishwar A, Shiva Keshava GB, Shukla PK. Monoclonal immunoglobulin G1 directed against Aspergillus fumigatus cell wall glycoprotein protects against experimental murine aspergillosis. Clin Diagn Lab Immunol. 2005;12(9):1063–8.
23. Choi JH, Brummer E, Kang YJ, Jones PP, Stevens DA. Inhibitor kappaB and nuclear factor kappaB in granulocyte-macrophage colony-stimulating factor antagonism of dexamethasone suppression of the macrophage response to Aspergillus fumigatus conidia. J Infect Dis. 2006;193(7):1023–8.
24. Cornely OA, Gachot B, Akan H, Bassetti M, Uzun O, Kibbler C, Marchetti O, de Burghgraeve P, Ramadan S, Pylkkanen L, Ameye L, Paesmans M, Donnelly JP, E. I. D. Group.

Epidemiology and outcome of fungemia in a cancer Cohort of the Infectious Diseases Group (IDG) of the European Organization for Research and Treatment of Cancer (EORTC 65031). Clin Infect Dis. 2015;61(3):324–31.
25. Cruz CR, Hanley PJ, Liu H, Torrano V, Lin YF, Arce JA, Gottschalk S, Savoldo B, Dotti G, Louis CU, Leen AM, Gee AP, Rooney CM, Brenner MK, Bollard CM, Heslop HE. Adverse events following infusion of T cells for adoptive immunotherapy: a 10-year experience. Cytotherapy. 2010;12(6):743–9.
26. Cunha C, Aversa F, Lacerda JF, Busca A, Kurzai O, Grube M, Loffler J, Maertens JA, Bell AS, Inforzato A, Barbati E, Almeida B, Santos e Sousa P, Barbui A, Potenza L, Caira M, Rodrigues F, Salvatori G, Pagano L, Luppi M, Mantovani A, Velardi A, Romani L, Carvalho A. Genetic PTX3 deficiency and aspergillosis in stem-cell transplantation. N Engl J Med. 2014;370(5):421–32.
27. Cunha C, Kurzai O, Loffler J, Aversa F, Romani L, Carvalho A. Neutrophil responses to aspergillosis: new roles for old players. Mycopathologia. 2014;178(5–6):387–93.
28. Danion F, Aguilar C, Catherinot E, Alanio A, DeWolf S, Lortholary O, Lanternier F. Mucormycosis: new developments into a persistently devastating infection. Semin Respir Crit Care Med. 2015;36(5):692–705.
29. de Sousa Mda G, Belda Jr W, Spina R, Lota PR, Valente NS, Brown GD, Criado PR, Benard G. Topical application of imiquimod as a treatment for chromoblastomycosis. Clin Infect Dis. 2014;58(12):1734–7.
30. Delsing CE, Gresnigt MS, Leentjens J, Preijers F, Frager FA, Kox M, Monneret G, Venet F, Bleeker-Rovers CP, van de Veerdonk FL, Pickkers P, Pachot A, Kullberg BJ, Netea MG. Interferon-gamma as adjunctive immunotherapy for invasive fungal infections: a case series. BMC Infect Dis. 2014;14:166.
31. Dignani MC, Rex JH, Chan KW, Dow G, deMagalhaes-Silverman M, Maddox A, Walsh T, Anaissie E. Immunomodulation with interferon-gamma and colony-stimulating factors for refractory fungal infections in patients with leukemia. Cancer. 2005;104(1):199–204.
32. Dornbusch HJ, Urban CE, Pinter H, Ginter G, Fotter R, Becker H, Miorini T, Berghold C. Treatment of invasive pulmonary aspergillosis in severely neutropenic children with malignant disorders using liposomal amphotericin B (AmBisome), granulocyte colony-stimulating factor, and surgery: report of five cases. Pediatr Hematol Oncol. 1995;12(6):577–86.
33. Feuchtinger T, Matthes-Martin S, Richard C, Lion T, Fuhrer M, Hamprecht K, Handgretinger R, Peters C, Schuster FR, Beck R, Schumm M, Lotfi R, Jahn G, Lang P. Safe adoptive transfer of virus-specific T-cell immunity for the treatment of systemic adenovirus infection after allogeneic stem cell transplantation. Br J Haematol. 2006;134(1):64–76.
34. Flynn TN, Kelsey SM, Hazel DL, Guest JF. Cost effectiveness of amphotericin B plus G-CSF compared with amphotericin B monotherapy. Treatment of presumed deep-seated fungal infection in neutropenic patients in the UK. PharmacoEconomics. 1999;16(5 Pt 2):543–50.
35. Garlanda C, Hirsch E, Bozza S, Salustri A, De Acetis M, Nota R, Maccagno A, Riva F, Bottazzi B, Peri G, Doni A, Vago L, Botto M, De Santis R, Carminati P, Siracusa G, Altruda F, Vecchi A, Romani L, Mantovani A. Non-redundant role of the long pentraxin PTX3 in anti-fungal innate immune response. Nature. 2002;420(6912):182–6.
36. Gaundar SS, Clancy L, Blyth E, Meyer W, Gottlieb DJ. Robust polyfunctional T-helper 1 responses to multiple fungal antigens from a cell population generated using an environmental strain of Aspergillus fumigatus. Cytotherapy. 2012;14(9):1119–30.
37. Gaziano R, Bozza S, Bellocchio S, Perruccio K, Montagnoli C, Pitzurra L, Salvatori G, De Santis R, Carminati P, Mantovani A, Romani L. Anti-Aspergillus fumigatus efficacy of pentraxin 3 alone and in combination with antifungals. Antimicrob Agents Chemother. 2004;48(11):4414–21.
38. Gil-Lamaignere C, Simitsopoulou M, Roilides E, Maloukou A, Winn RM, Walsh TJ. Interferon- gamma and granulocyte-macrophage colony-stimulating factor augment the

activity of polymorphonuclear leukocytes against medically important zygomycetes. J Infect Dis. 2005;191(7):1180–7.
39. Gill S, Olson JA, Negrin RS. Natural killer cells in allogeneic transplantation: effect on engraftment, graft- versus-tumor, and graft-versus-host responses. Biol Blood Marrow Transplant. 2009;15(7):765–76.
40. Graybill JR, Bocanegra R, Najvar LK, Loebenberg D, Luther MF. Granulocyte colony-stimulating factor and azole antifungal therapy in murine aspergillosis: role of immune suppression. Antimicrob Agents Chemother. 1998;42(10):2467–73.
41. Hamza NS, Lisgaris M, Yadavalli G, Nadeau L, Fox R, Fu P, Lazarus HM, Koc ON, Salata RA, Laughlin MJ. Kinetics of myeloid and lymphocyte recovery and infectious complications after unrelated umbilical cord blood versus HLA-matched unrelated donor allogeneic transplantation in adults. Br J Haematol. 2004;124(4):488–98.
42. Hebart H, Bollinger C, Fisch P, Sarfati J, Meisner C, Baur M, Loeffler J, Monod M, Latge JP, Einsele H. Analysis of T-cell responses to Aspergillus fumigatus antigens in healthy individuals and patients with hematologic malignancies. Blood. 2002;100(13):4521–8.
43. International Chronic Granulomatous Disease Cooperative Study Group. A controlled trial of interferon-gamma to prevent infection in chronic granulomatous disease. N Engl J Med. 1991;324:509–16.
44. Jarvis JN, Meintjes G, Rebe K, Williams GN, Bicanic T, Williams A, Schutz C, Bekker LG, Wood R, Harrison TS. Adjunctive interferon-gamma immunotherapy for the treatment of HIV-associated cryptococcal meningitis: a randomized controlled trial. AIDS. 2012;26(9):1105–13.
45. Kadri SS, Remy KE, Strich JR, Gea-Banacloche J, Leitman SF. Role of granulocyte transfusions in invasive fusariosis: systematic review and single-center experience. Transfusion. 2015;55(9):2076–85.
46. Klaesson S, Ringden O, Ljungman P, Aschan J, Hagglund H, Winiarski J. Does high-dose intravenous immune globulin treatment after bone marrow transplantation increase mortality in veno-occlusive disease of the liver? Transplantation. 1995;60(11):1225–30.
47. Kumaresan PR, Manuri PR, Albert ND, Maiti S, Singh H, Mi T, Roszik J, Rabinovich B, Olivares S, Krishnamurthy J, Zhang L, Najjar AM, Huls MH, Lee DA, Champlin RE, Kontoyiannis DP, Cooper LJ. Bioengineering T cells to target carbohydrate to treat opportunistic fungal infection. Proc Natl Acad Sci U S A. 2014;111(29):10660–5.
48. Larsen RA, Pappas PG, Perfect J, Aberg JA, Casadevall A, Cloud GA, James R, Filler S, Dismukes WE. Phase I evaluation of the safety and pharmacokinetics of murine-derived anti-cryptococcal antibody 18B7 in subjects with treated cryptococcal meningitis. Antimicrob Agents Chemother. 2005;49(3):952–8.
49. Lehrnbecher T, Chanock SJ. Myeloid growth factors in supportive care of cancer and marrow transplant therapies. In: Holland SM, editor. Cytokine therapeutics in infectious diseases. Philadelphia: Lippincott Williams & Williams; 2001. p. 251–93.
50. Lehrnbecher T, Foster C, Vazquez N, Mackall CL, Chanock SJ. Therapy-induced alterations in host defense in children receiving therapy for cancer. J Pediatr Hematol Oncol. 1997;19(5):399–417.
51. Lehrnbecher T, Groll AH, Chanock SJ. Treatment of fungal infections in neutropenic children. Curr Opin Pediatr. 1999;11(1):47–55.
52. Lehrnbecher T, Koehl U, Wittekindt B, Bochennek K, Tramsen L, Klingebiel T, Chanock SJ. Changes in host defence induced by malignancies and antineoplastic treatment: implication for immunotherapeutic strategies. Lancet Oncol. 2008;9(3):269–78.
53. Lehrnbecher T, Welte K. Haematopoietic growth factors in children with neutropenia. Br J Haematol. 2002;116(1):28–56.
54. Lewis R, Hogan H, Howell A, Safdar A. Progressive fusariosis: unpredictable posaconazole bioavailability, and feasibility of recombinant interferon-gamma plus granulocyte macrophage-colony stimulating factor for refractory disseminated infection. Leuk Lymphoma. 2008;49(1):163–5.

55. Maitta RW, Datta K, Chang Q, Luo RX, Witover B, Subramaniam K, Pirofski LA. Protective and nonprotective human immunoglobulin M monoclonal antibodies to Cryptococcus neoformans glucuronoxylomannan manifest different specificities and gene use profiles. Infect Immun. 2004;72(8):4810–8.
56. Matthews RC, Rigg G, Hodgetts S, Carter T, Chapman C, Gregory C, Illidge C, Burnie J. Preclinical assessment of the efficacy of mycograb, a human recombinant antibody against fungal HSP90. Antimicrob Agents Chemother. 2003;47(7):2208–16.
57. Mikulska M, Raiola AM, Bruno B, Furfaro E, Van Lint MT, Bregante S, Ibatici A, Del Bono V, Bacigalupo A, Viscoli C. Risk factors for invasive aspergillosis and related mortality in recipients of allogeneic SCT from alternative donors: an analysis of 306 patients. Bone Marrow Transplant. 2009;44(6):361–70.
58. Montagna MT, Lovero G, Coretti C, Martinelli D, Delia M, De Giglio O, Caira M, Puntillo F, D'Antonio D, Venditti M, Sambri V, Di Bernardo F, Barbui A, Lo Cascio G, Concia E, Mikulska M, Viscoli C, Maximova N, Candoni A, Oliveri S, Lombardi G, Pitzurra L, Sanguinetti M, Masciari R, Santantonio T, Andreoni S, Barchiesi F, Pecile P, Farina C, Viale P, Specchia G, Caggiano G, Pagano L. SIMIFF study: Italian fungal registry of mold infections in hematological and non-hematological patients. Infection. 2014;42(1):141–51.
59. Montagnoli C, Bozza S, Bacci A, Gaziano R, Mosci P, Morschhauser J, Pitzurra L, Kopf M, Cutler J, Romani L. A role for antibodies in the generation of memory antifungal immunity. Eur J Immunol. 2003;33(5):1193–204.
60. Montesinos P, Rodriguez-Veiga R, Boluda B, Martinez-Cuadron D, Cano I, Lancharro A, Sanz J, Arilla MJ, Lopez-Chulia F, Navarro I, Lorenzo I, Salavert M, Peman J, Calvillo P, Martinez J, Carpio N, Jarque I, Sanz GF, Sanz MA. Incidence and risk factors of post-engraftment invasive fungal disease in adult allogeneic hematopoietic stem cell transplant recipients receiving oral azoles prophylaxis. Bone Marrow Transplant. 2015;50(11):1465–72.
61. Moragues MD, Omaetxebarria MJ, Elguezabal N, Sevilla MJ, Conti S, Polonelli L, Ponton J. A monoclonal antibody directed against a Candida albicans cell wall mannoprotein exerts three anti-C. albicans activities. Infect Immun. 2003;71(9):5273–9.
62. Morgan J, Wannemuehler KA, Marr KA, Hadley S, Kontoyiannis DP, Walsh TJ, Fridkin SK, Pappas PG, Warnock DW. Incidence of invasive aspergillosis following hematopoietic stem cell and solid organ transplantation: interim results of a prospective multicenter surveillance program. Med Mycol. 2005;43(Suppl 1):S49–58.
63. Morrison BE, Park SJ, Mooney JM, Mehrad B. Chemokine-mediated recruitment of NK cells is a critical host defense mechanism in invasive aspergillosis. J Clin Invest. 2003;112(12):1862–70.
64. Mousset S, Hermann S, Klein SA, Bialleck H, Duchscherer M, Bomke B, Wassmann B, Bohme A, Hoelzer D, Martin H. Prophylactic and interventional granulocyte transfusions in patients with haematological malignancies and life-threatening infections during neutropenia. Ann Hematol. 2005;84(11):734–41.
65. Nagai H, Guo J, Choi H, Kurup V. Interferon-gamma and tumor necrosis factor-alpha protect mice from invasive aspergillosis. J Infect Dis. 1995;172(6):1554–60.
66. Nencioni A, Brossart P. Cellular immunotherapy with dendritic cells in cancer: current status. Stem Cells. 2004;22(4):501–13.
67. Neofytos D, Horn D, Anaissie E, Steinbach W, Olyaei A, Fishman J, Pfaller M, Chang C, Webster K, Marr K. Epidemiology and outcome of invasive fungal infection in adult hematopoietic stem cell transplant recipients: analysis of Multicenter Prospective Antifungal Therapy (PATH) Alliance registry. Clin Infect Dis. 2009;48(3):265–73.
68. Nierman WC, Pain A, Anderson MJ, Wortman JR, Kim HS, Arroyo J, Berriman M, Abe K, Archer DB, Bermejo C, Bennett J, Bowyer P, Chen D, Collins M, Coulsen R, Davies R, Dyer PS, Farman M, Fedorova N, Fedorova N, Feldblyum TV, Fischer R, Fosker N, Fraser A, Garcia JL, Garcia MJ, Goble A, Goldman GH, Gomi K, Griffith-Jones S, Gwilliam R,

Haas B, Haas H, Harris D, Horiuchi H, Huang J, Humphray S, Jimenez J, Keller N, Khouri H, Kitamoto K, Kobayashi T, Konzack S, Kulkarni R, Kumagai T, Lafon A, Latge JP, Li W, Lord A, Lu C, Majoros WH, May GS, Miller BL, Mohamoud Y, Molina M, Monod M, Mouyna I, Mulligan S, Murphy L, O'Neil S, Paulsen I, Penalva MA, Pertea M, Price C, Pritchard BL, Quail MA, Rabbinowitsch E, Rawlins N, Rajandream MA, Reichard U, Renauld H, Robson GD, Rodriguez de Cordoba S, Rodriguez-Pena JM, Ronning CM, Rutter S, Salzberg SL, Sanchez M, Sanchez-Ferrero JC, Saunders D, Seeger K, Squares R, Squares S, Takeuchi M, Tekaia F, Turner G, Vazquez de Aldana CR, Weidman J, White O, Woodward J, Yu JH, Fraser C, Galagan JE, Asai K, Machida M, Hall N, Barrell B, Denning DW. Genomic sequence of the pathogenic and allergenic filamentous fungus Aspergillus fumigatus. Nature. 2005;438(7071):1151–6.

69. Nosanchuk JD, Steenbergen JN, Shi L, Deepe Jr GS, Casadevall A. Antibodies to a cell surface histone-like protein protect against Histoplasma capsulatum. J Clin Invest. 2003;112(8):1164–75.
70. O'Donghaile D, Childs RW, Leitman SF. Blood consult: granulocyte transfusions to treat invasive aspergillosis in a patient with severe aplastic anemia awaiting mismatched hematopoietic progenitor cell transplantation. Blood. 2012;119(6):1353–5.
71. Orange JS, Grossman WJ, Navickis RJ, Wilkes MM. Impact of trough IgG on pneumonia incidence in primary immunodeficiency: a meta-analysis of clinical studies. Clin Immunol. 2010;137(1):21–30.
72. Pachl J, Svoboda P, Jacobs F, Vandewoude K, van der Hoven B, Spronk P, Masterson G, Malbrain M, Aoun M, Garbino J, Takala J, Drgona L, Burnie J, Matthews R. A randomized, blinded, multicenter trial of lipid-associated amphotericin B alone versus in combination with an antibody-based inhibitor of heat shock protein 90 in patients with invasive candidiasis. Clin Infect Dis. 2006;42(10):1404–13.
73. Pagano L, Caira M, Nosari A, Van Lint MT, Candoni A, Offidani M, Aloisi T, Irrera G, Bonini A, Picardi M, Caramatti C, Invernizzi R, Mattei D, Melillo L, de Waure C, Reddiconto G, Fianchi L, Valentini CG, Girmenia C, Leone G, Aversa F. Fungal infections in recipients of hematopoietic stem cell transplants: results of the SEIFEM B-2004 study – Sorveglianza Epidemiologica Infezioni Fungine Nelle Emopatie Maligne. Clin Infect Dis. 2007;45(9):1161–70.
74. Papadopoulou A, Kaloyannidis P, Yannaki E, Cruz CR. Adoptive transfer of Aspergillus-specific T cells as a novel anti-fungal therapy for hematopoietic stem cell transplant recipients: progress and challenges. Crit Rev Oncol Hematol. 2016;98:62–72.
75. Park SJ, Hughes MA, Burdick M, Strieter RM, Mehrad B. Early NK cell-derived IFN-{gamma} is essential to host defense in neutropenic invasive aspergillosis. J Immunol. 2009;182(7):4306–12.
76. Perruccio K, Tosti A, Burchielli E, Topini F, Ruggeri L, Carotti A, Capanni M, Urbani E, Mancusi A, Aversa F, Martelli MF, Romani L, Velardi A. Transferring functional immune responses to pathogens after haploidentical hematopoietic transplantation. Blood. 2005;106:4397–406.
77. Pham HP, Rogoza K, Stotler B, Duffy D, Parker-Jones S, Ginzburg Y, Bhatia M, Cairo M, Schwartz J. Granulocyte transfusion therapy in pediatric patients after hematopoietic stem cell transplantation: a 5-year single tertiary care center experience. J Pediatr Hematol Oncol. 2012;34(8):e332–6.
78. Polak-Wyss A. Protective effect of human granulocyte colony-stimulating factor (hG-CSF) on Cryptococcus and Aspergillus infections in normal and immunosuppressed mice. Mycoses. 1991;34(5–6):205–15.
79. Price TH, Boeckh M, Harrison RW, McCullough J, Ness PM, Strauss RG, Nichols WG, Hamza TH, Cushing MM, King KE, Young JA, Williams E, McFarland J, Holter Chakrabarty J, Sloan SR, Friedman D, Parekh S, Sachais BS, Kiss JE, Assmann SF. Efficacy of transfusion with granulocytes from G-CSF/dexamethasone-treated donors in neutropenic patients with infection. Blood. 2015;126(18):2153–61.

80. Raad II, Chaftari AM, Al Shuaibi MM, Jiang Y, Shomali W, Cortes JE, Lichtiger B, Hachem RY. Granulocyte transfusions in hematologic malignancy patients with invasive pulmonary aspergillosis: outcomes and complications. Ann Oncol. 2013;24(7):1873–9.
81. Richie DL, Ghannoum MA, Isham N, Thompson KV, Ryder NS. Nonspecific effect of Mycograb on amphotericin B MIC. Antimicrob Agents Chemother. 2012;56(7):3963–4.
82. Roilides E, Blake C, Holmes A, Pizzo PA, Walsh TJ. Granulocyte-macrophage colony-stimulating factor and interferon-gamma prevent dexamethasone-induced immunosuppression of antifungal monocyte activity against Aspergillus fumigatus hyphae. J Med Vet Mycol. 1996;34(1):63–9.
83. Roilides E, Holmes A, Blake C, Venzon D, Pizzo PA, Walsh TJ. Antifungal activity of elutriated human monocytes against Aspergillus fumigatus hyphae: enhancement by granulocyte-macrophage colony-stimulating factor and interferon-gamma. J Infect Dis. 1994;170(4):894–9.
84. Roilides E, Uhlig K, Venzon D, Pizzo PA, Walsh TJ. Enhancement of oxidative response and damage caused by human neutrophils to Aspergillus fumigatus hyphae by granulocyte colony-stimulating factor and gamma interferon. Infect Immun. 1993;61(4):1185–93.
85. Roilides E, Uhlig K, Venzon D, Pizzo PA, Walsh TJ. Prevention of corticosteroid-induced suppression of human polymorphonuclear leukocyte-induced damage of Aspergillus fumigatus hyphae by granulocyte colony-stimulating factor and gamma interferon. Infect Immun. 1993;61(11):4870–7.
86. Romani L. Immunity to fungal infections. Nat Rev Immunol. 2004;4(1):1–23.
87. Romani L. Immunity to fungal infections. Nat Rev Immunol. 2011;11(4):275–88.
88. Romani L, Bistoni F, Gaziano R, Bozza S, Montagnoli C, Perruccio K, Pitzurra L, Bellocchio S, Velardi A, Rasi G, Di Francesco P, Garaci E. Thymosin alpha 1 activates dendritic cells for antifungal Th1 resistance through toll-like receptor signaling. Blood. 2004;103(11):4232–9.
89. Safdar A. Immunotherapy for invasive mold disease in severely immunosuppressed patients. Clin Infect Dis. 2013;57(1):94–100.
90. Safdar A, Hanna HA, Boktour M, Kontoyiannis DP, Hachem R, Lichtiger B, Freireich EJ, Raad II. Impact of high-dose granulocyte transfusions in patients with cancer with candidemia: retrospective case-control analysis of 491 episodes of Candida species bloodstream infections. Cancer. 2004;101(12):2859–65.
91. Safdar A, Rodriguez G, Ohmagari N, Kontoyiannis DP, Rolston KV, Raad II, Champlin RE. The safety of interferon-gamma-1b therapy for invasive fungal infections after hematopoietic stem cell transplantation. Cancer. 2005;103(4):731–9.
92. Safdar A, Rodriguez G, Rolston KV, O'Brien S, Khouri IF, Shpall EJ, Keating MJ, Kantarjian HM, Champlin RE, Raad II, Kontoyiannis DP. High-dose caspofungin combination antifungal therapy in patients with hematologic malignancies and hematopoietic stem cell transplantation. Bone Marrow Transplant. 2007;39(3):157–64.
93. Safdar A, Rodriguez G, Zuniga J, Al Akhrass F, Pande A. Use of healthy-donor granulocyte transfusions to treat infections in neutropenic patients with myeloid or lymphoid neoplasms: experience in 74 patients treated with 373 granulocyte transfusions. Acta Haematol. 2014;131(1):50–8.
94. Schmidt S, Schneider A, Demir A, Lass-Florl C, Lehrnbecher T. Natural killer cell-mediated damage of clinical isolates of mucormycetes. Mycoses. 2016;59(1):34–8.
95. Schmidt S, Tramsen L, Hanisch M, Latge JP, Huenecke S, Koehl U, Lehrnbecher T. Human natural killer cells exhibit direct activity against Aspergillus fumigatus hyphae, but not against resting conidia. J Infect Dis. 2011;203(3):430–5.
96. Schmidt S, Tramsen L, Perkhofer S, Lass-Florl C, Hanisch M, Roger F, Klingebiel T, Koehl U, Lehrnbecher T. Rhizopus oryzae hyphae are damaged by human natural killer (NK) cells, but suppress NK cell mediated immunity. Immunobiology. 2013;218(7):939–44.
97. Schmidt S, Tramsen L, Perkhofer S, Lass-Florl C, Roger F, Schubert R, Lehrnbecher T. Characterization of the cellular immune responses to rhizopus oryzae with potential impact

on immunotherapeutic strategies in hematopoietic stem cell transplantation. J Infect Dis. 2012;206(1):135–9.
98. Seidel MG, Peters C, Wacker A, Northoff H, Moog R, Boehme A, Silling G, Grimminger W, Einsele H. Randomized phase III study of granulocyte transfusions in neutropenic patients. Bone Marrow Transplant. 2008;42(10):679–84.
99. Sionov E, Mendlovic S, Segal E. Experimental systemic murine aspergillosis: treatment with polyene and caspofungin combination and G-CSF. J Antimicrob Chemother. 2005;56(3):594–7.
100. Small CL, McCormick S, Gill N, Kugathasan K, Santosuosso M, Donaldson N, Heinrichs DE, Ashkar A, Xing Z. NK cells play a critical protective role in host defense against acute extracellular Staphylococcus aureus bacterial infection in the lung. J Immunol. 2008;180(8):5558–68.
101. Stern M, Passweg JR, Meyer-Monard S, Esser R, Tonn T, Soerensen J, Paulussen M, Gratwohl A, Klingebiel T, Bader P, Tichelli A, Schwabe D, Koehl U. Pre-emptive immunotherapy with purified natural killer cells after haploidentical SCT: a prospective phase II study in two centers. Bone Marrow Transplant. 2013;48(3):433–8.
102. Stevens DA, Brummer E, Clemons KV. Interferon- gamma as an antifungal. J Infect Dis. 2006;194(Suppl 1):S33–7.
103. Stratta RJ, Shaefer MS, Cushing KA, Markin RS, Reed EC, Langnas AN, Pillen TJ, Shaw Jr BW. A randomized prospective trial of acyclovir and immune globulin prophylaxis in liver transplant recipients receiving OKT3 therapy. Arch Surg. 1992;127(1):55–63. discussion 63-54
104. Stuehler C, Kuenzli E, Jaeger VK, Baettig V, Ferracin F, Rajacic Z, Kaiser D, Bernardini C, Forrer P, Weisser M, Elzi L, Battegay M, Halter J, Passweg J, Khanna N. Immune reconstitution after allogeneic hematopoietic stem cell transplantation and association with occurrence and outcome of invasive aspergillosis. J Infect Dis. 2015;212(6):959–67.
105. Stuehler C, Nowakowska J, Bernardini C, Topp MS, Battegay M, Passweg J, Khanna N. Multispecific Aspergillus T cells selected by CD137 or CD154 induce protective immune responses against the most relevant mold infections. J Infect Dis. 2015;211(8):1251–61.
106. Terszowski G, Passweg JR, Stern M. Natural killer cell immunity after transplantation. Swiss Med Wkly. 2012;142:w13700.
107. Tomblyn M, Young JA, Haagenson MD, Klein JP, Trachtenberg EA, Storek J, Spellman SR, Cooley S, Miller JS, Weisdorf DJ. Decreased infections in recipients of unrelated donor hematopoietic cell transplantation from donors with an activating KIR genotype. Biol Blood Marrow Transplant. 2010;16(8):1155–61.
108. Tramsen L, Beck O, Schuster FR, Hunfeld KP, Latge JP, Sarfati J, Roger F, Klingebiel T, Koehl U, Lehrnbecher T. Generation and characterization of anti-Candida T cells as potential immunotherapy in patients with Candida infection after allogeneic hematopoietic stem-cell transplant. J Infect Dis. 2007;196(3):485–92.
109. Tramsen L, Koehl U, Tonn T, Latge JP, Schuster FR, Borkhardt A, Uharek L, Quaritsch R, Beck O, Seifried E, Klingebiel T, Lehrnbecher T. Clinical-scale generation of human anti-Aspergillus T cells for adoptive immunotherapy. Bone Marrow Transplant. 2009;43(1):13–9.
110. Tramsen L, Schmidt S, Boenig H, Latge JP, Lass-Florl C, Roeger F, Seifried E, Klingebiel T, Lehrnbecher T. Clinical-scale generation of multi-specific anti-fungal T cells targeting Candida, Aspergillus and mucormycetes. Cytotherapy. 2013;15(3):344–51.
111. Tramsen L, Schmidt S, Koehl U, Huenecke S, Latge JP, Roeger F, Schubert R, Klingebiel T, Lehrnbecher T. No effect of antifungal compounds on functional properties of human antifungal T-helper type 1 cells. Transpl Infect Dis. 2013;15:430–4.
112. Tramsen L, Schmidt S, Roeger F, Schubert R, Salzmann-Manrique E, Latge JP, Klingebiel T, Lehrnbecher T. Immunosuppressive compounds exhibit particular effects on functional properties of human anti-Aspergillus Th1 cells. Infect Immun. 2014;82(6):2649–56.

113. Voigt J, Hunniger K, Bouzani M, Jacobsen ID, Barz D, Hube B, Loffler J, Kurzai O. Human natural killer cells acting as phagocytes against Candida albicans and mounting an inflammatory response that modulates neutrophil antifungal activity. J Infect Dis. 2014;209(4):616–26.
114. Walsh TJ, Anaissie EJ, Denning DW, Herbrecht R, Kontoyiannis DP, Marr KA, Morrison VA, Segal BH, Steinbach WJ, Stevens DA, van Burik JA, Wingard JR, Patterson TF. Treatment of aspergillosis: clinical practice guidelines of the Infectious Diseases Society of America. Clin Infect Dis. 2008;46(3):327–60.
115. Walsh TJ, Groll A, Hiemenz J, Fleming R, Roilides E, Anaissie E. Infections due to emerging and uncommon medically important fungal pathogens. Clin Microbiol Infect. 2004;10(Suppl 1):48–66.
116. Wan L, Zhang Y, Lai Y, Jiang M, Song Y, Zhou J, Zhang Z, Duan X, Fu Y, Liao L, Wang C. Effect of granulocyte-macrophage colony-stimulating factor on prevention and treatment of invasive fungal disease in recipients of allogeneic stem-cell transplantation: a prospective multicenter randomized phase IV trial. J Clin Oncol. 2015;33(34):3999–4006.
117. Wharton RE, Stefanov EK, King RG, Kearney JF. Antibodies generated against streptococci protect in a mouse model of disseminated aspergillosis. J Immunol. 2015;194(9):4387–96.

Vaccination Against Fungal Diseases: Lessons from *Candida albicans*

10

Paula Sampaio and Célia Pais

Abstract

The advances in medicine have achieved great benefits by improving or even eliminating various debilitating diseases or malignancies, expanding life expectancy. However, it has also originated the development of a compromised population susceptible to opportunistic diseases. A global major concern is the emergence and spread of life-threatening invasive infections in immunocompromised patients, in which the opportunistic fungal infections have greatly increased in the last decades. The high mortality rates associated with these infections, which remain as high as 40%, are due to the limited therapeutic options and the emergence of drug-resistant fungi, but also due to the lack of efficient early diagnosis. Consequently, these facts led to the opinion that new approaches are needed to improve the outcome of these patients, such as immunopreventive strategies that could even be combined with standard antifungal treatment. In view of the proven effectiveness of various antibacterial and antiviral vaccines in preventing the respective diseases, several works have been developed to induce protective immunity against fungal infections as well. The better understanding of how the immune system works against fungal pathogens has made possible to explore immunomodulatory strategies that can protect both immunocompetent and immunocompromised hosts and generate memory. Recently, two fungal vaccines against *Candida* have advanced through clinical trials. However, there are still many challenges in the development of an efficient vaccine against invasive fungal infections. We will provide an update on the progress made in immunization against fungal infections, reviewing host-fungi interactions, antigens, and adjuvants exploited in vaccine strategies, and discuss concerns that need to be overcome to further advance in the area of fungal vaccines.

P. Sampaio (✉) • C. Pais
Centre of Molecular and Environmental Biology (CBMA), Department of Biology, University of Minho, Braga, Portugal
e-mail: psampaio@bio.uminho.pt

A. Carvalho (ed.), *Immunogenetics of Fungal Diseases*,
DOI 10.1007/978-3-319-50842-9_10

10.1 *Candida* and Its Relation with the Host

In healthy individuals, *Candida* colonization, as part of the normal human microbiota, remains generally benign without any symptoms of disease [1, 2]. Tolerance of the immune system toward commensal species and maintenance of a homeostatic balance at the mucosal surfaces reflect a series of strategies such as avoidance of immune recognition, active suppression of the host response, and regulation of the immune response by the host, as well as the normal mucosal microbiota, confining microbes to this surface [2, 3]. However, when tissue homeostasis is disrupted, *Candida* might penetrate the forbidden compartments of host tissues and cells, causing pathologies, ranging from recalcitrant skin/mucosal infections to life-threatening systemic infections. The deep-seated or the disseminated infections have increased in frequency particularly in patients with medical conditions and treatments that affect natural barriers of the body or negatively impact the competence of the immune system. Such treatments include the use of broad-spectrum antibiotics, prosthetic devices and grafts, burn injuries, or surgery, and medical conditions refer to patients with leukemia, neutropenia, or under chemo and immunosuppressive therapies and patients with HIV infection [4]. The current methods to protect susceptible individuals from these opportunistic infections include prophylactic use of antifungal agents or protective environments such as rooms with controlled air flow. Although it is accepted that early, presumptive treatment of patients with invasive candidiasis is a major determinant of survival, such strategies have not been validated by prospective studies [5].

In intensive care units (ICU), *Candida* spp. colonization may occur in up to 80% of critically ill patients, but curiously, the proportion of invasive candidiasis is less than 10% [6, 7]. Therefore, the immune system is important for the maintenance of integrity at the mucosal surface, and, even in an immunocompromised state, *Candida* species remain in the benign commensal state rather than in the invasive pathogenic one. Indeed, some studies suggest that *C. albicans* may evolve to avoid confrontation with the host, favoring commensalism [8, 9]. How the immune system distinguishes these dual behaviors, commensal vs pathogenic, is a fundamental question in the development of immune-preventive strategies against commensal species and particularly *Candida* species.

The development of new immunotherapies, including vaccines, is driven by the progress made in the understanding of the molecular pathogenic mechanisms of the infectious agent. Understanding how mucosal homeostasis is established, maintained, or disrupted during fungal exposure and/or colonization should help to guide the development of new immunotherapies. Knowledge about the immune response against *Candida* infections has greatly increased in this last decade, with new data and reviews emerging frequently [10–16]. Thus, a brief review to the immune responses to *Candida* developed at the mucosa surface will be presented.

10.1.1 Within the Mucosal Layers: Interaction of *Candida albicans* with the Epithelium

The mucosal epithelium is a critical barrier and the frontline of sensing microbes. Due to its commensal nature, the initial interaction of *Candida* with the human immune system is frequently via epithelial cells of the mucosa [17, 18]. There are multiple ways to contain *C. albicans* in the mucosa, such as the microbial flora or the active role of epithelial cells that produce antimicrobial peptides [15]. In addition, epithelial cells secrete mucins that establish a protective film, forming a dense lattice close to the epithelial surface in which secreted antimicrobial molecules are embedded [19]. Curiously, it has been described that in the gastric mucosa, this mucin film is organized into two layers, an inner layer (50 μm thick) that is densely packed, firmly attached to the epithelium, and devoid of microbes, in contrast to the outer layer (100 μm thick) that is movable, has an expanded volume due to proteolytic cleavages of the mucins, and is colonized by microbes [20]. Recently, it was described that mucin induces an oval-shaped morphology in *C. albicans* in which genes related to adhesion, filamentation, and biofilm formation are downregulated [21] and that mucin has an inherent direct candidacidal activity [22]. Mucosal epithelial cells express innate immune receptors or pattern-recognition receptors (PRRs) that recognize microbe-associated molecular patterns (MAMPs), allowing the immune system to detect attachment of microbes and act accordingly. However, the PRR that mediates recognition of fungi in epithelial cells are still largely unknown or undefined. The major known PRRs involved in the recognition of *Candida* cells were identified in the phagocytic cells and include the Toll-like receptors (TLRs), C-type lectin receptors (CLRs), NOD-like receptors (NLRs), and RIG-I-like receptors (RLRs) [15]. Among the 13 TLRs discovered, expression of TLR1 through TLR9 has been identified in human intestinal epithelial cells (IECs) [23], but its expression varies in different organisms and different mucosal surfaces (oral, vaginal, or gastric) [17]. In addition, TLR2 and TLR4 that are important for host anti-*Candida* defenses [14, 24] have demonstrated hyporesponsiveness to their ligands in human IECs [23]. Furthermore, using a model of oral reconstituted human epithelium (RHE) TLR2, and particularly TLR4, seems to be highly responsive to *Candida* MAMPs [25]. Expression of CLR in epithelial cells seems to be restricted to dectins. Human IECs express functional Dectin-1 that recognizes fungal β-glucans [26], and bronchial epithelial cells also express Dectin-1, which plays an important role in the control of *Aspergillus fumigatus* infections [27]. As a result of the long coevolution of fungi, and particularly *C. albicans* with mucosal surfaces having particular environments, the cross talk between fungi in the different mucosal surfaces has evolved in multiple ways under the double constraints of sensing microbes and adjusting the immune response to the perceived degree of threat while maintaining homeostasis at the mucosa.

Fungal cells differ from animal cells primarily due to the cell wall that surrounds their plasma membrane. The *Candida* cell wall structure has two distinct layers, an outer layer mainly composed of mannan and mannoproteins (O- and N-linked glycoproteins) and an inner layer that contains the skeletal polysaccharides chitin, β-1,3-glucan, and β-1,6-glucan, which confer strength and shape to the yeast cells [28]. These cell wall molecules, which are absent from the human body, are the major source of MAMPs for recognition by host PRRs. However, much of these molecules are expressed in both the commensal state and in the pathogenic state. Recently it was suggested that the pathogenic state may be recognized by "patterns of pathogenesis" or POP rather than only by microbial molecular structures [29]. In this hypothesis, MAMPs are delivered along with additional information that can be used by the host to distinguish pathogenic from nonpathogenic state and thereby guide the ensuing innate immune response. During such pathogenic behaviors, MAMPs access forbidden compartments of host tissues and cells, being recognized by PRRs as genuine pathogen-associated molecular patterns (PAMPs), and elicit an appropriate immune response. This POP hypothesis does not define a pathogen but a pathogenic behavior that can be adopted by any microbe. This allows a particular microbe to be considered a commensal or a pathogen, depending on time and context. Its pathogenicity is determined by its interaction with the host and can change with host, location in the host, and the immune state of the host [3]. The cross talk between *Candida albicans* and the immune system can also be integrated into this hypothesis. It is well established that *Candida* show different behaviors, the pathogenic (invasive) and the nonpathogenic (commensal) [1, 15, 30], but favoring commensalism [8, 9].

One sign of POP that has been defined is the microbial overgrowth in their host [3]. Epithelial cells are able to actively monitor the density of resident microbiota by sampling microbial molecules through PRRs [23]. It is of particular significance that mucosal epithelial cells are able to discriminate between the commensal and the pathogenic behavior of *C. albicans* cells, and there are several ways to control yeast overgrowth [11, 31, 32]. The majority of the epithelial TLRs and Dectin-1 signal through MyD88 adaptor, leading to a transcriptional response primarily dependent on the transcription factor NF-κB [15, 23]. In commensalism the presence of *C. albicans* yeast or hyphae triggers the NF-κB signaling pathway and an early response of the mitogen-activated protein kinase (MAPK) activation through ERK1/2 and JNK signaling. At the mucosal surfaces, this response leads to the secretion of IL-22, by innate and adaptive immune cells, that stimulates the proliferation of epithelial cells and, together with IL-17, the production of antimicrobial peptides, controlling fungal growth and tissue homeostasis [12, 31]. However, when *C. albicans* outgrows and a high fungal hyphal burden is present, the threshold level of the MAPK activation is reached and a second pathway, the MAPK/MKP-1/c-Fos, is activated [31]. Activation of this second response results in the production of proinflammatory cytokines, such as interleukin 1α/β (IL-1α/β), IL-6, GM-CSF, TNF-α and chemokines, RANTES, IL-8, and CCL20 that induce the recruitment, differentiation, and activation of various immune cells, including phagocytes [11, 31]. This immune activation results in reduction of fungal burdens back down below the threshold level of activation and thus to the commensal state. One additional way to modulate *C. albicans* population density is through quorum sensing, in which molecules produced during continuous *C. albicans* growth act as inhibitors of the yeast-to-hypha transition [1, 33], and both morphological forms are known to be required for virulence [34]. Curiously, the recently described non-lytic expulsion of internalized hyphal *Candida* cells by macrophage after phagocytosis benefits not only the immune cells, avoiding their own lysis, but also the fungus as it escapes from intracellular death [35]. This suggests that reestablishment of homeostasis does not implicate the complete elimination of the fungus, but rather reduction of its burden to the commensal state. Thus, at the mucosal surface, there is a constant cross talk between *C. albicans* and host mucosal immune system in order to keep the fungal burden below a certain threshold and maintain homeostasis [31].

Another POP behavior is cytosolic invasion, as many pathogens deliver active proteins, or virulence factors to access forbidden compartments of host tissues [3]. When perturbations at the mucosa surface occur, such as the composition of the competitive commensal bacteria that may result from antibiotic use, or when the immune system becomes severely weakened by factors such as HIV infection, chemotherapy, or chirurgic interventions, the proper restriction of *C. albicans* may fail as well as the capacity to control its overgrowth, predisposing individuals to *Candida* invasion. If containment at the mucosa is breached, the yeast proliferates and penetrates forbidden compartments of the host tissues. *Candida albicans* has the ability to invade host epithelial cells by two routes: via active penetration and via induced endocytosis [36, 37]. The active penetration is exclusively a fungal attribute and includes the physical pressure applied by the advancing hyphal growth in combination with the secretion of extracellular hydrolases like proteases, phospholipases, and lipases [15, 38]. The induced endocytosis is the passive uptake of *C. albicans* cells through yeast surface proteins Als3p and Hgc1p by the E-cadherin receptor in host epithelial cells [38].

As stated above, the epithelial cells actively monitor resident microbes by sampling microbial molecules and channels that transport microbial cell wall components into epithelial cells [23]. To aid in the consequent epithelial response, several PRRs are intracellular and cytoplasmic and are involved in pathogen recognition, antigen processing and presentation, production of antimicrobial β-defensins, and activation of the inflammasomes. The inflammasome is a multiprotein complex that triggers the posttranslational activation of caspase-1 that in turn cleaves and activates the secretion of a variety of substrates, including pro-interleukin-1β and pro-interleukin-18, leading to an inflammatory response [15]. These PRR receptors are not exposed to pathogens unless they get into the cells, when invading mucosa, like TLR3 and TLR9 that recognize fungi nucleic acids or NOD2 that recognize fungal chitin [39, 40]. It has also been reported that this activation may induce the maintenance of a minimal level of "physiological inflammation" by activating NOD proteins in the cytoplasm of gut epithelial and immune cells. Curiously, recognition of fungal chitin by NOD2, together with TLR9 and the mannose receptor, is essential for the selective secretion of the anti-inflammatory cytokine IL-10 by phagocytic cells [41]. This exerts a collaborative control in which TLR signaling is required for the transcription of pro-IL-1β and pro-IL-18, and the posttranslational inflammasome response is then required for subsequent cleavage and secretion of the active cytokine. This dual control may be an important regulatory mechanism to limit inappropriate or unnecessary production of cytokines that trigger potent responses that may be potentially damaging to the host, particularly concerning commensal organisms. Thus, the immune system can initiate responses based not only on whether PAMPs are present but also on where those PAMPs are presented, allowing the epithelium to adjust the response to the perceived degree of threat and return to the homeostatic state once the pathogen has been controlled.

10.1.2 Beyond the Mucosal Layers: Overview of the Immune Response Against *Candida* Infections

At the mucosal epithelium, *Candida* may assume a fully pathogenic behavior, invading deeper tissues, gaining access to the bloodstream and causing invasive infections [11, 12]. One of the causes of this drastic rupture of homeostasis is a too weak immune system. The life-threatening opportunistic *Candida* infections occur particularly in immunocompromised patients in which the immune forces that normally contain *C. albicans* and establish equilibrium are at risk of being overwhelmed.

The host immune system responds with the innate immune attack as the immediately acting primary line of defense against fungi penetration. Recognition of fungal-associated PAMPs will lead to the initiation of a host defense that is mandatory to limit fungal burden in order to clear the invading fungus from non-authorized sites [11, 15]. The cell populations that orchestrate this initial response include the phagocytic cells: neutrophils, macrophages, and dendritic cells (DCs) [10, 13, 15].

Macrophages are considered the first line of defense since they are distributed in various tissues as resident cells. Macrophages exhibit a considerable phenotypic diversity and functional plasticity that confer them the ability to efficiently respond to stimuli. The fungal cell wall is a dynamic structure that is continuously changing throughout the fungus cell cycle and during morphological transition. During tissue invasion, macrophages readily ingest the round yeast form of *C. albicans* as well as the relatively short filaments. The development of hyphae triggers the recognition of cell wall β-glucans via the Dectin-1/inflammasome pathway. Engagement of Dectin-1 induces not only direct macrophage activation and internalization of the fungus but it also has a synergistic effect on TLR2 and TLR4 responses, via NF-κB activation, leading to IL-1β production and T-helper cell 17 (Th17 cell) activation [32, 42, 43]. However, upon hyphal growth, *C. albicans* is able to shield β-glucans with surface mannans as a mechanism to evade cellular phagocytosis [18]. Thus, other PAMPs, such as mannans and mannoproteins, are also recognized by several CLRs, including mannose receptor, Dectin-2, dendritic cell DC-SIGN, and MINCLE [14, 44]. Dectin-2, mainly expressed on dendritic cells, macrophages, and neutrophils, recognizes *Candida* α-mannan and, together with Dectin-3, has been reported to form heterodimers, mediating *Candida* uptake by the phagocyte and leading to proinflammatory responses during *C. albicans* infection, also via NF-κB activation [10, 45].

In consequence of the inflammatory response, neutrophils migrate to the site of infection, and after the recognition of *Candida* cells, they can directly kill the yeast cells and inhibit their growth and the yeast-to-hyphal transition, limiting in this way the progression of fungus [46]. The importance of these phagocytes is highlighted by the observation that the depletion of mononuclear phagocytes results in accelerated fungal proliferation in tissues and increased mortality [47] and that neutropenic patients or patients with impaired neutrophil function are more susceptible to systemic fungal infections [46]. Phagocytic clearance of *C. albicans* involves the accumulation of phagocytes at the site where the yeast cells are located and engulfment and killing of fungal cells after the recognition of cell-surface fungal PAMPs [48]. These innate immune cells damage or kill *C. albicans* cells by using a combination of oxidative and non-oxidative mechanisms that includes the production of antimicrobial peptides and degradative enzymes and the generation of antimicrobial reactive oxygen species (ROS)/nitric oxide synthase (iNOS) [49, 50]. Human neutrophils and macrophages express constitutively chitotriosidase (CHIT-1), an enzyme that promotes digestion of fungal cell wall chitin and whose expression increases significantly during the end/late phase of infection [41]. Curiously, low concentrations of small chitin particles have been shown to induce IL-10 secretion, via NOD2 and TLR9 signaling [41]. This mechanism has been proposed to contribute to the resolution of the infection when the pathogen has been defeated by the immune system, promoting the attenuation of inflammatory-mediated diseases and consequent immune homeostasis.

The innate immune system not only specifically recognizes diverse microorganisms but also initiates and modulates the subsequent adaptive responses that are delivered by T cells and B cells through their interactions with antigen-presenting cells. Phagocytic DCs play an essential role in the activation of adaptive immune responses, being one of the most efficient antigen-presenting cells (APCs). DCs are important for processing and presenting fungal antigens, but, due to the dual nature of *C. albicans*, their reaction to this fungus must be flexible in order to shape T-cell responses accordingly. Th1 responses involving proinflammatory cytokines, such as IFN-γ and TNF-α, were considered protective against fungal infections, whereas Th2 responses, with the secretion of IL-4 and IL-10, were believed to enhance host susceptibility [16]. However, with the identification of Th17 response, involving proinflammatory cytokines IL-17 and IL-22, this is now considered a major pathway for protection against fungal infections [12]. These cytokines induce neutrophil recruitment and activation, as well as the activation of epithelial cells and release of antifungal β-defensins, being important at the mucosal surface. The importance of Th17 in anti-*Candida* response was confirmed by the identification of functionally specific Th17 clones that respond to *C. albicans* by releasing IL-17 and IFN-γ, but not IL-10 [51]. Indeed, patients with defects in Th17 immunity have been directly linked to increased susceptibility to chronic mucocutaneous candidiasis (CMC) [52]. After recognition of *Candida*, the plasticity of DCs is reflected into distinct signaling pathways that are translated into different in vivo adaptive immune responses [53]. Inflammatory DCs initiate antifungal Th17/Th2 cell responses to yeast through signaling pathways that involve adaptor MyD88, whereas tolerogenic

DCs activate Th1/Treg (T regulatory) cell responses to hypha through TRIF adaptor [16, 53].

The balance between proinflammatory and anti-inflammatory signals is essential for successful host/pathogen interaction in fungal infections in which Treg cells play a critical role [53]. Treg cells, essentially via production of IL-10, are able to inhibit components of innate and adaptive immunity in order to regulate the host's immune defense to an adequate level, a protective response without total elimination of the fungus and preventing an exacerbated level of tissue damage [16, 53]. However, overly potent Treg suppression can inhibit protective immunity, favoring the pathogen. Nevertheless, since Treg cells control the quality and magnitude of innate and adaptive effector responses, the outcomes may range from protective tolerance to overt immunosuppression, determining the balance between commensalism and pathogenicity. At the mucosa, a local anti-inflammatory/tolerogenic response through secretion of IL-10 and TGF-β would allow for the fungus persistence, whereas beyond the mucosa, an appropriate inflammatory immune response is necessary to eliminate the fungus and return to a homeostasis state.

The role of Th17 responses in systemic fungal infection is somehow controversial since, on one hand, it is described that IL-17RA−/− and IL-17A−/− mice have elevated susceptibility to disseminated candidiasis [54, 55] and IL-17A mediates vaccine-induced protection in mice [56]. On the other hand, humans with mutations in the IL-17 pathway typically do not develop disseminated disease [55], and candidemic patients showed significantly higher levels of IL-17A than patients without invasive candidiasis [57]. The idea that elevated Th17 and Treg responses are harmful in disseminated candidiasis seemingly contrasts with the apparent protective role of IL-17 in mice. In disseminated candidiasis, it has been reported that *C. albicans* drives expansion of a complex Treg cell population that by depletion of IL-2 promotes the development of Th17 responses that are associated with immune pathology and with *C. albicans* survival and dissemination [55], [58].

Th17 and Treg subsets are reciprocally regulated during naïve T-cell differentiation. However, it is clear that IL-17/Th17 and Treg cells have a complex relationship and that the outcome of the response to *Candida* depends on the site of infection in which the corresponding microenvironment is able to shape these responses. At the intestinal mucosa, high levels of transforming growth factor beta (TGF-β) and retinoic acid have been found that together with short-chain fatty acids (SCFAs) from commensal microbes, fermentation supports tolerogenic Tregs, favoring *C. albicans* commensalism. In contrast, internal organs are shielded from the external environment, and thus inflammation induced during disseminated *C. albicans* infection is more likely to go unchecked, resulting in collateral tissue damage by Th17 responses [55, 58]. Together, these data underline the importance of the balance between proinflammatory and anti-inflammatory responses for both susceptibility to acquire invasive candidiasis and ability to clear the infection, once it has disseminated.

In addition to the cellular responses, adaptive B cell, by inducing antibody-mediated memory responses, may neutralize adherence and spread on and/or through epithelial and endothelial tissues. The role of antibodies in the defense against candidiasis has been controversial due to the belief that immunocompromised patients, the main targets of opportunistic fungal infections, were unable to develop adequate adaptive B-cell response. In addition, due to the fact that *Candida* are commensal organisms, natural anti-*Candida* antibodies may be present in the serum of normal individuals, but no correlation with these antibodies and protection to a subsequent infection has been observed.

There is now substantial evidence for the important role of antibody-mediated immunity in clearance of infectious agents, including host resistance to systemic candidiasis. Regarding the class of immunoglobulins, it has been proposed that IgM titers against intracellular proteins that are not localized to the cell wall would be higher in patients with systemic candidiasis than in controls, which suggests that these antigens might be less visible to the humoral immune system during commensal growth [59]. However, regarding the subclass, a recent study evaluated how the IgG subclass of an anti-*Candida* antibody influences its biological functions, using the mouse model [60]. Four IgG subclass variants of the human antimannan antibody, Mg1, M1g2, M1g3, and M1g4, equivalent to IgG1, IgG2, IgG3, and IgG4, were constructed and evaluated. They found that the four IgG subclasses differ in protection against hematogenously disseminated candidiasis in mice, with IgG1, IgG3, and IgG4 being more effective than IgG2. This difference has been attributed to the lower capacity of IgG2 to mediate FcγR-dependent phagocytic clearance. All variants promoted deposition of both murine and human complement C3 onto the yeast cell surface; however, IgG4 was less potent in activating the complement system. The fact that IgG4 was less potent in activating the complement system but induced similar levels of protection than IgG1 and IgG3 and was even more protective than IgG2 suggests that the role of the complement system in mediating protection may not be that determinant. Indeed, in a murine model of cryptococcosis, it was found that complement-nonactivating human IgG2- or IgG4-mouse chimeric antibodies are protective, while complement-activating human IgG1- or IgG3-mouse chimeric antibodies are nonprotective [61].

The study of the immunoglobulins present in the serum of human subjects without signs of infection in comparison with patients with proven systemic candidiasis has also contributed to the identification of proteins that could be specifically recognized in each situation. The antibodies identified specifically in subjects without infection were considered as natural anti-*Candida* antibodies and are believed to arise from the commensal relation with the host. Some of the natural anti-*Candida* antibodies identified *Candida,* Eno1p, Pgk1p, Adh1p, and Pdc11p, are abundant metabolic enzymes present in the yeast cell wall [62]. However, only antibodies against Pgk1p and Adh1p seem to differentiate patients with systemic candidiasis from noninfected subjects. Antibodies against glyceraldehyde-3-phosphate dehydrogenase (Gap1p), phosphoglycerate kinase (Pgk1p), phosphoglycerate mutase (Gpm1p), enolase (Eno1p), pyruvate kinase (Cdc19p), aconitase (Aco1p), methionine synthase (Met6p), hyphal wall protein (Hwp1), and mannan, among others, have been identified specifically in patients with systemic candidiasis. However, conditions that make the molecular targets available to the immune system to induce antibodies differ according to many variables, including the morphology changes of the pathogens, the competence of the immune system at the entry port, the composition of the commensals and their similarity of epitopes, and the history of antimicrobial treatments that have different modes of action, among others. All these mechanisms contribute to expose antigenic molecules to the immune system, and some treatments will increase/alter exposure of certain antigenic molecules. This may be one of the reasons why it has been so difficult to identify antibodies/antigenic molecules that would be useful for immunoglobulin-based prophylactics and therapeutics. Nevertheless, Mycograb (NeuTec Pharma), a human recombinant antibody anti-Hsp90p, was found to be therapeutically effective in combination with amphotericin B in patients with systemic candidiasis in a randomized, blinded, multicenter trial [63].

These studies evidence that the role of antibody-mediated resistance to fungal infections is important and may be exploited as new therapeutic approaches; however, the isotypes that could be more effective in a response that involves antibodies must be carefully chosen to mimicking the host's natural protective antibody and balance between its disease-causing effects, as exacerbated complement activation, and its effects on clearance of microbes.

Intense investigation of immunological mechanisms involved in fungal infections means that we are closer to understanding the processes involved in the identification and clearance of pathogens from the human body and in establishing immune memory to respond to future exposure. The ideal vaccine would initiate an innate immune response capable of directing the adaptive immune response toward efficient inactivation and removal of the specific pathogen from non-allowed sites, followed by the development of adequate immune memory. In the next section, an update of the studies toward the development of vaccination strategies will be presented.

10.2 Induction of Immunity in Experimental Models

10.2.1 Concerns About the Development of Preventive Strategies

The increasing incidence and severity of invasive fungal infections coupled with diagnostic difficulties and high cost of treatments prompted the investigation on vaccination [64]. However, for years the development of fungal vaccines has lagged behind that of vaccines against bacteria and viruses because of the idea that most patients who develop life-threatening fungal infections have profound defects in their immune systems and are unable to respond to vaccination. Indeed invasive *Candida* infections often take place in hospital settings; however, it is has been estimated that only 10–20% of patients who develop bloodstream infection from *Candida* are seriously immunocompromised. The large majority develop the infection after patient's normal bacterial flora is disrupted by antibiotics or when their skin or gut mucosa are breached by burns, central venous catheters, or surgery [4, 5, 65]. Furthermore, several studies confirmed the immunogenicity and efficacy of vaccines in seriously immunocompromised patients, such as those with active leukemia, HIV infections, or cancer patients [66–68]. Thus, immunocompromised patients are able to respond to vaccination, and vaccination has been recommended to patients with HIV and cancer despite their weakened immune systems [69–71]. It has been assumed that acutely ill hospitalized patients whose primary host defense defect is anatomical will also respond to vaccination [65]. In the case of *Candida* systemic infections, the various medical procedures that are identified as risk factors, such as exposure to broad-spectrum antibiotics, central venous catheters, or major surgery, are perfectly recognized, opening a window of opportunity to vaccinate at-risk patients even before the onset of infection [72–74]. In addition, prevention of infectious disease in the elderly has become a priority in the twenty-first century as the proportion of older individuals increases globally. Fungal infections due to *Candida, Aspergillus,* and *Cryptococcus* are known to be more frequent in the extreme of the ages, children and elder patients.

Consistent with Benjamin Franklin's dictum "an ounce of prevention is worth a pound of cure," preventive therapies against invasive candidiasis may reduce the severity of these infections. A vaccine that could prevent or improve the outcome of fungal infections would not only benefit the at-risk patients but also be of major benefit for national healthcare systems by reducing hospital costs.

10.2.2 Evidences from Systemic Candidiasis in the Human Host

Several studies were undertaken to identify *Candida albicans* immunogenic proteins specifically recognized by antibodies produced during the natural course of systemic *Candida* infection and that could be exploited for vaccine development or even as useful biomarkers for diagnosis. One of the earliest studies evaluated, by immunoblotting, 201 sequential serum samples from 45 patients with systemic candidiasis in which 13 were involved in an outbreak at London Hospital [75]. This study showed a high heterogeneity in antibody response but was able to identify an antibody against a 47-kD antigen present in all patients that recovered from the systemic infection. Later, the 47-kD antigen was identified as a breakdown product of heat-shock protein (Hsp) 90 from *C. albicans*. The presence of antibodies against a 47-kD antigen in serum of other patients with systemic candidemia with a favorable outcome has also been identified by other independent studies. Serum from these patients passively transferred to mice infected with a lethal dose of *C. albicans* was able to induce protection, and a monoclonal antibody raised against a synthesized conserved epitope (LKVIRK) of Hsp90p reduced mice mortality when given 24 h before an i.v. challenge [76]. This antibody seems to protect through neutralization of the protein-binding activity of *Candida* circulating Hsp90p or by inhibition of *Candida* growth [77]. However, an epitope mapping analysis indicated that antibodies reacting to epitopes of this protein showed 100% direct homology with comparable sites on human Hsp90p, raising the concern of development of autoimmune reactions. These studies showed that patients who recover from systemic candidiasis may produce autoantibodies against self-epitopes.

More recently another study used a highly sensitive proteomic approach to identify potential candidate markers for diagnosis and follow-up of systemic candidiasis [62]. This study identified immunoreactive protein species that were present in patients with proven candidemia and also in patients with no apparent *Candida* infection. In patients with invasive candidiasis, the authors were able to unambiguously identify 42 different *C. albicans* protein targets of the human immune response. The abundance of housekeeping enzymes, most of them (65%) metabolic enzymes, was discussed, as among other possibilities, being part of a universal signal for infection. Since these are ubiquitous and highly conserved enzymes, their epitopes can be shared by several infectious agents and allow the development of a natural resistance to infection. The identifications of these proteins by the immune system may be considered as part of the "patterns of pathogenesis" response. Among the metabolic enzymes that are also present on the *C. albicans* cell surface, antibodies against glyceraldehyde-3-phosphate dehydrogenase (Gap1p), phosphoglycerate kinase (Pgk1p), phosphoglycerate mutase (Gpm1p), enolase (Eno1p), pyruvate kinase (Cdc19p), aconitase (Aco1p), and methionine synthase (Met6p) had already been identified in human serum previously. Several other proteins, including Hxk2p (hexokinase) and Pgi1p and 6-phosphofructokinase, were identified as antigens of the immune system for the first time in this study. Curiously, antibodies against *C. albicans* proteins Eno1p, Fba1p, Tkl1p, Ino1p, Met6p, Sah1p, Ilv5p, Ade17p, and Qcr2p increased in response to antifungal treatment, indicating that their exposure to the immune system increased with the antifungal treatment. From this survey, 14% of the identified targets were chaperons and heat-shock proteins, including Ssa1p and Ssb1p identified in previous studies as antigens and Ssc1p and Sse1p newly identified as antigens in this study. Curiously, the 47-kDa fragments of Hsp90p identified previously [75] were not identified in this analysis, only the 82-kDa fragment of the same protein. The *C. albicans* elongation factor 1 (Eft1p) and Eft2p, known to be located in the cell wall and proposed as potential antigens for vaccine development, were also found in this study.

The protein targets identified in the serum of subjects with no infection were considered as targets of natural anti-*Candida* antibodies. These natural antibodies identified *Candida* Eno1p, Pgk1p, Adh1p, and Pdc11p, which corresponded to abundant glycolytic and fermentative enzymes. The natural antibodies were considered to be elicited during commensal colonization by *C. albicans* or against other homologue protein from different commensals or infectious agents that cross-react with *C. albicans* proteins. This study also identified targets that could be correlated with recovery from systemic candidiasis in humans, like high serum levels of anti-Eno1p antibodies, the appearance or maintenance of anti-Hsp90p, anti-Tpi1p, or the disappearance of serum anti-Met6p or anti-Pgk1p antibody levels.

Another study measured IgG and IgM titers in the serum of human systemic *Candida* infections against 15 specific recombinant *C. albicans* antigens [59]. It is documented that patients with systemic candidiasis already exhibit significantly high IgG titers against a wide range of antigens (ENO1, HWP1, mannan, and CGTA) before or at the time that the diagnosis is confirmed by a positive blood culture. This study suggests that invasive candidemia may be preceded by low-level systemic exposure to *Candida* spp., possibly due to "leakage" from mucosal sites of colonization.

10.2.3 Exploited Protection Strategies Against Candidiasis

10.2.3.1 Whole-Cell Vaccines

The need for therapeutic or preventive use of a vaccine in candidiasis, particularly in certain groups of at risk patients, is reflected in the huge number of experimental investigations designed to attempt induction of protection (Fig. 10.1). The early studies trace back to the decade of the 1950s.

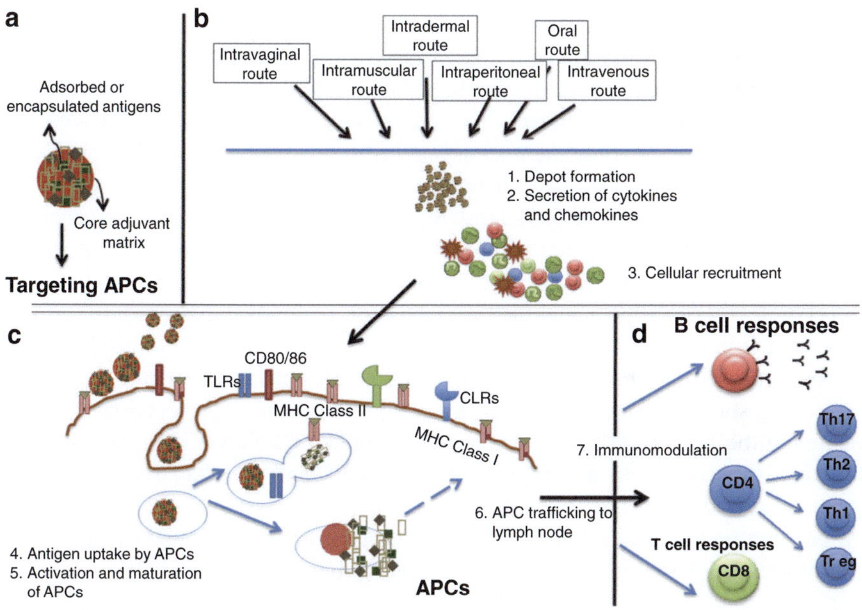

Fig. 10.1 Overview of innate and immune responses to pathogen/adjuvant actions. (**a**) A schematic of a vaccine formulation with the antigen (that could be live attenuated/low virulent cells, killed cells, disrupted cells, ribosomal extracts, cell wall extracts, glycoconjugates, or recombinant proteins/peptide) and adjuvant (including aluminum compounds, MF59 Freund's adjuvants, AS03 and AS04, virosomes, or liposomes). (**b**) Vaccine formulation is delivered into the body through different route of entry. Some adjuvants presumably form a depot at the site of injection (*1*), which is associated with slow release of antigen. Other adjuvants are associated with secretion of cytokines and chemokines (*2*), which may induce the recruitment of various immune cells to the injection site, including APCs (*3*). (**c**) APCs express various PRRs on the surface (including TLRs, CLRs) and intracellularly (TLRs, NLRs, and RLRs), which enhances antigen uptake (*4*) and favors activation and maturation (*5*) of APCs. Mature APCs increase the capacity for antigen processing and presentation and upregulate the expression of MHC (class I and II) and co-stimulatory (CD80, CD86) molecules. (**d**) Mature APCs then migrate to the draining lymph nodes (*6*) to interact with antigen-specific B or T cell to activate antibody secretion and B cells and/or effector $CD8^+$ T and $CD4^+$ T-cell responses (*7*)

One of the early documented studies repeatedly immunized rabbits intravenously (i.v.) with heat-killed *C. albicans* prior to infection and then assessed survival, histopathology of infected organs, and passive immunization. The authors concluded that this immunization did not result in protection and that the anti-*Candida* antibodies induced by vaccination did not protect the animals [78]. Latter, by using the same model but immunizing with heat-killed and heat-weakened *Candida*, protection was only observed in rabbits immunized with viable *Candida*, and histological analysis indicated that cellular immunity was important [79]. These observations point to the active action of the pathogen in the immunization process. In the murine model, low virulent *Candida* strains, modified in the filamentation capacity and stress response, were shown to provide protection against a subsequent intravenous systemic *Candida* infection [80–82]. The efficacy of these strategies reached 100% for all strains at least in one evaluated condition. Other study, using the mouse model, also observed the importance of fungal pathogenicity on priming of mice with *Candida* [83]. Naïve BALB/c mice were intraperitoneally (i.p.) primed with a low inoculum of *Candida* yeast cells that were heat-killed, deliberately attenuated, or in its pathogenic native form. One month later, mice were infected with the pathogenic strains, and only the mice primed with the pathogenic native form were able to clear the infection. Live-attenuated pathogens or in its pathogenic native form have been shown to be especially immunostimulatory when used as vaccines. This may be explained by the hypothesis that the immune system also responds to POP and suggest why killed strains failed to elicit protection [29]. However, due to the complexity of antigens and the inexistence of generalizable procedure for how best to attenuate pathogens for their use as vaccines, attenuated strains challenge safety requirements. However, changing to a subcutaneous (s.c.) immunization with a *Candida* sonicate, Mourad and Friedman [84] were able to protect 50% of mice, obtaining the best result in comparison with viable or killed *C. albicans* cells. In addition, they observed that transferring passively anti-*Candida* serum to naïve mice conferred them protection against a subsequent systemic candidiasis [84]. After these results, subcellular antigens have been further exploited as candidates for augmenting host defense and vaccine development against candidiasis.

10.2.3.2 Ribosomal Vaccines

Ribosomal subcellular vaccines derived from both prokaryotic and eukaryotic pathogens were widely exploited as protectors and afforded high levels of protection at small dose levels, being the duration of the immunity they provided greater than the ones obtained with previous antigens used. Thus, ribosomal fractions were also used to try to induce protection against candidemia. Studies documented that it was possible to induce protection by immunization with *C. albicans* ribosomes, not only against heterologous *C. albicans* strains, with 30–78% of survival, but also cross protection against *C. tropicalis* isolates, with 57–64% of survival rate from a systemically administered lethal infection [85]. Ribosomal vaccine was also exploited in experimentally induced cell-mediated immunocompromised mice, resulting in a survival rate that reached 76% [86]. This vaccine was also exploited in tumor-bearing mice, and although the survival rate did not change, it was able to expand the median survival time [87]. These results showed that vaccination of immunocompromised and tumor-bearing hosts with *Candida* ribosome could provide enhanced resistance to disseminated candidiasis. These works encouraged the continuing studies in immunization against candidiasis and revealed the immunogenicity of subcellular components and the role of antibodies in the protection. A variety of cell constituents, routes of administration, and protocols have been tested, and despite the degree of variability in the results observed, induction of protection was considered possible. However, due to the complexity of the antigen that would probably include mRNA, rRNA, and ribosomal proteins, newly synthesized polypeptides along with other cell components from the extraction procedure, the identification of the moiety to fully describe the protective immunity mechanism was difficult, and other more defined antigens have been exploited.

10.2.3.3 Cell Wall Component Vaccines

Fungal cell wall constituents are excellent candidates for vaccine development since the cell wall is a unique microbial feature with an important role in antigen presentation and immunomodulation [28]. *Candida albicans* cell wall is composed mainly of carbohydrates (80–90%), such as mannans, β-glucans, and chitin, while proteins and lipids are a minority. β-glucans and chitin are located at the innermost layer of the cell wall, providing structural rigidity and strength, while mannans are abundant in the outer layer. Purified polysaccharide vaccines are poorly immunogenic and largely ineffective, due to the inability of the polysaccharide to induce T-cell responses. Thus, in glycan-based vaccines, it is common to conjugate the polysaccharide to a carrier molecule such as the tetanus or diphtheria bacterial toxoid [88], which are accepted for human use, or to peptides derived from the infectious agent of interest [89]. Nevertheless, glycopeptides may still be poorly immunogenic, and adjuvant has been also included, like the complete Freund's adjuvant [89]. Previous studies have shown that the major cell wall components that elicit a host immune system response are proteins and mannoproteins, in which both the carbohydrate and protein moieties are important [89, 90]. *Candida* surface mannans were used either alone or encapsulated [91] or even conjugated with protein to induce protection against experimental disseminated candidiasis [92]. The formulations of mannans conjugated with BSA showed high levels of protection with 100% survival in a disseminated murine model. This study also suggested that di- and trisaccharides of mannans were more efficient than tetra-, penta-, or hexasaccharides in inducing protective antibodies. In order to avoid the controversy of results that might be influenced by the distinct methods of mannan extraction, the new approaches developed fully synthetic mannan conjugated vaccines. In this view, a synthetic trisaccharide mannan-tetanus toxoid conjugated vaccine was used in experimental immunization protocol that was designed to simulate the clinical situation in which vaccination can be performed before a patient becomes immunocompromised by treatment with immunosuppressive drugs to induce leukopenia [93]. Although no survival rate was quantified in this study, this conjugate vaccine achieved a statistically significant reduction of fungal burden in the kidney and liver of immunized rabbits, when compared to controls, and this was attributed to the high titer of specific IgG antibody capable of opsonizing the surface of *C. albicans* cells. This model indicated that even in leukocytopenic animals, a previous vaccination is able to induce resistance against disseminated candidiasis.

Xin and collaborators [89] selected *C. albicans* cell-surface proteins previously identified as inducers of antibodies during human candidiasis [62] to conjugate with β-mannan. The selected proteins were fructose-bisphosphate aldolase (Fba), methyltetrahydropteroyltriglutamate (Met6), hyphal wall protein-1 (Hwp1), glyceraldehyde-3-phosphate dehydrogenase (Gap1), and phosphoglycerate kinase (Pgk1). By using an antigen-pulsed DC-based vaccine strategy, immunization with β-(Man)3-Hwp1, β-(Man)3-Fba, or β-(Man)3-Met6 conjugates showed 80–100% survival rate, while with β-(Man)3-Enol or β-(Man)3-Gap1, the survival rate was 40% or 80%, respectively. Curiously, in this study β-(Man)3-Pgk1 slightly enhanced disease. The β-(Man)3-Fba conjugate vaccine, which induced the highest protection, showed similar results against disseminated candidiasis in two different mouse strains, BALB/c and C57BL/6 mice. However, the immunization protocol utilizing dendritic cells is cost prohibitive. Thus, β-(Man)3-Fba has been exploited in a subcutaneous immunization protocol using different adjuvants. After several approaches using of β-(Man)3-Fba with alum or MPL (lipid A, monophosphoryl) with no significant protection, the use of tetanus toxoid was able to restore protection previously observed and even protect 100% outbred mice [94].

The protective responses against *Candida* mannan components appeared to be mainly by induction of protective antibodies specific against the fungal peptide epitopes and the conjugated polysaccharides, which enabled the production of anti-polysaccharide IgG antibodies in vivo. The switch from IgM to IgG, the activation of the complement system, and the rapid deposition of high amounts of factor C3b onto the yeast cell wall are mechanisms that contribute to inhibit *Candida* growth in vitro [89, 94, 95]. These results substantiate the role of antibody in protection against systemic candidiasis in the animal model, evidenced by high survival rates and reduced organ fungal burden.

Although mannoproteins are the major components of the cell wall in eliciting immune responses, β-glucans were also exploited. However, due to their poor immunogenicity, β-glucans must be also conjugated with other molecules. The brown alga *Laminaria digitata* β-1,3-glucans, the laminarin, has been exploited as immunizing antigen conjugated with the diphtheria toxoid, and results showed it was protective against both mucosal and systemic candidiases in mice, with a protective rate around 70% [88]. Remarkably, this laminarin vaccine strategy conferred cross protection to mice lethally challenged with the major fungal pathogens *C. albicans*, *Aspergillus fumigatus*, and *Cryptococcus neoformans* [96]. The bacterial calreticulin (Crt) protein is functionally similar to heat-shock proteins, and one of the main characteristics of this HSP family is that they possess a potent immunostimulatory activity. This characteristic was exploited as an effective carrier or adjuvant for β-glucans in assisting the production of glycotope-specific IgG antibodies in healthy as well as in immunocompromised mice. Laminarin conjugated with a peptide from calreticulin (LAM-CRT) induced proliferation of B lymphocytes and production of specific laminarin and β-1,3-glucans IgG1 antibodies, even in athymic (T-cell-deficient) nude mice [97]. Vaccination with LAM-CRT protected mice against systemic *C. albicans* challenge with a survival rate around 60%.

10.2.3.4 Vaccines for Neutralizing Virulence Factors

The previous approaches of vaccination were mainly based on the stimulation of the immune system with whole microbes or with constitutive microbial epitopes present at the surface of the infectious organism. However, the most effective human vaccines, which prevent tetanus and diphtheria, are directed against the bacterial toxins rather than against the structural epitopes. Thus, another approach in the development of immunoprotective therapies against fungal infections is the development of strategies that focused on the neutralization of virulence factors, either present in the cell wall or secreted that should be produced by microorganisms in their pathogenic form [83]. Virulence factors include proteins involved in the adhesion to and invasion of host tissues, secreted lytic enzymes, the morphogenetic yeast-to-hyphae switching, the maintenance of cellular integrity, or the avoidance of the host immune response.

In this view, vaccines based on the adhesins Als1p and Als3p were exploited. Als1p allows binding of *C. albicans* to human vascular endothelial cells, and Als3p is a hypha-specific surface protein that also mediates attachment to epithelial and endothelial cells. In addition, Als3p is one of the adhesion molecules that is responsible for the binding to host cell receptors, such as E-cadherin, and induce passive endocytose of *C. albicans* by host epithelial cells [38]. Intraperitoneal immunization of BALB/c mice with a recombinant N-terminal peptide of Als1p (rAls1p-N) induced modest protection against invasive candidiasis, protecting 25% of the infected mice [98]. However, when a subcutaneous route of infection was tested, the protection rate was much higher, around 50–57% of immunocompetent mice survive the lethal infection [99]. This vaccination regime was also applied to neutropenic mice that were challenged with a ten-time lower inoculum, with and overall survival of 88% versus 38% of the controls, as well as in a mucosal oropharyngeal candidiasis model, with results showing a clear reduction on invasive tongue lesions. The recombinant N-terminal peptide of Als3p (rAls3p-N) was also exploited and compared with rAls1p-N [100]. Results indicated that rAls3p-N is as effective as rAls1p-N against disseminated candidiasis, with similar survival rates, around 40–50%, but was more effective than rAls1p-N against oropharyngeal or vaginal candidiasis. This high effectiveness in mucosal models may be due to the fact that Als3p mediated superior adhesion to epithelial cells than Als1p.

These data showed promising results, and rAls3p-N stands out as a candidate for further development of an anti-candidal vaccine. However, these vaccines used Freund's adjuvant to enhance immunogenicity, which is not allowed for human use. In order to switch to an adjuvant approved for human use, these vaccines were tested with alum (Alhydrogel), but the efficacy was lower than with Freund's adjuvant even using a higher dose of the recombinant proteins. The survival rate using Freund's adjuvant ranged from 100% to 50% using 20 μg of rAls1p-N, while with Alhydrogel diluted in phosphate-buffered saline (PBS) was of only 10% using 100 μg of rAls1p-N [101]. Regarding rAls3p-N, the protection of around 40–50%

with Freund's adjuvant shifted to around 35% with 300 μg of antigen with Alhydrogel [102]. Interestingly, Als3p is structurally similar to the *Staphylococcus aureus* surface clumping factor (ClfA) that is also involved in adhesion, so these authors also tested for a cross-reactivity of rAls3p-N vaccine against *S. aureus* infection in mice. Results showed that vaccination with rAls3p-N in Alhydrogel improved the survival of mice subsequently infected with multiple clinical isolates of *S. aureus* (40–70% of survival rate) [103]. Although rAls1p-N and rAls3p-N vaccines induced broader antibody-based responses, antibody titers did not significantly correlate with survival in both recombinant peptides. Thus, the protective mechanism of these recombinant peptides was not correlated with protective antibodies but was associated to enhancing cell-mediated immunity. In concordance with these observations, B-cell-deficient mice showed the same pattern of resistance, while in T-cell deficient (nude), the protection against systemic candidiasis previously observed was abolished.

More recently, the efficacy of rAls3p-N vaccine with alum as adjuvant in protecting against vulvovaginal candidiasis was evaluated in a murine VVC model [56]. In this model, rAls3p-N induced a strong immune humoral response with high anti-rAls3p-N serum IgG and vaginal IgA titers. In addition, ex vivo killing of opsonized *C. albicans* by neutrophils was correlated with significant decrease in vaginal fungal burden both in inbred and outbred mice infected with different clinical *C. albicans* isolates. As in previous studies, the role of B and T cells in vaccine-mediated protection was evaluated in B-cell-deficient and nude mice, respectively, showing that contrary to the systemic model, rAls3p-N efficacy in the VVC model requires both B and T cells.

Other virulence factors that were thought to be neutralized were the secreted aspartyl proteinases (SAPs), an enzyme family with ten members, from Sap1p to Sap10p. While Sap1p and Sap8p are secreted and released to the surrounding medium, Sap9p and Sap10p remain bound to the cell surface [2]. These enzymes are involved in the degradation of mucous substrates and defensive factors, promoting *Candida* damage to epithelial and endothelial cells and helping the fungal cells to elude the host immune response. One of the early studies presented results of immunization against a secreted unidentified 43,000-MW protein, named p43, that resulted in the complete neutralization of its immunomodulatory effects and was very efficient in protecting mice, i. e., no CFUs were observed in the kidney of vaccinated mice in comparison with the controls [104]. The mechanism of protection involved the production of protective specific antibodies against p43 evaluated by passive administration. In latter studies, the same authors used *C. albicans* Sap2p, a 41,000-MW secreted protein that they believed to mediate some of the effects observed with p43. However, they concluded that although an immunomodulatory role for Sap2p on *C. albicans* was also observed, it appeared unlikely that p43 activities previously described were caused by Sap2p alone [105]. Nevertheless, this study assessed the potential of an intradermal (i.d.) vaccination with 10 μg Sap2p inoculum incorporated in alum adjuvant in preventing systemic candidiasis in BALB/c mice. After a lethal inoculum of *C. albicans*, an effective protection was obtained in Sap2p-immunized mice with a survival rate of around 75%. The immune protection against systemic candidiasis in mice immunized with Sap2p is antibody mediated as indicated by the correlation of survival with an increase in serum antibodies to Sap2p and by the passive transfer of anti-Sap2 IgG that significantly decreased yeast burden in the kidneys of *C. albicans*-infected mice.

Meanwhile, intravaginal (i.v.g.) and intranasal (i.n.) immunizations with a Sap preparation, mainly consisting of Sap2p, showed that neutralization of these secreted proteins could also be effective in conferring protection against vaginal candidiasis in the rat model. An inoculum of 100 μg of Sap with cholera toxin as adjuvant induced a high degree of protection against vaginal challenge with *C. albicans*. This study showed that the i.n. route is as efficient as the i.v.g. in inducing protection against mucosal candidiasis, and it is recognized that i.n. route is much more easy to subject compliance to self-administration [106]. In order to specify the antigen to propose a candidate vaccine against mucosal candidiasis, a recombinant and truncated Sap2 protein (rSap2t) was produced, and the immunization with this recombinant protein induced antibody-mediated protection against *Candida* infection in an experimental model of rat vaginitis, confirming the previous results [107].

Hyr1p is an important virulence factor for *C. albicans*, a mannoprotein on the cell wall implicated in the resistance to phagocyte killing, and another approach to induce protection used this protein [108]. Mice were immunized with a recombinant fragment (rHyr1p-N) in complete Freund's adjuvant or in Alhydrogel and then infected with *C. albicans*. The results showed that vaccination with rHyr1p-N mixed with both adjuvants markedly improved survival in a range of 60% or 70%. The mechanism of resistance included the action of polyclonal antibodies specific to anti-rHyr1p that enhanced mouse neutrophil killing activity evidenced by the lower organ fungal burden [108]. In order to expand these findings to both immunocompetent and neutropenic mice and to evaluate if this vaccination strategy also protects against non-*albicans Candida* spp., immunizations with rHyr1p-N in alum were tested. Results showed a dose-dependent improved survival rates in immunocompetent mice compared to mice receiving adjuvant alone, with the best results observed with 33 μg of rHyr1p-N in alum (survival rate of around 40%). Vaccination with the highest dose also reduced the tissue fungal burden by approximately 16-fold when compared to control mice. This vaccine effectively protected neutropenic mice against candidiasis (survival rate of around 20%) and significantly increased the mouse immune response as determined by detection of increased anti-rHyr1p-N antibody titers and reduced CFUs in the kidneys. The rHyr1p-N vaccine also induced a significant reduction of tissue fungal burden of vaccinated mice and then infected with *C. glabrata*, *C. parapsilosis*, and *C. tropicalis*. The mechanism of protection rendered by rHyr1p-N appears to be attributed, at least in part, to protective antibody response as evidenced by the results obtained with passive immunization with purified rabbit anti-Hyr1p IgG prolonged survival of mice infected with *C. albicans*.

Evidence has accumulated that antibodies specific for certain yeast cell-surface epitopes may be protective and, thus, screens for antibodies against those epitopes expressed during pathogenesis in human disseminated candidiasis have been performed [59]. From these studies, some of the antigens responsible for the induction of antibodies identified during the convalescent phase or that could be correlated with higher probability of recovery were tested. Anti-wall enolase antibodies stand out as protective antibody, and thus enolase was tested to evaluate if it would induce protection against a systemic infection in the mice model. One hundred micrograms of purified recombinant enolase (rEno1p) in complete Freund's adjuvant were evaluated in an immunization protocol, and results indicated to be effective in reducing the CFUs of organs of immunized mice [109]. The immune protection appeared to be mainly antibody mediated as indicated by the increased titers of enolase-specific IgG1 and IgG2a in serum of immunized mice that enhanced opsonization-mediated yeast killing by neutrophils. Passive transfer of anti-rEno1p also reduced fungal burden of non-immunized infected mice.

Antibodies against heat-shock proteins, particularly anti-Hsp90p, have also been detected in sera from patients that recovered from invasive candidiasis in contrast to those that did not survived, and consequently Hsp90p, a cell wall protein, has been suggested as an important target for protective studies. In addition, Mycograb (NeuTec Pharma) a monoclonal antibody binds to the immunodominant epitope of *C. albicans*. Hsp90p has been applied in combined therapies with positive results [63]. Two strategies have been exploited, an Hsp90-expressing DNA vaccine and a recombinant Hsp90 protein vaccine [110, 111]. However, and although particularly the recombinant protein induced significant increases in both serum and vaginal hsp90-CA-specific IgG and IgA antibodies when compared to the control group, these vaccination approaches did not elicit sufficient protection.

In sum, the best protective effects observed to date have been stimulated by immunization with viable cells from virulent or avirulent *C. albicans* strains. Killed cells or subcellular components have been moderately successful and even less efficient in subunit vaccines. However, in the last years, the focus on the development of fungal vaccines has been placed on subunit vaccines that are easily controlled in terms of preparation and composition, enabling a more precise evaluation of their mechanism of action and good manufacturing practices. Although expectations for these vaccines are high, some authors think that for invasive candidiasis univalent vaccines are unlikely to be successful [64]. The reasons for these disbelieve are mainly due to the fact that the most effective vaccines developed are against known virulence factors with inducing of protective antibodies. One of the main characteristic features of *C. albicans* is its extraordinary range of virulence factors that are expressed by families of genes. Most of these gene families are composed of at least ten different members that in their action facilitate tissue invasion by enabling the fungus to escape from, modulate, or even exacerbate host immunity and in most situations play redundant roles. Thus, the univalent vaccines confer a considerable probability that the fungus can escape from immune responses induced by the vaccination strategy by compensatory expression of other virulence traits. Taking into account these observations, the use of at least two unrelated virulence-associated fungal immunogens was recommended to be present in the vaccine formulation, such as the Als3p and the Sap2p.

Other approach to reduce the chances of immune evasion is to go back to the use of a more complex immunization antigen. A recent study used dithiothreitol

(DTT)-extracted *C. albicans* cell wall surface proteins (CWSP) as antigens incorporated into cationic liposomes as adjuvant/delivery system. The cationic surfactant dioctadecyldimethylammonium bromide (DODAB) and monoolein, 1-monooleoyl-rac-glycerol (MO), were used to develop a DODAB:MO lipid-based delivery system loaded with CWSP and determined its immunogenicity for the development of a vaccine against systemic *Candida* infection [112]. Results showed that immunized mice displayed strong humoral response, with high levels of IgGs against specific cell wall proteins, and restimulated splenocytes derived from immunized mice secreted high levels of IFN-γ and IL-17. This vaccine strategy was able to protect around 70% of mice [113]. The main advantage of this system is that liposomes, as particulate carriers, entrap and protect the specific protein(s) against degradation, enhancing APC uptake of the liposomes and activation.

Many positive results have been achieved in the last years in the development of fungal vaccines. Technological developments have allowed for a rapid expansion of the number of general strategies for making new vaccines, and studies will continue, based on more comprehensive understanding of the immunobiology of pathogen, the type and specificity of immune response required for persistent protection against disease, the attainment of mucosal immunity, and the optimal vaccination strategy to achieve protection. From all these studies, several candidate vaccines have been proposed, and an important outcome is that the selection of antigens and the complexation method of conjugation are critical since it may result in the development of potentially useful protective vaccine candidates, or it may enhance disease susceptibility. Problems associated with conjugated vaccines such as variation in antigen loading, immunogenic linkers, and antigenic carrier proteins must be considered. The important point, from the standpoint of antibody-mediated protection, is that the enormous antigenic complexity of the *Candida* cell should not be expected to reliably induce production of protective antibodies, as defined by specificity, titer, isotype, and effector function. *Candida albicans* antigens that appeared to have potential immunoprotective responses seem to be protein or glycoprotein components that play their structural/physiological role outside the plasma membrane, belonging to the cell wall, or that are secreted to the exocellular environment.

In recent years, advancement of vaccines has focused on improving immune adjuvant and the use of novel vaccine carriers. Some of these particulate carriers also show adjuvant properties. Herein, we will present the adjuvant carriers that are used in commercial vaccines and the carriers that are being used in the development of fungal vaccines.

10.2.4 Licensed Adjuvant Carriers

The main goal of vaccination is the induction of a protective immunity against a particular disease, and in some subunit vaccines, this can only be achieved by addition of an adjuvant or adjuvant combinations. Subunit, highly purified antigens may lack PAMPs needed to activate the innate immune system and downstream adaptive responses. It is thought that the use of adjuvants (Latin word adjuvare, meaning "to help or aid") may help to overcome this first step on the innate immune response [114]. Thus, the choice of adjuvant/s is important since it can direct the type of adaptive immune response to the administered antigen, preferentially activating specific T-cell responses. Adjuvants may also improve immune responses in populations where responses to vaccines are typically reduced, such as infants, the elderly, and the immunocompromised, which is the more vulnerable population for acquiring fungal infections.

Although adjuvants are important components of the vaccine strategy, their mechanisms of action only recently are being revealed [115]. Latest evidence suggest that adjuvants may have one or more of the following mechanisms of action: (1) depot effect (sustained release of antigen at the site of injection), (2) secretion of cytokines and chemokines, (3) cellular recruitment at the site of injection, (4) increase antigen uptake and presentation to APCs, (5) upregulation of MHC II and co-stimulatory molecules, (6) migration to the draining lymph nodes, and (7) modulation of the immune adoptive responses (Fig. 10.1) [115]. The most widely recognized vaccine adjuvants are aluminum-based mineral salts, emulsions, virosomes, and liposomes, which are also considered delivery systems.

The most well-known adjuvants in vaccination strategies are aluminum-based mineral salts, also known as alum. Aluminum salts consist of crystalline nanoparticles that aggregate to form a heterogeneous dispersion of particles of several microns. They are highly charged and conducive, which allows the binding between the antigens or immunomodulatory molecules to alum due to strong electrostatic interactions [116, 117]. Regardless the progress in understanding aluminum salts, its mode of action is still poorly understood. It is described that in the peritoneal cavity of mice, alum induces recruitment of immune cells through induction of chemoattractants like CCL2 the neutrophil chemotaxin KC (CXCL1) and eosinophil chemotaxin eotaxin (CCL11) [118]. Eosinophils appear to have a crucial role in priming and differentiation of B cells, resulting in robust antibody production and Th2-type immune responses [119]. However, there is evidence suggesting that injection of alum leads to tissue damage and cell death with the release of endogenous danger signals and inflammasome activation, which leads to the release of IL-1β and IL-18, in a caspase-1-dependent manner [120]. There are some conflicting results with regard to the role of inflammasomes in adjuvant activity of alum, but the most recent idea is that inflammasome activation by alum might play an important role in activating innate immunity, but the contribution of inflammasomes in the activation of adaptive immunity remains unclear [119]. Aluminum adjuvants act primarily to increase antibody production and are therefore suitable for vaccines targeting pathogens in which the antibodies mediated killing is important and therefore may not be suitable for vaccine strategies where a strong cellular immunity is essential.

An emulsion is a mixture of two nonmiscible liquids and an emulsifier that is required to stabilize the emulsion by increasing its kinetic stability. Depending on the water-to-oil ratio, the type of emulsifier, and the mixing procedure, a water-in-oil (W/O) or an oil-in-water (O/W) emulsion may be produced [121]. The MF59 was the first oil-in-water adjuvant to be developed and approved for use in human vaccines, and it is the second most frequently used in licensed vaccines after alum. It is composed by squalene, polysorbate 80, and sorbitan trioleate. Similar to alum, MF59 also induces the release of the chemokines such as CCL2, CCL3, CCL4, and CXCL8, which are involved in cell recruitment from blood into peripheral tissue. MF59 also accelerates and enhances monocyte differentiation into DCs, augments Ag uptake, and facilitates migration of DCs into tissue-draining lymph nodes to prime adaptive immune responses [122]. MF59 does not seem to be correlated with enhanced antibodies titers, and it seems to induce balanced Th1/Th2 responses [115].

Freund's adjuvants were the earlier used emulsion adjuvants. Freund's complete adjuvant (FCA) is a mixture of 85% mineral oil (Marco 52) and 15% emulsifier (Arlacel A, mannide monooleate) prepared with 500 μg/ml of heat-killed and dried *Mycobacterium tuberculosis*. Incomplete Freund's adjuvant (IFA) lacks the mycobacterial component, making it safer but less potent. However, Freund's adjuvants were considered too reactogenic for continued use in humans [123].

More recently two new emulsions, adjuvant systems 03 (AS03) and 04 (AS04), were developed. AS03 is composed of squalene, α-tocopherol, and polysorbate 80, while adjuvant AS04 is composed of monophosphoryl lipid A preparation (MPL) and aluminum salt. AS04 was shown to induce optimal immune responses only when co-localized with antigen, providing a depot effect [124]. The depot effect at the injection site is the most widely recognized mechanism of action of adjuvants. This slow release of antigens ensures constant stimulation of the immune system and has been correlated with production of high antibody titers. Recent evidence indicates that this is not the main mechanism of action of alum or MF59. AS04 was also found to induce maturation of DCs (via TLR4), which then trafficks to the draining lymph nodes to activate antigen-specific T cells [124]. AS03 was found to upregulate cytokines, such as colony-stimulating factor 3 (CSF3) and IL-6 and chemokines as CCL2, CCL3, and CCL5, which then leads to cellular recruitment at the injection. The mononuclear cells after taking up antigen traffick to draining lymph nodes [125]. These data suggest that the direct effects of AS04 and AS03 adjuvants are on innate immune cells and effectors, activating of APCs and trafficking to draining lymph node, and also inducing secretion of cytokines and chemokines. It is described that these effects will enhance antibody responses and Th1 responses [115, 124, 125].

Virosomes are spherical unilamellar vesicles of phospholipid carrying envelope virus proteins on their surface or encapsulated within the lumen [126]. Influenza virosomes have been used in the first vaccine to use an adjuvant other than aluminum, a vaccine against hepatitis A licensed in 1994 [126]. Influenza virosome ensures robust and long-lasting immune responses against subunit antigens with an excellent safety profile. The adjuvant effect of virosomes is once more related to their ability to enhance antigen processing and presentation by APCs. Through fusion of the virosome membrane with the membrane of endosomes or phagosomes, the encapsulated protein antigens gain direct access to the MHC class I presentation pathway [127]. In addition, virosomes can also deliver their contents to DCs and

MHC class I and class II molecules and induce maturation of DCs, being able to activate T-helper cells [128]. This phenomenon of presentation of antigen located in the MHC class II pathway to MHC class I pathway is called "cross presentation" and helps the development of both T-helper and T cytotoxic responses, against the antigen [129]. This cross presentation has been considered a major focus to the success of producing an effective immune response to a vaccine, particularly against intracellular parasites. The cytokine profile induced by virosomes, including TNF-α, GM-CSF, IFN-γ, and IL-2, is consistent with a Th1 response.

Liposomes are double or multilayered, biodegradable carrier vesicles made up of phospholipids and/or synthetic lipids that consist of a lipid bilayer shell with an aqueous core. Liposomal formulations can be tailored in terms of the lipid composition, the liposomal charge, the size/lamellarity, and/or the membrane fluidity in order to obtain optimal retention of different types of antigens, including adjuvants, and enhancement of the desired vaccine-specific immune responses [130]. The conjugation of hydrophilic molecules in the surface of liposomes is also possible and further facilitates the uptake by phagocytes [131]. In addition, liposomes are highly acceptable by the human body and present low toxicity. From these characteristics, liposomes are, without any doubt, the most studied carrier system, and the interest for liposome-based vaccines has markedly increased over the last decades.

The lipids selected for liposomal system will ultimately determine their properties and ability of inducing maturation of DCs, which is important to achieve an optimized vaccine carrier. The particle size governs cellular trafficking to secondary lymph nodes, antigen uptake, and cellular responses, and it has been described that small particles (20–200 nm) drain freely toward lymph nodes, while large particles (500, 1,000 nm) are dependent on DCs for transport to the lymph nodes [132]. The selection of the type of lipids also determines liposomal membrane fluidity, which is linked to cellular trafficking and antigen presentation to APCs. It has been determined that rigid, saturated dimethyl dioctadecyl ammonium (DDA) lipid greatly enhances priming ability of Th1-directed immune response, compared with a fluid unsaturated lipid [133]. The surface charge of the liposome, the zeta potential value, is also determined by their lipid composition and dictates the colloidal stability of the formulation. The surface charge of liposomes has a major importance in the immune response, with cationic liposomes having an advantage over their neutral and anionic counterparts [131]. Indeed, the high surface density of positive charges offers an important platform for antigen adsorption due to electrostatic interactions. Moreover, the interaction between the positively charged liposomes and the negatively charged membranes of APCs facilitates liposome uptake, increasing the vaccine potency without the need to increase the concentration of antigen [134]. In addition, the depot effect at the site of injection has also been described for the cationic adjuvant formulation (CAF) 01, a combination of DDA/TDB (trehalose-6,6-dibehenate) which is currently in phase I clinical trial [115, 135].

In sum, an essential point in the investigation of modern adjuvants is not only the initiation of a potent adequate immune response but mainly targeting APC receptors to achieve such response avoiding as much as possible the toxicity associated. Moreover, the ideal adjuvant should be able to promote an antigen-specific immune response and should be nontoxic, biocompatible, readily biodegraded and eliminated, inexpensive to produce, stable before administration, and physicochemically well defined to facilitate quality control important to ensure reproducible manufacturing and activity.

10.2.5 Vaccine Strategies Against *Candida* Infections that Advanced to Clinical Trials

Many positive results have been achieved in the development of fungal vaccines in the last years. However, few vaccine formulations directed against *C. albicans* have successfully completed phase I clinical trials, and although the majority of the studies are concerned with the development of vaccines against systemic candidiasis, the only approaches that enter clinical trials were against recurrent vulvovaginal candidiasis (VVC). The first study described in the literature is the phase II study of D.651, an oral vaccine designed to prevent VVC prepared with *C. albicans* ribosomes and membrane proteoglycan from a nonencapsulated *Klebsiella pneumoniae* as adjuvant [136]. Latter, the PEV7 from Pevion Biotech (Ittigen, Switzerland) composed of an antigen fragment of Sap2p embedded in a virosomal formulation with intrinsic adjuvanticity was proposed against VVC infection. Finally, the NDV-3 from NovaDigm Therapeutics (USA) based on a recombinant protein fragment from Als3 with alum as the adjuvant is also in phase 1b/2a clinical trial to evaluate NDV-3 again in patients diagnosed with VVC.

The preliminary phase II study of D.651 vaccine was conducted in 22 women with a history of frequent recurrences of vulvovaginal candidiasis. Vaccine was taken orally and administered intermittently over 6 months in capsules. The vaccine was well tolerated and reduced an average of 3.59 attacks of VVC per 6 months to an average of 0.55 attacks per 6 months. However, this trial was conducted without placebo, and no further studies on this vaccine have been documented.

The PEV7 vaccine is based on a truncated and enzymatically inactive recombinant aspartyl proteinase-2 (rSap2) of *C. albicans* presented on the surface of influenza virosomes [106, 107, 137]. PEV7 was considered to be safe in a repeated-dose toxicological study in rats and generated a robust serum IgG and IgA anti-Sap2 antibody response in mouse and rat models after intramuscular and intravaginal immunizations. Phase I clinical trial used lyophilized virosome formulations for intramuscular and intravaginal application with the intention to assess the safety and immunogenicity of PEV7 via a systemic prime/mucosal boost regime in 48 healthy volunteers. Half of the women received intramuscular injections, while the other half received intravaginal capsules. This capsular formulation for intravaginal application represents an innovation with the advantage of an easier administration, favoring patient compliance. Results showed that 100% of the vaccinated women developed specific and functional B-cell memory. Both routes of vaccination induced a rapid and specific production of antibodies either in serum and/or cervicovaginal secretion, which was very encouraging with regard to the therapeutic potential of the vaccine [138]. A summary of the study can be found at clinicaltrials.gov website, identifier number NCT01067131.

The NDV-3 trial is a multicenter, double-blind, randomized, placebo-controlled study to evaluate the safety, tolerability, immunogenicity, and efficacy of this vaccine. Due to previous results, this vaccine was developed to treat and prevent infections caused by *Candida* but also to *Staphylococcus aureus*, being the first vaccine to demonstrate preclinical cross kingdom potential [103]. This phase 1b/2a trial involved 188 patients from multiple centers in the United States with the aim to study and estimate the effect of a single, intramuscularly administered dose of NDV-3, as compared to placebo, by evaluating safety and tolerability, as well as humoral and cellular immune responses. The study will also summarize recurrence of VVC over six- and 12-month period, time-to-onset of first VVC episode, and severity of subsequent VVC episodes. A summary of the study can be found at clinicaltrials.gov website, identifier number NCT01926028.

10.2.6 Concerns to Overcome to Further Advance in Fungal Vaccines

The development of innovative vaccines to protect patients from fungal and bacterial infections that can be recurrent, drug resistant, and in some cases life-threatening is still necessary. Other vaccines are ready to enter clinical trials if industrial interest and sufficient monetary support can be raised. Nevertheless, there are still some crucial points to solve such as (1) the majority of the studies that were performed in animal models that have limitations, (2) further understanding of the mechanisms of the *C. albicans*-host interaction in mucosal and systemic infections, and (3) the development of autoimmunity.

The majority of the studies have been developed in animal models that although very useful do not fully recapitulate infection by the opportunistic commensal *C. albicans*. Mice and humans are undoubtedly substantially different regarding their innate immune response to *Candida*. One of the main limitations is that, unlike humans, mice do not have a *C. albicans* GI flora and they lack *Candida* serum antibodies. Several attempts to develop a more real model have been made, and there have been indications that *Candida*-colonized mice were able to developed fungal-specific antibodies in the serum due to the colonization and that these animals, if immunized with a specific protein, were able to develop specific antibodies to that immunogen [139]. However, the information that can be gained from using such mice is still limited. The consequences may be that vaccines that are very efficient in the animal model could be less effective in human, and the protection of the vaccine is not persistent or high grade or cause unacceptable toxicity. Thus, in preclinical trials, the effectiveness of vaccines should be tested in different species of animals, including mice, rabbits, and monkeys. The infection models could include immune-normal animals and immune-deficient animals and could involve variations in the symbiotic bacteria.

To design any vaccine, the mechanisms that confer protective immunity in the host against fungi must be fully understood. This knowledge is important in the selection for constituents from the fungus that elicit the particular type of immune response. In addition, there is little control of the *C. albicans* strain used in the studies, the dose of the inocula to produce the intended outcome of death or tissue infection, the dosage and delivery time of the vaccines to produce the greatest protection effect, the information regarding the different outcomes form various routes of *Candida* infection, or the multiple parameters tested, such as tissue CFU and survival rates. This is further complicated in the development of a multivalent vaccine. Although substantial advances have been made in the understanding of host-*Candida* interactions, the current paradigm of *C. albicans*-specific immunity suggests that pathogenic growth of the fungus is prevented by a combination of innate and adaptive Th1/Th17 responses, which activates phagocytes as the major candidacidal effectors [33, 58]. However, despite the idea that Th17 cells are protective against fungal infections, recent studies suggest that inflammatory Th17 and Treg responses are protective at mucosal surfaces, but in systemic candidiasis, a time-dependent and coordinated Th17/Treg response is fundamental for a positive outcome [63]. The balance between protective versus pathogenic immunity is crucial in determining the disease outcome. This is one of the reasons that justify why vaccines against mucosal candidiasis have advanced to clinical trials. Another concern in the development of subunit vaccines is the adjuvant used. Adjuvants have been used for long time, but their mechanisms of action are not fully understood. They may act by a combination of various mechanisms to create a local immunocompetent environment at the injection site. Many of the preclinical studies were conducted using adjuvants that are not recommended for human use such as the Freund's adjuvant, and when switched to an adjuvant recommended, the results were not the same and in many cases were lower than expected. In addition, and probably due to the lack of knowledge about their mechanism of action, adjuvants are selected just taking into consideration what is in use. Adjuvants should be selected depending on the type of innate responses that are needed to be activated, because they may alter the quality and quantity of adaptive immune responses. That is why just changing the adjuvant without considering its mechanism of action may not produce the expected results. Thus, more studies should be developed in order to better understand the mechanisms of action of adjuvants, providing critical information that will help in a rational design of vaccines and inform on adjuvant safety. These informations will lead to the recommendation of new adjuvants for human use.

The development of autoimmunity was always an important concern, particularly in the case of commensal species as *C. albicans*. Keeping the balance of the immune system in eliminating invading pathogens, while still maintaining self-tolerance to avoid autoimmunity, is critical for the body's health. In this balance, the mucosa microbiota provides benefits to the host by actively participating in the regulation of immune homeostasis. These evidences are confirmed by the consequences of altering the gut microbial communities, termed dysbiosis, such as the autoimmune disorders. The mucosa microbiota has a profound effect on both the innate and adaptive immune system so it is not surprising that some members of the microbiota have been linked to autoimmune diseases. It has been determined that the microflora of mice with colitis fails to metabolize tryptophan into metabolites that act as aryl hydrocarbon receptor (AHR) ligands, modulating production of IL-22, an important cytokine for intestinal homeostasis [140]. Intestinal inflammation is attenuated after inoculation of mice with three *Lactobacillus* strains capable of metabolizing tryptophan or by treatment with an AHR agonist. Despite difficulties in fungal DNA extraction methods and fungal identification methods, the gut, oral, lung, and skin niches presented four genera in common: *Aspergillus*, *Candida*, *Cryptococcus*, and *Penicillium* [141]. Fungi have long been suspected to be involved in inflammatory bowel disease (IBD) pathogenesis since many genes involved in the immune response against fungi have associated single nucleotide polymorphisms (SNPs) in IBD patients, such as in DECTIN-1, CARD9, or NFkBp105 genes in the signaling pathways of antigen-presenting cells and IL12p40, IL23R, or IL-6ST, cytokines and cytokine receptors involved in Th17 and Th1 polarization, among others [142]. These findings suggest a role of fungi in inflammatory pathogenesis. Thus, it is not surprising to find that fungi, and particularly *C. albicans*, are more abundant in the gut microbiota of these patients. But this enhancement in the fungal population is particularly related to a genetic defect in microbial sensing in the susceptible human population. Using animal models, gut inflammation induced by dextran sodium sulfate (DSS) promoted *C. albicans* growth, and this growth enhances inflammation. Thus, it seems that there is a vicious circle in which intestinal inflammation induces *C. albicans* proliferation, which itself enhances the inflammatory process. That is why it is described that *C. albicans* has a negative impact on inflammation. Thus, any factor that significantly alters the local microbiota such as prolonged use of broad-spectrum antibiotics enhances the fungal population in the microbiota and augments intestinal inflammation, contributing to the initiation of the vicious circle and enhancing the changes of fungi translocation and systemic infection. But this predisposition to increased inflammation may not be a direct action of *Candida* in inducing the autoimmune dysfunction, unless patients present genetic defect in fungi sensing. Indeed, host genes affect the composition and function of the gut microbiota.

In order to induce an autoimmune dysfunction, vaccination against *C. albicans* either enhances chronic inflammation, particularly at the mucosa, or develops an adaptive response against an epitope similar to a human molecule. Antibodies against *Saccharomyces cerevisiae* mannan as well as against other fungal cell wall components, such as anti-laminarin that identifies β-1,3-glucans and against β-1,4-N-acetylglucosamine, present in the chitin layers, have been shown to be associated with Crohn's disease [141, 143]. But once more, the existence of these antibodies may be due to the fact that in susceptible individuals, intestinal inflammation induces *C. albicans* proliferation, enhancing the changes of fungi translocation and being seen by the immune system. There is no evidence that in normal individuals the presence of these antibodies enhances the probability of mucosa inflammation. On the contrary, from the vaccination studies against *Candida* vaginal infections, a reduction in the inflammation sign as well as a local reduced fungal burden is documented [144]. However, regarding vaccine development studies against systemic candidiasis, mucosal inflammation is not a parameter that is frequently included in these studies. Thus, the study of the induction of inflammatory at the mucosa should also be included in the studies addressing systemic candidiasis.

In terms of cross-reactions responses against molecules/epitopes with homology to human molecules, epitope mapping analysis has showed that some heat-shock proteins epitopes from *C. albicans* may have as much as 100% direct homology with human heat-shock proteins [76]. Thus, antibodies developed against the heat-shock proteins, particularly Hsp90p, raise the concern of development of autoimmune reactions. In children idiopathic short stature with *C. albicans* and/or *H. pylori* gut colonization, it was reported that the incidence of autoantibodies against selected neuropeptides is high due to molecular mimicry between antigens of these microbiota and the selected neuropeptides [145]. However, further studies are necessary to elucidate this issue. To avoid induction of these autoantibodies by vaccination, the selection of target molecules is essential, molecules that are unique to the fungi should be addressed, and an epitope mapping analysis should always be performed.

In summary, despite the advances in our knowledge and understanding in pathogenesis and immune responses, invasive fungal infections continue to result in significant morbidity and mortality in critically ill patients. The traditional antifungal chemotherapy has met some limitations, such as the toxicity and emergence of resistance, limiting their effectiveness. Therefore, there is an urgent need to improve treatment options for these patients, and vaccines can represent novel approaches against fungal infections. Although the currently available vaccines have demonstrated good protection, there is still a long way to go before a vaccine to be applied in patients with predisposing factors to systemic fungal infections will be achieved.

References

1. Gow NA et al. *Candida albicans* morphogenesis and host defence: discriminating invasion from colonization. Nat Rev Microbiol. 2012;10(2):112–22.
2. Mayer FL, Wilson D, Hube B. *Candida albicans* pathogenicity mechanisms. Virulence. 2013;4(2):119–28.
3. Eberl G. A new vision of immunity: homeostasis of the superorganism. Mucosal Immunol. 2010;3(5):450–60.
4. Paramythiotou E et al. Invasive fungal infections in the ICU: how to approach, how to treat. Molecules. 2014;19(1):1085–119.
5. Kullberg BJ, Arendrup MC. Invasive Candidiasis. N Engl J Med. 2015;373(15):1445–56.
6. Eggimann P, Pittet D. Candida colonization index and subsequent infection in critically ill surgical patients: 20 years later. Intensive Care Med. 2014;40(10):1429–48.
7. Kett DH et al. Candida bloodstream infections in intensive care units: analysis of the extended prevalence of infection in intensive care unit study. Crit Care Med. 2011;39(4):665–70.
8. Sampaio P et al. Virulence attenuation of *Candida albicans* genetic variants isolated from a patient with a recurrent bloodstream infection. PLoS One. 2010;5(4):e10155.

9. Hirakawa MP et al. Genetic and phenotypic intra-species variation in *Candida albicans*. Genome Res. 2015;25(3):413–25.
10. Becker KL et al. Antifungal innate immunity: recognition and inflammatory networks. Semin Immunopathol. 2015;37(2):107–16.
11. Cheng SC et al. Interplay between *Candida albicans* and the mammalian innate host defense. Infect Immun. 2012;80(4):1304–13.
12. De Luca A et al. IL-22 defines a novel immune pathway of antifungal resistance. Mucosal Immunol. 2010;3(4):361–73.
13. Duhring S et al. Host-pathogen interactions between the human innate immune system and *Candida albicans*-understanding and modeling defense and evasion strategies. Front Microbiol. 2015;6:625.
14. Netea MG et al. An integrated model of the recognition of *Candida albicans* by the innate immune system. Nat Rev Microbiol. 2008;6(1):67–78.
15. Netea MG et al. Immune defence against Candida fungal infections. Nat Rev Immunol. 2015;15(10):630–42.
16. Romani L. Immunity to fungal infections. Nat Rev Immunol. 2011;11(4):275–88.
17. Naglik JR, Moyes D. Epithelial cell innate response to *Candida albicans*. Adv Dent Res. 2011;23(1):50–5.
18. Luo S et al. Complement and innate immune evasion strategies of the human pathogenic fungus *Candida albicans*. Mol Immunol. 2013;56(3):161–9.
19. Lievin-Le Moal V, Servin AL. The front line of enteric host defense against unwelcome intrusion of harmful microorganisms: mucins, antimicrobial peptides, and microbiota. Clin Microbiol Rev. 2006;19(2):315–37.
20. Johansson ME et al. The inner of the two Muc2 mucin-dependent mucus layers in colon is devoid of bacteria. Proc Natl Acad Sci U S A. 2008;105(39):15064–9.
21. Kavanaugh NL et al. Mucins suppress virulence traits of *Candida albicans*. MBio. 2014;5(6):e01911.
22. Bobek LA, Situ H. MUC7 20-Mer: investigation of antimicrobial activity, secondary structure, and possible mechanism of antifungal action. Antimicrob Agents Chemother. 2003;47(2):643–52.
23. Fukata M, Arditi M. The role of pattern recognition receptors in intestinal inflammation. Mucosal Immunol. 2013;6(3):451–63.
24. Netea MG et al. Immune sensing of *Candida albicans* requires cooperative recognition of mannans and glucans by lectin and Toll-like receptors. J Clin Invest. 2006;116(6):1642–50.
25. Weindl G et al. Human epithelial cells establish direct antifungal defense through TLR4-mediated signaling. J Clin Invest. 2007;117(12):3664–72.
26. Cohen-Kedar S et al. Human intestinal epithelial cells respond to beta-glucans via Dectin-1 and Syk. Eur J Immunol. 2014;44(12):3729–40.
27. Sun WK et al. Dectin-1 is inducible and plays a crucial role in Aspergillus-induced innate immune responses in human bronchial epithelial cells. Eur J Clin Microbiol Infect Dis. 2012;31(10):2755–64.
28. McKenzie CG et al. Contribution of *Candida albicans* cell wall components to recognition by and escape from murine macrophages. Infect Immun. 2010;78(4):1650–8.
29. Vance RE, Isberg RR, Portnoy DA. Patterns of pathogenesis: discrimination of pathogenic and nonpathogenic microbes by the innate immune system. Cell Host Microbe. 2009;6(1):10–21.
30. Li M et al. The expression of beta-defensin-2, 3 and LL-37 induced by *Candida albicans* phospholipomannan in human keratinocytes. J Dermatol Sci. 2011;61(1):72–5.
31. Moyes DL et al. A biphasic innate immune MAPK response discriminates between the yeast and hyphal forms of *Candida albicans* in epithelial cells. Cell Host Microbe. 2010;8(3):225–35.

32. Cheng SC et al. The dectin-1/inflammasome pathway is responsible for the induction of protective T-helper 17 responses that discriminate between yeasts and hyphae of *Candida albicans*. J Leukoc Biol. 2011;90(2):357–66.
33. Hornby JM et al. Quorum sensing in the dimorphic fungus *Candida albicans* is mediated by farnesol. Appl Environ Microbiol. 2001;67(7):2982–92.
34. Lowman DW et al. Novel structural features in *Candida albicans* hyphal glucan provide a basis for differential innate immune recognition of hyphae versus yeast. J Biol Chem. 2014;289(6):3432–43.
35. Bain JM et al. Non-lytic expulsion/exocytosis of *Candida albicans* from macrophages. Fungal Genet Biol. 2012;49(9):677–8.
36. Filler SG, Sheppard DC. Fungal invasion of normally non-phagocytic host cells. PLoS Pathog. 2006;2(12):e129.
37. Mech F et al. Epithelial invasion outcompetes hypha development during *Candida albicans* infection as revealed by an image-based systems biology approach. Cytometry A. 2014;85(2):126–39.
38. Wilson D et al. Identifying infection-associated genes of *Candida albicans* in the postgenomic era. FEMS Yeast Res. 2009;9(5):688–700.
39. Nahum A et al. The biological significance of TLR3 variant, L412F, in conferring susceptibility to cutaneous candidiasis. CMV Autoimmun Autoimmun Rev. 2012;11(5):341–7.
40. Kasperkovitz PV et al. Toll-like receptor 9 modulates macrophage antifungal effector function during innate recognition of *Candida albicans* and *Saccharomyces cerevisiae*. Infect Immun. 2011;79(12):4858–67.
41. Wagener J et al. Fungal chitin dampens inflammation through IL-10 induction mediated by NOD2 and TLR9 activation. PLoS Pathog. 2014;10(4):e1004050.
42. Brown GD et al. Dectin-1 is a major beta-glucan receptor on macrophages. J Exp Med. 2002;196(3):407–12.
43. Ferwerda G et al. Dectin-1 synergizes with TLR2 and TLR4 for cytokine production in human primary monocytes and macrophages. Cell Microbiol. 2008;10(10):2058–66.
44. Saijo S et al. Dectin-2 recognition of alpha-mannans and induction of Th17 cell differentiation is essential for host defense against *Candida albicans*. Immunity. 2010;32(5):681–91.
45. Zhu LL et al. C-type lectin receptors Dectin-3 and Dectin-2 form a heterodimeric pattern-recognition receptor for host defense against fungal infection. Immunity. 2013;39(2):324–34.
46. Koh AY et al. Mucosal damage and neutropenia are required for *Candida albicans* dissemination. PLoS Pathog. 2008;4(2):e35.
47. Qian Q et al. Elimination of mouse splenic macrophages correlates with increased susceptibility to experimental disseminated candidiasis. J Immunol. 1994;152(10):5000–8.
48. Erwig LP, Gow NA. Interactions of fungal pathogens with phagocytes. Nat Rev Microbiol. 2016;14(3):163–76.
49. Aratani Y et al. Critical role of myeloperoxidase and nicotinamide adenine dinucleotide phosphate-oxidase in high-burden systemic infection of mice with *Candida albicans*. J Infect Dis. 2002;185(12):1833–7.
50. Bain JM et al. *Candida albicans* hypha formation and mannan masking of beta-glucan inhibit macrophage phagosome maturation. MBio. 2014;5(6):e01874.
51. Zielinski CE et al. Pathogen-induced human TH17 cells produce IFN-gamma or IL-10 and are regulated by IL-1beta. Nature. 2012;484(7395):514–8.
52. Puel A et al. Chronic mucocutaneous candidiasis in humans with inborn errors of interleukin-17 immunity. Science. 2011;332(6025):65–8.
53. Bonifazi P et al. Balancing inflammation and tolerance in vivo through dendritic cells by the commensal *Candida albicans*. Mucosal Immunol. 2009;2(4):362–74.
54. Huang W et al. Requirement of interleukin-17A for systemic anti-*Candida albicans* host defense in mice. J Infect Dis. 2004;190(3):624–31.

55. Whibley N, Gaffen SL. Brothers in arms: Th17 and Treg responses in *Candida albicans* immunity. PLoS Pathog. 2014;10(12):e1004456.
56. Ibrahim AS et al. NDV-3 protects mice from vulvovaginal candidiasis through T- and B-cell immune response. Vaccine. 2013;31(47):5549–56.
57. Krause R et al. Elevated levels of interleukin 17A and kynurenine in candidemic patients, compared with levels in noncandidemic patients in the intensive care unit and those in healthy controls. J Infect Dis. 2015;211(3):445–51.
58. Whibley N et al. Expansion of Foxp3(+) T-cell populations by *Candida albicans* enhances both Th17-cell responses and fungal dissemination after intravenous challenge. Eur J Immunol. 2014;44(4):1069–83.
59. Clancy CJ et al. Immunoglobulin G responses to a panel of *Candida albicans* antigens as accurate and early markers for the presence of systemic candidiasis. J Clin Microbiol. 2008;46(5):1647–54.
60. Nishiya CT et al. Influence of IgG subclass on human antimannan antibody-mediated resistance to hematogenously disseminated Candidiasis in mice. Infect Immun. 2015;84(2):386–94.
61. Beenhouwer DO et al. Human immunoglobulin G2 (IgG2) and IgG4, but not IgG1 or IgG3, protect mice against *Cryptococcus neoformans* infection. Infect Immun. 2007;75(3):1424–35.
62. Pitarch A et al. Proteomics-based identification of novel *Candida albicans* antigens for diagnosis of systemic candidiasis in patients with underlying hematological malignancies. Proteomics. 2004;4(10):3084–106.
63. Pachl J et al. A randomized, blinded, multicenter trial of lipid-associated amphotericin B alone versus in combination with an antibody-based inhibitor of heat shock protein 90 in patients with invasive candidiasis. Clin Infect Dis. 2006;42(10):1404–13.
64. Cassone A. Development of vaccines for *Candida albicans*: fighting a skilled transformer. Nat Rev Microbiol. 2013;11(12):884–91.
65. Spellberg B. Vaccines for invasive fungal infections. F1000 Med Rep. 2011;3:13.
66. Kintu K et al. Feasibility and safety of ALVAC-HIV vCP1521 vaccine in HIV-exposed infants in Uganda: results from the first HIV vaccine trial in infants in Africa. J Acquir Immune Defic Syndr. 2013;63(1):1–8.
67. Skorka K et al. Indirect induction of regulatory T cells accompanies immune responses during peptide vaccination of chronic lymphocytic leukaemia patients. Br J Haematol. 2015;174:155–7.
68. Berglund A et al. The response to vaccination against influenza A(H1N1) 2009, seasonal influenza and Streptococcus pneumoniae in adult outpatients with ongoing treatment for cancer with and without rituximab. Acta Oncol. 2014;53(9):1212–20.
69. Ariza-Heredia EJ, Chemaly RF. Practical review of immunizations in adult patients with cancer. Hum Vaccin Immunother. 2015;11(11):2606–14.
70. Centers for Disease, C. and Prevention. Prevention and control of influenza with vaccines: recommendations of the Advisory Committee on Immunization Practices (ACIP) – United States, 2012-13 influenza season. MMWR Morb Mortal Wkly Rep. 2012;61(32):613–8.
71. Flowers CR et al. Antimicrobial prophylaxis and outpatient management of fever and neutropenia in adults treated for malignancy: American Society of Clinical Oncology clinical practice guideline. J Clin Oncol. 2013;31(6):794–810.
72. Wisplinghoff H et al. Nosocomial bloodstream infections in US hospitals: analysis of 24,179 cases from a prospective nationwide surveillance study. Clin Infect Dis. 2004;39(3):309–17.
73. Pfaller MA, Diekema DJ. Epidemiology of invasive candidiasis: a persistent public health problem. Clin Microbiol Rev. 2007;20(1):133–63.
74. Andes DR et al. Impact of treatment strategy on outcomes in patients with candidemia and other forms of invasive candidiasis: a patient-level quantitative review of randomized trials. Clin Infect Dis. 2012;54(8):1110–22.

75. Matthews RC, Burnie JP, Tabaqchali S. Immunoblot analysis of the serological response in systemic candidosis. Lancet. 1984;2(8417–8418):1415–8.
76. Matthews RC et al. Autoantibody to heat-shock protein 90 can mediate protection against systemic candidosis. Immunology. 1991;74(1):20–4.
77. Matthews R, Hodgetts S, Burnie J. Preliminary assessment of a human recombinant antibody fragment to hsp90 in murine invasive candidiasis. J Infect Dis. 1995;171(6):1668–71.
78. Hurd RC, Drake CH. *Candida albicans* infections in actively and passively immunized animals. Mycopathol Mycol Appl. 1953;6(4):290–7.
79. Balogh E et al. Experimental investigation of immunreactivity against *Candida albicans*. 1. Reaction of rabbits immunized with *Candida albicans* and challenged with living *Candida albicans*. Mykosen. 1971;14(8):385–92.
80. Bistoni F et al. Evidence for macrophage-mediated protection against lethal *Candida albicans* infection. Infect Immun. 1986;51(2):668–74.
81. Saville SP et al. Efficacy of a genetically engineered *Candida albicans* tet-NRG1 strain as an experimental live attenuated vaccine against hematogenously disseminated candidiasis. Clin Vaccine Immunol. 2009;16(3):430–2.
82. Fernandez-Arenas E et al. Contribution of the antibodies response induced by a low virulent *Candida albicans* strain in protection against systemic candidiasis. Proteomics. 2004;4(4):1204–15.
83. Tavares D, Ferreira P, Arala-Chaves M. Increased resistance in BALB/c mice to reinfection with *Candida albicans* is due to immunoneutralization of a virulence-associated immunomodulatory protein. Microbiology. 2003;149(Pt 2):333–9.
84. Mourad S, Friedman L. Passive immunization of mice against *Candida albicans*. Sabouraudia. 1968;6(2):103–5.
85. Segal E, Nussbaum S, Barr-Nea L. Protection against systemic infections with various Candida species elicited by vaccination with *Candida albicans* ribosomes. Sabouraudia. 1985;23(4):275–85.
86. Segal E, Sandovsky-Losica H. Experimental vaccination with *Candida albicans* ribosomes in cyclophosphamide-treated animals. Sabouraudia. 1981;19(4):267–73.
87. Segal E et al. Induction of protection against candidiasis in tumor-bearing mice by vaccination with *Candida albicans* ribosomes. J Med Vet Mycol. 1987;25(6):355–63.
88. Torosantucci A et al. A novel glyco-conjugate vaccine against fungal pathogens. J Exp Med. 2005;202(5):597–606.
89. Xin H et al. Synthetic glycopeptide vaccines combining beta-mannan and peptide epitopes induce protection against candidiasis. Proc Natl Acad Sci U S A. 2008;105(36):13526–31.
90. Lopez-Ribot JL et al. Antibody response to *Candida albicans* cell wall antigens. FEMS Immunol Med Microbiol. 2004;41(3):187–96.
91. Han Y, Rhew KY. Comparison of two Candida mannan vaccines: the role of complement in protection against disseminated candidiasis. Arch Pharm Res. 2012;35(11):2021–7.
92. Han Y, Ulrich MA, Cutler JE. *Candida albicans* mannan extract-protein conjugates induce a protective immune response against experimental candidiasis. J Infect Dis. 1999;179(6):1477–84.
93. Lipinski T et al. A beta-mannan trisaccharide conjugate vaccine aids clearance of *Candida albicans* in immunocompromised rabbits. Vaccine. 2012;30(44):6263–9.
94. Xin H et al. Self-adjuvanting glycopeptide conjugate vaccine against disseminated candidiasis. PLoS One. 2012;7(4):e35106.
95. Cutler JE. Defining criteria for anti-mannan antibodies to protect against candidiasis. Curr Mol Med. 2005;5(4):383–92.
96. Torosantucci A et al. Protection by anti-beta-glucan antibodies is associated with restricted beta-1,3 glucan binding specificity and inhibition of fungal growth and adherence. PLoS One. 2009;4(4):e5392.
97. Li WJ et al. Adjuvanticity of a recombinant calreticulin fragment in assisting anti-beta-glucan IgG responses in T cell-deficient mice. Clin Vaccine Immunol. 2013;20(4):582–9.

98. Ibrahim AS et al. Vaccination with recombinant N-terminal domain of Als1p improves survival during murine disseminated candidiasis by enhancing cell-mediated, not humoral, immunity. Infect Immun. 2005;73(2):999–1005.
99. Spellberg BJ et al. The anti-*Candida albicans* vaccine composed of the recombinant N terminus of Als1p reduces fungal burden and improves survival in both immunocompetent and immunocompromised mice. Infect Immun. 2005;73(9):6191–3.
100. Spellberg BJ et al. Efficacy of the anti-Candida rAls3p-N or rAls1p-N vaccines against disseminated and mucosal candidiasis. J Infect Dis. 2006;194(2):256–60.
101. Ibrahim AS et al. The anti-Candida vaccine based on the recombinant N-terminal domain of Als1p is broadly active against disseminated candidiasis. Infect Immun. 2006;74(5): 3039–41.
102. Lin L et al. Considerable differences in vaccine immunogenicities and efficacies related to the diluent used for aluminum hydroxide adjuvant. Clin Vaccine Immunol. 2008;15(3):582–4.
103. Spellberg B et al. The antifungal vaccine derived from the recombinant N terminus of Als3p protects mice against the bacterium *Staphylococcus aureus*. Infect Immun. 2008;76(10):4574–80.
104. Tavares D et al. Immunoprotection against systemic candidiasis in mice. Int Immunol. 1995;7(5):785–96.
105. Vilanova M et al. Protection against systemic candidiasis in mice immunized with secreted aspartic proteinase 2. Immunology. 2004;111(3):334–42.
106. De Bernardis F et al. Intravaginal and intranasal immunizations are equally effective in inducing vaginal antibodies and conferring protection against vaginal candidiasis. Infect Immun. 2002;70(5):2725–9.
107. Sandini S et al. A highly immunogenic recombinant and truncated protein of the secreted aspartic proteases family (rSap2t) of *Candida albicans* as a mucosal anticandidal vaccine. FEMS Immunol Med Microbiol. 2011;62(2):215–24.
108. Luo G et al. *Candida albicans* Hyr1p confers resistance to neutrophil killing and is a potential vaccine target. J Infect Dis. 2010;201(11):1718–28.
109. Li W et al. Immunisation with the glycolytic enzyme enolase confers effective protection against *Candida albicans* infection in mice. Vaccine. 2011;29(33):5526–33.
110. Raska M et al. Comparison of protective effect of protein and DNA vaccines hsp90 in murine model of systemic candidiasis. Folia Microbiol (Praha). 2005;50(1):77–82.
111. Raska M et al. Systemic and mucosal immunization with *Candida albicans* hsp90 elicits hsp90-specific humoral response in vaginal mucosa which is further enhanced during experimental vaginal candidiasis. Med Mycol. 2008;46(5):411–20.
112. Carneiro C et al. DODAB:monoolein liposomes containing *Candida albicans* cell wall surface proteins: a novel adjuvant and delivery system. Eur J Pharm Biopharm. 2015;89:190–200.
113. Carneiro C et al. Protective effect of antigen delivery using monoolein-based liposomes in experimental hematogenously disseminated candidiasis. Acta Biomater. 2016;39:133–45.
114. Coffman RL, Sher A, Seder RA. Vaccine adjuvants: putting innate immunity to work. Immunity. 2010;33(4):492–503.
115. Awate S, Babiuk LA, Mutwiri G. Mechanisms of action of adjuvants. Front Immunol. 2013;4:114.
116. Ferreira SA, Gama FM, Vilanova M. Polymeric nanogels as vaccine delivery systems. Nanomedicine. 2013;9(2):159–73.
117. Morefield GL et al. Role of aluminum-containing adjuvants in antigen internalization by dendritic cells in vitro. Vaccine. 2005;23(13):1588–95.
118. Kool M et al. Alum adjuvant boosts adaptive immunity by inducing uric acid and activating inflammatory dendritic cells. J Exp Med. 2008;205(4):869–82.
119. Oleszycka E, Lavelle EC. Immunomodulatory properties of the vaccine adjuvant alum. Curr Opin Immunol. 2014;28:1–5.

120. Li H, Nookala S, Re F. Aluminum hydroxide adjuvants activate caspase-1 and induce IL-1beta and IL-18 release. J Immunol. 2007;178(8):5271–6.
121. Schijns VE, Strioga M, Ascarateil S. Oil-based emulsion vaccine adjuvants. Curr Protoc Immunol. 2014;106(2 18):1–7.
122. Seubert A et al. The adjuvants aluminum hydroxide and MF59 induce monocyte and granulocyte chemoattractants and enhance monocyte differentiation toward dendritic cells. J Immunol. 2008;180(8):5402–12.
123. Jensen FC et al. Adjuvant activity of incomplete Freund's adjuvant. Adv Drug Deliv Rev. 1998;32(3):173–86.
124. Didierlaurent AM et al. AS04, an aluminum salt- and TLR4 agonist-based adjuvant system, induces a transient localized innate immune response leading to enhanced adaptive immunity. J Immunol. 2009;183(10):6186–97.
125. Morel S et al. Adjuvant system AS03 containing alpha-tocopherol modulates innate immune response and leads to improved adaptive immunity. Vaccine. 2011;29(13):2461–73.
126. Moser C et al. Influenza virosomes as vaccine adjuvant and carrier system. Expert Rev Vaccines. 2013;12(7):779–91.
127. Bungener L et al. Virosome-mediated delivery of protein antigens in vivo: efficient induction of class I MHC-restricted cytotoxic T lymphocyte activity. Vaccine. 2005;23(10):1232–41.
128. Bungener L et al. Virosome-mediated delivery of protein antigens to dendritic cells. Vaccine. 2002;20(17–18):2287–95.
129. Amigorena S, Savina A. Intracellular mechanisms of antigen cross presentation in dendritic cells. Curr Opin Immunol. 2010;22(1):109–17.
130. Tan LS. Liposomes as antigen vehicles to increase immunogenicity: effects of variation of structural characteristics. Ann Acad Med Singapore. 1991;20(1):78–83.
131. Vartak A, Sucheck SJ. Recent advances in subunit vaccine carriers. Vaccines (Basel). 2016;4(2):12.
132. Manolova V et al. Nanoparticles target distinct dendritic cell populations according to their size. Eur J Immunol. 2008;38(5):1404–13.
133. Christensen D et al. Cationic liposomes as vaccine adjuvants. Expert Rev Vaccines. 2011;10(4):513–21.
134. Hafez IM, Maurer N, Cullis PR. On the mechanism whereby cationic lipids promote intracellular delivery of polynucleic acids. Gene Ther. 2001;8(15):1188–96.
135. Henriksen-Lacey M et al. Liposomes based on dimethyldioctadecylammonium promote a depot effect and enhance immunogenicity of soluble antigen. J Control Release. 2010;142(2):180–6.
136. Levy DA et al. Phase II study of D.651, an oral vaccine designed to prevent recurrences of vulvovaginal candidiasis. Vaccine. 1989;7(4):337–40.
137. De Bernardis F et al. A virosomal vaccine against candidal vaginitis: immunogenicity, efficacy and safety profile in animal models. Vaccine. 2012;30(30):4490–8.
138. De Bernardis F et al. Studies of immune responses in Candida vaginitis. Pathogens. 2015;4(4):697–707.
139. Cutler JE et al. Horizontal transmission of *Candida albicans* and evidence of a vaccine response in mice colonized with the fungus. PLoS One. 2011;6(7):e22030.
140. Lamas B et al. CARD9 impacts colitis by altering gut microbiota metabolism of tryptophan into aryl hydrocarbon receptor ligands. Nat Med. 2016;22:598–605.
141. Richard ML et al. Gut fungal microbiota: the Yin and Yang of inflammatory bowel disease. Inflamm Bowel Dis. 2015;21(3):656–65.
142. Jostins L et al. Host-microbe interactions have shaped the genetic architecture of inflammatory bowel disease. Nature. 2012;491(7422):119–24.
143. Quinton JF et al. Anti-*Saccharomyces cerevisiae* mannan antibodies combined with antineutrophil cytoplasmic autoantibodies in inflammatory bowel disease: prevalence and diagnostic role. Gut. 1998;42(6):788–91.

144. Pericolini E et al. Secretory aspartyl proteinases cause vaginitis and can mediate vaginitis caused by *Candida albicans* in Mice. MBio. 2015;6(3):e00724.
145. Stawerska R et al. Prevalence of autoantibodies against some selected growth and appetite-regulating neuropeptides in serum of short children exposed to *Candida albicans* colonization and/or Helicobacter pylori infection: the molecular mimicry phenomenon. Neuro Endocrinol Lett. 2015;36(5):458–64.

MIX
Papier aus verantwortungsvollen Quellen
Paper from responsible sources
FSC® C105338

If you have any concerns about our products,
you can contact us on
ProductSafety@springernature.com

In case Publisher is established outside the EU,
the EU authorized representative is:
Springer Nature Customer Service Center GmbH
Europaplatz 3, 69115 Heidelberg, Germany

Printed by Libri Plureos GmbH
in Hamburg, Germany